Quick Look Nursing:

Obstetric and Pediatric Pathophysiology

BERNADETTE MADARA, BC, APRN
Associate Professor
Southern Connecticut State University

CAROL T. AVERY, EDD, RN, C
Professor, Department of Nursing
Western Connecticut State University

VANESSA POMARICO-DENINO, MSN, APRN
Family Nurse Practitioner, Women's Health
Medical Associates of North Haven, LLC

LINDA WAGNER, EDD, MSN
Associate Professor of Nursing
Southern Connecticut State University

JONES AND BARTLETT PUBLISHERS
Sudbury, Massachusetts
BOSTON   TORONTO   LONDON   SINGAPORE

World Headquarters
Jones and Bartlett Publishers
40 Tall Pine Drive
Sudbury, MA 01776
978-443-5000
info@jbpub.com
www.jbpub.com

Jones and Bartlett Publishers Canada
6339 Ormindale Way
Mississauga, Ontario L5V 1J2
Canada

Jones and Bartlett Publishers International
Barb House, Barb Mews
London W6 7PA
UK

Jones and Bartlett's books and products are available through most bookstores and online booksellers. To contact Jones and Bartlett Publishers directly, call 800-832-0034, fax 978-443-8000, or visit our website, www.jbpub.com.

Substantial discounts on bulk quantities of Jones and Bartlett's publications are available to corporations, professional associations, and other qualified organizations. For details and specific discount information, contact the special sales department at Jones and Bartlett via the above contact information or send an email to specialsales@jbpub.com.

The authors, editor, and publisher have made every effort to provide accurate information. However, they are not responsible for errors, omissions, or for any outcomes related to the use of the contents of this book and take no responsibility for the use of the products and procedures described. Treatments and side effects described in this book may not be applicable to all people; likewise, some people may require a dose or experience a side effect that is not described herein. Drugs and medical devices are discussed that may have limited availability controlled by the Food and Drug Administration (FDA) for use only in a research study or clinical trial. Research, clinical practice, and government regulations often change the accepted standard in this field. When consideration is being given to use of any drug in the clinical setting, the health care provider or reader is responsible for determining FDA status of the drug, reading the package insert, and reviewing prescribing information for the most up-to-date recommendations on dose, precautions, and contraindications, and determining the appropriate usage for the product. This is especially important in the case of drugs that are new or seldom used.

Production Credits
Executive Editor: Kevin Sullivan
Acquisitions Editor: Emily Ekle
Associate Editor: Amy Sibley
Editorial Assistant: Patricia Donnelly
Production Director: Amy Rose
Production Editor: Carolyn F. Rogers
Senior Marketing Manager: Katrina Gosek
Associate Marketing Manager: Rebecca Wasley
Manufacturing and Inventory Coordinator: Amy Bacus
Compositor: Graphic World
Cover Illustrator: Cara Judd
Cover Layout Artist: Timothy Dziewit
Printing and Binding: Malloy, Inc.
Cover Printing: Malloy, Inc.

Library of Congress Cataloging-in-Publication Data
Obstetric and pediatric pathophysiology / Bernadette Madara ... [et al.].
    p. ; cm. -- (Quick look nursing)
  Includes bibliographical references and index.
  ISBN-13: 978-0-7637-4117-4 (pbk. : alk. paper)
  ISBN-10: 0-7637-4117-5 (pbk. : alk. paper)
  1. Gynecologic nursing. 2. Maternity nursing. 3. Pediatric nursing. I. Madara, Bernadette. II. Series.
  [DNLM: 1. Female Urogenital Diseases--physiopathology--Handbooks. 2. Female Urogenital Diseases--physiopathology--Nurses' Instruction. 3. Pregnancy Complications--physiopathology--Handbooks. 4. Pregnancy Complications--physiopathology--Nurses' Instruction. 5. Pediatrics--Handbooks. 6. Pediatrics--Nurses' Instruction. 7. Reproduction--Handbooks. 8. Reproduction--Nurses' Instruction. WQ 39 O14 2008]
  RG105.O33 2008
  618.2'0231--dc22
                        2007022557
6048

Printed in the United States of America
11 10 09 08 07   10 9 8 7 6 5 4 3 2 1

• • • •

We dedicate this book to our students and patients
who have inspired us
and to all users of this book
who continue to move the nursing profession forward.

• • • •

CONTENTS

PREFACE

This book is intended for use by students and practicing nurses who work in maternal–child healthcare settings. Our aim is to provide a quick overview of normal physiology of conception, pregnancy, and the birth process along with pathophysiology related to common maternal and pediatric health issues. We hope you find this reference book useful in your educational journey and practice.

ACKNOWLEDGMENTS

It is with my deepest appreciation and gratitude to the following people who have made this venture possible:

Bunny Madara: For asking me to be part of this book and for your faith in my expertise and skills.

Stephanie Esposito, APRN, Lillian Falko, APRN, Patricia Gatcomb, APRN, and Barbara Stone, RN: Your collective expertise in your specialized fields is so greatly appreciated. You keep me inspired!

To Mom and Dad; my sisters, Karen, Susan, and Liz; and my nieces, Alana and Demi, for being so supportive of my career and for keeping David entertained and well-fed as I spent my weekends at the computer.

And to my wonderful husband, David: For always believing in me in all that I do. I would not have been able to accomplish all that I have without your constant love and support!

Vanessa

Sincere thanks to the coauthors of this book who worked so well together to complete this project. Their dedication to teaching is apparent. A special thank you to Linda who took on added responsibility to help make this project a success.

Thank you to all of the students whom I have had the pleasure to teach. You have inspired me!

Thank you also to my family who supported me during this project.

And finally, thank you to the staff at Jones and Bartlett, especially Amy Sibley, Associate Editor, who believed in this project and helped it to become a reality.

Bernadette

I wish to thank Bunny Madara for asking me to participate in this project and Vanessa Denino whose cooperation made writing this a joy.

Carol

I wish to acknowledge my children, Lisa and Ben, and my partner, Rick, for their inspiration and support and their gift of laughter, love, and passion that enriches my life.

Linda

ABOUT THE AUTHORS

Bernadette Madara, BC, APRN
Dr. Bernadette Madara is an associate professor of nursing at Southern Connecticut State University in New Haven, Connecticut. She is an APRN with Board Certification in medical–surgical nursing. Dr. Madara has taught on both the undergraduate and graduate levels.

Carol T. Avery, EdD, RN, C
Carol T. Avery is a tenured professor at Western Connecticut State University Department of Nursing in Danbury, Connecticut. Her expertise is in maternal-newborn nursing and women's health. She graduated from St. Vincent's Hospital School of Nursing, a three-year diploma school, and completed her bachelor's degree at the University of Bridgeport in Bridgeport, Connecticut. Carol earned her master's degree at Hunter College of the City University of New York and her doctorate at Teacher's College, Columbia University. Achievements include the presidency of Kappa Alpha chapter of Sigma Theta Tau International Nursing Honor Society and the vice presidency of the American Assembly for Men in Nursing. In addition, Dr. Avery produced a video exploring the opinions and predictions of nurse leader Dr. Luther Christman, entitled *A Conversation with Luther.*

Vanessa Pomarico-Denino, MSN, APRN
Vanessa Pomarico-Denino is a family nurse practitioner specializing in women's health at Medical Associates of North Haven, LLC. She received an associate's degree in Nursing at the University of Bridgeport and went on to earn her bachelor's degree as well as her master's degree in Nursing at Southern Connecticut State University. Vanessa taught both undergraduate and graduate nursing at SCSU and provided women's health services at their student health center for several years. She remains an active guest lecturer in their family nurse practitioner program. She is a clinical instructor and preceptor for SCSU family nurse practitioner students as well as at the Yale University School of Nursing.

Linda Wagner, EdD, MSN
Linda Wagner is a tenured associate professor of nursing at Southern Connecticut State University and has been involved with undergraduate, graduate, and RN-BSN students for over 18 years. Her specialty areas are

pediatrics and family nursing, leadership and nursing education, with a research interest in family transitions and caring in practice. She received her BSN from Western Connecticut State University, her MSN in nursing of children from the University of Pennsylvania, and her EdD in educational leadership from the University of Hartford.

I

Reproduction
and Family Health

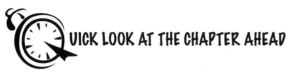

The menstrual cycle is thought of as an unending cycle, or a circle. A woman is continuously in one phase or another throughout her reproductive life.

There are four phases of the menstrual cycle:

- Follicular phase or proliferative phase

- Ovulatory phase

- Luteal phase or secretory phase

- Menstrual phase

The typical menstrual cycle lasts 26 to 35 days. Bleeding varies from 3 to 7 days, but the amount is usually no more than 2 to 4 ounces.

1

Menstrual Cycle

TERMS

- ☐ Corpus luteum
- ☐ Estrogenic phase
- ☐ Follicle-stimulating hormone
- ☐ Follicular phase
- ☐ Luteal phase
- ☐ Luteinizing hormone
- ☐ Menarche
- ☐ Menstrual phase
- ☐ Ovulatory phase
- ☐ Progestational phase
- ☐ Proliferative phase
- ☐ Secretory phase

The first menstrual period of puberty is called **menarche.** Bleeding during menarche may be irregular and unpredictable at the onset, but eventually the cycle becomes rhythmic until menopause. Menopause is the cessation of menstruation. The typical menstrual cycle lasts 26 to 35 days. Bleeding varies from 3 to 7 days, but the amount is usually no more than 2 to 4 ounces.

Menstrual blood contains mucus and destroyed cellular tissue from the endometrium that does not coagulate. However, when exposed to the air it has a fleshy odor and can become offensive.

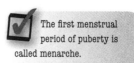
The first menstrual period of puberty is called menarche.

At the time of ovulation some women experience engorgement, tingling in the breasts, an increase in vaginal secretions, some spotting, and an increase in weight due to sodium and water retention. It has been found that a slight lowering with a decided sudden rise (biphasic) in basal temperature is significant in determining periods of greatest fertility.

At birth there are approximately 100,000 to 200,000 primordial or primitive follicles. Through the process of atresia (retrogression and disappearance of follicles in the mammalian ovary) the number at puberty becomes 30,000 to 40,000 follicles.

The menstrual cycle is thought of as an unending cycle, or a circle. A woman is continuously in one phase or another throughout her reproductive life. There are four phases of the menstrual cycle (Figure 1-1):

1. **Follicular phase** or **estrogenic phase** (refers to the ovarian function) or **proliferative phase** (refers to the uterine function)
2. **Ovulatory phase** (refers to the ovary)
3. **Luteal** or **progestational phase** (refers to the ovary) or **secretory phase** (refers to uterine function)
4. **Menstrual phase**

To understand the menstrual cycle it is necessary to trace the hormonal releasing factors. The hypothalamus has a vascular connection to the pituitary gland. The cyclic release of gonadotropins is brought about through the influence of the anterior lobe of the pituitary gland by hormonal agents released by the hypothalamus. These hormonal agents are called releasing factors because they directly affect the release of **follicle-stimulating hormone** and **luteinizing hormone** from the pituitary gland. The anterior lobe of the pituitary gland controls hormonal function of the menstrual cycle. These hormones stimulate the ovaries to produce estrogen and progesterone.

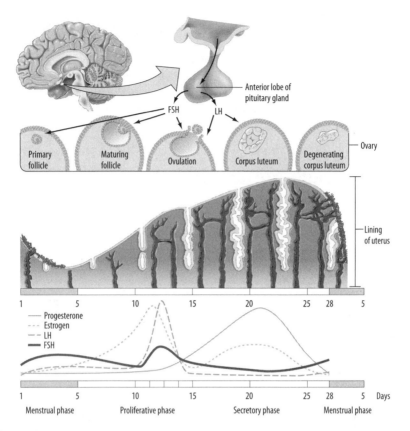

Figure 1-1 Phases of the menstrual cycle.

 FOLLICULAR PHASE

Under the influence of follicle-stimulating hormone a follicular fluid containing estrogen accumulates in the center of the follicle, the ovum increases in size, and the nucleus moves from the center of the cell to the periphery. There is a rise in the estrogen levels in the bloodstream, and the pituitary gland releases luteinizing hormone, which causes rupture of the follicle and extrusion of the ovum, which is called ovulation (ovulatory phase).

The follicular or proliferative phase is conditioned by estrogen and extends from the end of menstruation to ovulation (ovulation, middle cycle). During the proliferative (estrogenic) phase, the endometrium within the uterus becomes thickened, succulent, and extremely rich in blood supply.

OVULATORY PHASE

There are no marked changes that occur in the endometrium during the ovulatory process. There is a distinct fall and then a rise in the basal body temperature, which remains high until the onset of the menstrual period. The rise in the body temperature is attributed to the high titers of progesterone (thermogenic hormone) after ovulation.

LUTEAL (PROGESTATIONAL) PHASE

After ovulation, in which the ova has been extruded from the graafian follicle, the cavity of the ruptured graafian follicle becomes filled with a tissue known as the **corpus luteum**. This phase is also called the secretory phase, because it refers to uterine function. The luteinizing hormone stimulates the corpus luteum in the ovary to secrete small quantities of estrogen and large quantities of progesterone for a period of 8 days. The stroma of the endometrium becomes highly vascularized and edematous, the mucosa thickens, and the glands develop corkscrew and serrati (notched and toothed) features. At this time the progestational endometrium is optimum for implantation of a fertilized ovum.

MENSTRUAL PHASE

When an ovum is not fertilized by a sperm there is a reduction in progesterone, causing endometrial vascular stasis, vasoconstriction, and finally endometrial shedding with menstrual bleeding. Menstruation is a definite point-ending cycle; therefore the first day of the last menstrual period is noted in calculating the interval of cycles.

BASAL BODY TEMPERATURE

In women who are ovulating there is normally a rhythmic variation in the basal body temperature curve during the course of the menstrual cycle. The basal temperature is lower during the first part of the menstrual cycle (proliferative phase). It rises in association with ovulation and remains relatively higher during the luteal phase of the cycle. The rise in the basal temperature occurs as a result of the influence of progesterone, which is produced by the corpus luteum after ovulation. Progesterone causes this thermogenic effect through its influence on the central nervous system. The basal body temperature increases as much as 0.5 degrees Fahrenheit, and a relatively higher temperature is sustained until just before the onset of the menstrual period. If pregnancy occurs, the levels of progesterone are maintained and the basal temperature remains high past the expected time of the period. In the absence of a pregnancy, the basal body temperature decreases a day or so before the menstrual period.

The basal body temperature is often used when an infertility problem is suspected. It is a convenient and cost-effective way to determine whether a woman is ovulating. The woman is instructed to take her temperature each day immediately upon awakening and before getting out of bed. This easy method is then documented daily on a monthly chart for approximately 3 consecutive months. If ovulating, the temperature shows a slight dip, followed by a rise in the basal temperature. Another cost-effective method is observing daily variations in cervical mucus. Early in the cycle (preovulatory) the cervical mucus is scant and sticky, but just before ovulation it becomes abundant and transparent and is most receptive to sperm penetration. After ovulation, the cervical mucus again becomes scant and sticky.

LUNAR MONTHS

Most women consider themselves 1 month pregnant at the time of the first missed menstrual period and 2 months pregnant at the second missed period. But because conception does not take place until ovulation (14 days after the onset of menstruation in a 28-day cycle), obviously that embryo does not attain the age of 1 month until about 2 weeks after the first missed period (assuming a 28-day cycle). Therefore the embryo's "birthday" by months regularly falls 2 weeks or so after any numerically specified missed period.

When addressing the age of a pregnancy in months, the medical community refers to lunar months, that is, periods of 4 weeks. The normal length of gestation if taken from

 The normal length of gestation if taken from the first day of the last menstrual period is 10 lunar months, 40 weeks, or 280 days. If taken from the date of the fertilization, the length is 9½ months, 38 weeks, or 266 days.

the first day of the last menstrual period is 10 lunar months, 40 weeks, or 280 days. If taken from the date of the fertilization, the length is 9½ months, 38 weeks, or 266 days.

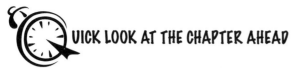

QUICK LOOK AT THE CHAPTER AHEAD

Infertility is the inability to conceive a child after one year of regular sexual intercourse without using any method of contraception. Included in this definition is also the inability to carry a pregnancy to term.

Infertility can affect both genders (females and males). There are many risk factors that can affect infertility in both men and women.

Laboratory and diagnostic tests as well as treatment modalities are available to the infertile couple.

2

Infertility

TERMS
- [ ] **Artificial insemination**
- [ ] **Basal body temperature (BBT)**
- [ ] **Endometriosis**
- [ ] **Gamete intrafallopian transfer**
- [ ] **Hysterosalpingogram**
- [ ] **Infertility**
- [ ] **In vitro fertilization**
- [ ] **Laparoscopy**
- [ ] **Ovulation predictor kit**
- [ ] **Postcoital test**
- [ ] **Semen analysis**
- [ ] **Surrogate embryo transfer**
- [ ] **Zygote intrafallopian transfer**

9

Infertility is defined as the inability to conceive a child after 1 year of regular sexual intercourse without using any method of contraception or the inability to carry a pregnancy to term. Secondary infertility is when a woman who has been pregnant previously cannot conceive. All infertility affects approximately 6.1 million Americans, or 10% of the population that has reached the reproductive age.

A normal fertile couple has a 20% chance of conceiving during each ovulatory cycle. As a woman ages, infertility increases; therefore women older than age 40 have a 50% decrease in fertility rate. The societal trend to delay pregnancy until later in life increases infertility because the prevalence of diseases such as ovulatory dysfunction and endometriosis increases.

In about 30% of the couples it is the male who is infertile. Another 20% of women have tubal, vaginal, or uterine problems as the cause of infertility. There can also be a combined infertility (both male and female factors) or unexplained infertility.

 RISK FACTORS

Some of the risk factors for infertility in women are as follows:

- Endometriosis
- History of pelvic inflammatory disease
- Hormonal imbalances leading to irregular ovulation
- Fallopian tube blockages
- Fibroid tumors
- Sexually transmitted infections
- Age older than 35
- Overweight or underweight (disrupts hormonal functions)
- Chronic diseases (diabetes and thyroid malfunction)
- Multiple abortions (miscarriages)
- Smoking and alcohol consumption
- Stress (psychological)
- Endocrine changes (begins 10 to 15 years before menopause)

 Endometriosis and sexually transmitted infections are two of the risk factors for female infertility.

Some of the infertility risk factors for men are as follows:

* Undescended testicles and testicular disorders (surgery and trauma)
* Tight jeans or other tight-fitting pants
* Overuse of hot tubs or saunas (high temperatures)
* Mumps after puberty
* Exposure to toxic substances (x-rays, mercury, and lead)
* Heavy alcohol consumption
* Sexually transmitted infections
* Cigarette smoking
* Extended periods of bike riding

 Heavy alcohol consumption is a risk factor for male infertility.

In the female any irregularities that lead to hormonal imbalance (hypothalamic–pituitary–ovarian cycle) may alter ovulation. Appropriate ovarian function may be affected by excessive exercise, stress, inadequate nutrition, poor health, and inappropriate levels of pituitary, thyroid, and adrenal hormones. Abnormalities in the structure of the fallopian tubes (narrowing, blockage, congenital defects, infections, and endometriosis) can lead to infertility or tubal pregnancies. Abnormalities in the uterus (fibroid tumors, congenital malformations, inadequate endometrium, and endometriosis) can also lead to infertility. Bicornuate uterus, septal uterus, and unicornuate uterus are examples of congenital malformations of the uterus. **Endometriosis** is the implantation of uterine endometrium outside the uterus. The most common sites for endometriosis are the lower pelvis and bowel. Inadequate endometrium (thinning of the uterine lining after surgical procedures and inadequate hormonal production) can lead to infertility.

 ## MALE DIAGNOSTIC TESTS

In the male there needs to be an adequate number of sperm, and the sperm need to be healthy and mature. After ejaculation, the sperm must be able to penetrate and fertilize the ovum. Therefore **semen analysis** is the primary indicator of male fertility.

To obtain a sample of semen, the male needs to abstain from sexual intercourse for 48 hours. Through masturbation semen is ejaculated into a sterile specimen container and delivered to the laboratory within 2 hours for analysis. The laboratory analysis comprises analyzing the sperm for volume, motility, number, viscosity, shape, and viability.

If the sperm analysis is normal, no further male evaluation is needed. However, a male physical examination needs to be included for the evaluation of fertility. The exam includes the penis, scrotum, testicles, vas deferens, epididymis, and normal development of external genitalia. Body hair distribution, muscle development, and Adam's apple development are needed for the assessment of normal male sexual characteristics. An internal prostrate exam is necessary to rule out tenderness and swelling.

 ## FEMALE DIAGNOSTIC TESTS

Testing the **basal body temperature (BBT)** is an inexpensive way to determine a woman's ovulation pattern. She must faithfully record her BBT each day for at least 3 months, because there is the possibility that in 1 month she may not ovulate. The woman is instructed to take her temperature each morning (using a special BBT or tympanic thermometer) before she arises, drinks any fluid, or eats. Her daily temperature is then plotted on a monthly graph. If she is sick (colds or infections), she is instructed to note this condition on the graph paper. During ovulation the basal temperature dips (about 0.5°F), and then it rises (to about 0.4–0.8°F) 24 to 72 hours after. The temperature stays elevated for approximately 11 to 16 days, or until 3 to 4 days before the next menstrual flow. This biphasic pattern indicates ovulation. The woman is instructed that the most fertile time is 3 to 4 days before ovulation and 1 to 2 days after. A good suggestion is to have sexual intercourse every other day during this time. Since the ovulation predictor kits have become available the BBT test has become less popular, because it is less accurate.

An **ovulation predictor kit** is a urine test used to predict ovulation based on the luteinizing hormone that is measured in the urine. Luteinizing hormone triggers ovulation, which occurs after the luteinizing hormone surge. Luteinizing hormone can be detected in the urine 8–12 hours after its peak levels. The woman should be instructed to test her urine at the same time each day.

Laparoscopy is a procedure using an endoscope to view the pelvic organs. The endoscope is inserted through a small incision in the anterior wall of the abdomen (near the umbilicus). It is usually done early in the menstrual cycle to visualize the peritoneal cavity. If a woman is infertile, it may reveal endometriosis, fibroids, pelvic adhesions, polycystic ovaries, and tubal occlusion. This method is also used in reproductive technology to retrieve eggs.

Hysterosalpingogram is an x-ray procedure performed to assess for tubal patency and health. This procedure is done 2–5 days after the end of menses. A dye (iodine) is passed through the fallopian tubes to determine whether blockage exists and, if so, to determine its location. Minor adhesions may be removed by this procedure because it can have a curative effect.

The **postcoital test** evaluates the cervical mucus to determine the receptivity of the cervical mucus to sperm and the ability of the sperm to travel within it. Cervical mucus is examined 2–8 hours after intercourse (during the ovulatory time) via a pelvic exam. Live sperm are examined for structure, number, and motility, whereas cervical mucus is examined for spinnbarkeit (stretchable mucus greater than 8 cm), viscosity, quantity, clarity, and pH.

 # MANAGEMENT

Depending on the infertility problem, laboratory and diagnostic test results are reviewed and different treatment modalities are suggested to the infertile couple. Usually, less invasive and less complex treatments are started first; if unsuccessful, then more invasive procedures and combined treatments are implemented. Surgery and drugs are some of the most common treatments for most infertile couples. Surgery is implemented to repair damaged reproductive organs, whereas various ovulation drugs are used for ovulatory problems.

Regardless of the treatment choice, a thorough explanation of the risks and benefits of the suggested treatments must be done. There are other ways of conceiving, such as with assisted reproductive techniques. These reproductive strategies include **artificial insemination, in vitro fertilization, gamete intrafallopian transfer, zygote intrafallopian transfer**, and **surrogate embryo transfer**.

SECTION I • REVIEW QUESTIONS

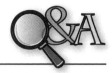

1. The first menstrual period at puberty is called:
   a. Menstrual phase
   b. Menarche
   c. Menopause
   d. Secretory phase

2. Infertility is defined as the inability to conceive a child after:
   a. One year of regular sexual intercourse without using any method of contraception
   b. One year of regular sexual intercourse using various methods of contraception
   c. Two years of regular sexual intercourse without using any method of contraception
   d. Two years of regular sexual intercourse using various methods of contraception

3. The hormonal agents that directly affect the release of follicle-stimulating hormone and luteinizing hormone from the pituitary gland are called:
   a. Estrogen hormones
   b. Progesterone hormones
   c. Releasing factors
   d. Ovulatory factors

4. The ovulation predictor kit is a urine test to predict ovulation based on the _____ hormone that is measured in the urine.
   a. Progesterone
   b. Estrogen
   c. Luteinizing
   d. Ovarian

5. During the menstrual cycle, there is a hormone that causes a rise in the basal body temperature. This hormone is produced by the corpus luteum after ovulation and is called:
   a. Estrogen
   b. Progesterone
   c. Follicle-stimulating hormone
   d. Luteinizing hormone

6. What is the primary indicator of male fertility?
   a. Postcoital test
   b. Semen analysis
   c. Spinnbarkeit
   d. Testicular exam

7. When managing the infertile couple, what treatments are started first?
   a. Invasive procedures
   b. Surgery and drugs
   c. Drugs only
   d. Less invasive procedures and less complex treatments

8. During this phase of the menstrual cycle, the endometrium within the uterus becomes thickened, succulent, and rich in blood supply. This phase is called the:
   a. Ovulatory phase
   b. Menstrual phase
   c. Secretory phase
   d. Proliferative phase

9. Which of the following female diagnostic tests is an inexpensive test to determine a woman's ovulation pattern?
   a. Basal body temperature (BBT)
   b. Postcoital test
   c. Laparoscopy
   d. Hysterosalpingogram

10. At what time during the menstrual cycle does the cervical mucus becomes abundant, transparent, and receptive to sperm penetration?
   a. Late in the cycle
   b. Early in the cycle
   c. After ovulation
   d. Just before ovulation

ANSWERS AND RATIONALES

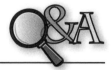

1. The answer is b.

2. The answer is a.

3. The answer is c.

4. The answer is c. Rationale: Luteinizing hormone triggers ovulation.

5. The answer is b.

6. The answer is b. Rationale: This laboratory analysis comprises analyzing the sperm for volume, motility, number, viscosity, shape, and viability. If normal, no further male evaluation is needed except for a physical exam of the male genitalia.

7. The answer is d. Rationale: In treating infertility the protocol is to start with the simple less invasive procedures and, if unsuccessful, to move to the more invasive and complex treatments.

8. The answer is d. Rationale: In this phase of the menstrual cycle the endometrium begins to thicken. In the secretory phase the endometrium becomes highly vascularized and edematous.

9. The answer is a. Rationale: All the other tests are more expensive and invasive and do not measure ovulation.

10. The answer is d. Rationale: Cervical mucus needs to be the most conductive to sperm penetration just before ovulation for fertilization to be most successful.

II

Family Planning

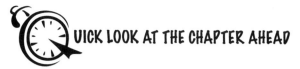

There are multiple choices for contraception available and is dependant upon the user's preference, cost, availability, safety, and convenience. Other issues that need to be taken into consideration are the cultural and religious beliefs of the patient and marital status. Different contraceptive choices are influenced by the patient's age and lifestyle.

Contraception may be barrier (such as condoms or a diaphragm), hormonal (such as oral contraceptive pills, Depo-Provera, vaginal ring), or based on fertility awareness or natural family planning. Permanent sterilization can be performed on both male and female patients.

3

Methods of Contraception

TERMS
☐ Barrier contraception
☐ Depot medroxyprogesterone acetate
☐ Fertility-awareness methods (FAMs)
☐ Intrauterine devices (IUDs)
☐ Oral contraceptives
☐ Sterilization
☐ Transdermal patch
☐ Tubal ligation
☐ Vaginal ring
☐ Vasectomy

19

Awareness for the need for birth control has been an issue since the early 1900s when a nurse, Margaret Sanger, began distributing contraception information to women. Her vision and dedication to the family planning movement eventually evolved into what is now known as Planned Parenthood Federation of America.

Today, in spite of the many choices available for contraception and family planning, in the United States more than 53% of pregnancies are unintended and there are 1.3 million terminations annually.

> ✓ Today, in spite of the many choices available for contraception and family planning, in the United States more than 53% of pregnancies are unintended and there are 1.3 million terminations annually.

Choosing a birth control method is an individual choice based on efficacy, safety, and convenience (Table 3-1). As a woman ages her birth control needs change. What was once easy and effective may no longer be the best choice. If a particular method requires thought and planning on the user's part, the rate of failure is much higher than one that is easier to use.

Selection is influenced by age, weight, marital status, and frequency of intercourse. When selecting a contraceptive method, one must consider several factors. A woman's advanced reproductive age may preclude her from taking hormonal contraception. If she is obese or smokes, a hormonal contraception may not be the best choice because it increases her risk for developing thromboembolic disorders.

Table 3-1 Birth Control Methods

Nonhormonal Methods	Hormonal Methods
Barrier methods	Combined oral contraceptives
Condoms: male and female	Depot medroxyprogesterone acetate
Vaginal spermicidal foams, films, or suppositories	Transdermal patch
Sponge	Vaginal ring
Diaphragm	Intrauterine device
Cervical cap	Hormonal implants
Fertility-awareness method or natural family planning	
Basal body temperature	
Billings or ovulation method	
Calendar or rhythm	
Sterilization	
Tubal ligation	
Vasectomy	

Cultural or religious beliefs must also be considered: Contraception may be contrary to a woman's beliefs. Marital status must be considered. A woman who is in a mutually monogamous relationship may not need protection against sexually transmitted infections (STIs), whereas a woman who is active with multiple partners or whose partner is not mutually monogamous needs a barrier contraception to protect her from STIs.

Frequency of intercourse influences the type of protection needed. If a woman is infrequently active, she may prefer to use a method that is more episodic than long term. Cost is another important factor because many health insurance carriers do not cover birth control. Efficacy is equally important. Method failure leads to an unintended pregnancy.

 ## TYPES OF CONTRACEPTION

Nonhormonal methods include barrier contraception, fertility-awareness methods (FAMs), and sterilization. Hormonal methods include combined oral contraceptives (COCs), progesterone-only contraceptive pills, the patch, the vaginal ring, depot medroxyprogesterone acetate injection, and the intrauterine device (IUD).

The withdrawal method, or coitus interruptus, has a high failure rate because of presence of sperm in preejaculatory fluid and the dependence on the male to predict when he will ejaculate.

Barrier contraception, which is coitus dependent, includes such methods as condom use (female or male condoms), cervical caps, diaphragms, the sponge, and spermicide. Condoms prevent sperm from entering the vagina and are 88% effective against pregnancy. They offer protection from STIs. Although they are inexpensive and easy to obtain, condoms require planning and about 1 in 200 break. Effectiveness is significantly increased (97%) if used in conjunction with a vaginal spermicide containing nonoxynol-9.

Female condoms have been available since the early 1990s and are approximately 95% effective. It is inserted vaginally and covers the vaginal walls. Like the male condom, it protects against human immunodeficiency virus infection and STIs. However, sheepskin condoms should be used if a person is latex allergic.

The vaginal sponge was removed from the general market in 1995 but has recently gained approval from the U.S. Food and Drug Administration for use again. It is a polyurethane sponge saturated with spermicide that is inserted into the vagina, covering the cervix. It provides immediate effectiveness and can remain in place for 24 hours with repeated acts of coitus. It must be left in place for 6 hours after the last act of intercourse. It provides contraception by the use of spermicide but also provides a physical barrier to sperm, which is absorbed by the sponge. It is available without a prescription via the Internet.

The diaphragm and cervical cap fit over the cervix and are inserted up to 6 hours before intercourse. Spermicide is placed inside the device before insertion with additional spermicide application inserted vaginally for repeated acts of coitus. The devices must remain in place for 6 to 8 hours after the last act of coitus. They are both made of latex and require an office visit for fitting by a health care professional. The diaphragm is about 94% effective against pregnancy, and the cervical cap is approximately 92% effective. There is a higher incidence of urinary tract infections with the use of both methods.

Oral contraceptives remain the most popular form of birth control in the United States. They contain hormones that inhibit ovulation and thicken cervical mucus and are 97–99% effective against pregnancy. Synthetic estrogen and progestin are the primary compounds used in COCs containing 20–35 µg of estrogen and 0.5–1.0 mg progestin. Monophasic pills contain the same amount of hormones daily, whereas triphasic or biphasic contain varying amounts of estrogen and progestin throughout the cycle. This type of contraception is taken daily for 28 days with a 7-day pill-free week to allow for a withdrawal bleed. Newer COCs today can be taken for 84 days continuously, allowing a woman to have her menses only four times per year.

Progesterone-only pills contain only progestin and are taken daily with no pill-free week. These thicken cervical mucus and are only slightly lower in their effectiveness as COCs. Progesterone-only pills are generally used by lactating women or those who cannot take estrogen.

In addition to providing contraception, COCs provide cycle control, decreased menstrual flow, and less cramping associated with menses.

The **transdermal patch** is a beige matrix patch with an adhesive that affixes to the skin. The patch is applied to the upper arm, abdomen, or buttocks weekly for 3 weeks and then removed to allow for a withdrawal bleed. A new patch is then applied after a 7-day patch-free week. It has many of the same noncontraceptive benefits as oral contraceptive pills and similarly does not offer any protection against STIs. Because of the adhesive, some patch wearers experience localized irritation. Its mechanism of action is similar to that of the vaginal ring. It is highly effective against pregnancy (99%). There is decreased effectiveness if used by a woman who weighs more than 198 pounds.

The **vaginal ring** is a flexible ring that contains both estrogen and progestin. It is inserted into the vagina for 3 weeks continuously and then removed for 1 week to allow for a withdrawal bleed. A new ring is then inserted. The time-released hormones are absorbed by the vaginal tissue, preventing pregnancy by inhibition of ovulation and cervical mucus thickening. It does not protect against STIs. It is associated with an increase in vaginal discharge known as leukorrhea.

Depot medroxyprogesterone acetate inhibits ovulation by suppressing follicle-stimulating hormone and luteinizing hormone production. It is administered intramuscularly every 12 weeks and has a pregnancy rate of less than 1%. It is safely used during lactation. The major disadvantage of this type of contraception is weight gain (approximately 8 pounds during the first year of use), irregular bleeding, and slow return of fertility. Recent studies also suggest osteoporosis with greater than 2 years use, and it is unknown at this time if bone loss is reversible.

Implanon is a single-rod subdermal implant containing progesterone that is inserted into the upper arm by a health care professional. It provides up to 3 years of contraception. It provides immediate protection against pregnancy upon insertion. Irregular bleeding is a common side effect. Its predecessor, Norplant, is no longer available.

IUDs (intrauterine devices) are gaining favor among women seeking long-term contraception. The IUD is a "T"-shaped device that is inserted into the uterus during the first 5 days of menses by a health care provider and provides immediate protection against pregnancy. The woman checks the string or filament for confirmation of placement before and after intercourse. The IUD is effective for 3–10 years depending on the type used. LNG-IUS and the Copper T 380 A are highly effective (99%) IUDs on the market today. They contain progestin that thickens cervical mucus. The IUD acts as a foreign body that alters the endometrial lining, making it an unsuitable environment for implantation. There is a higher risk of pelvic inflammatory disease among women with IUDs who are not in a mutually monogamous relationship because the filament acts as a wick in the presence of bacteria.

Sterilization is considered a permanent means of contraception. It can be performed on both men and women. Male sterilization, known as a **vasectomy**, is an in-office procedure performed by an urologist. The vas deferens is severed, preventing sperm from traveling from the testes to the penis. It is not considered successful until three ejaculate specimens reveal no sperm. Once successful, its failure rate is less than 1%.

Tubal ligation, or female sterilization, involves surgical severance and electrocoagulation or suturing of the fallopian tubes. This is a laparoscopic procedure performed under general anesthesia. The severed portion of the tube can also be clipped or banded with silastic or titanium rings. A newer nonsurgical sterilization procedure is done by the insertion of microfibers transcervically into the fallopian tubes, causing scarring after several months. This prohibits fertilization.

Fertility-awareness methods (FAMs), or natural family planning, is a nonhormonal method of birth control. This method requires familiarity of bodily changes during the menstrual cycle and periodic abstinence or use of barrier methods during ovulation if pregnancy is not desirable.

The FAM technique uses the calendar method to predict ovulation. It is also known as the rhythm method. This is based on the assumption that ovulation occurs on day 14 of the menstrual cycle and that sperm are viable for 3 days. The patient must chart her menstrual cycle for at least 6–8 months for accuracy.

The ovulation method, or Billings method, uses cervical mucus to evaluate hormonal changes during the menstrual cycle to determine ovulation. The differences in the texture of the cervical mucus (thick and sticky to clear and slippery) correspond with ovulation.

The basal body temperature (BBT) method requires a woman to measure and record her temperature with a special BBT thermometer upon awakening daily. The BBT is the lowest temperature reached by a healthy person before rising. Hormonal changes cause the BBT to rise slightly (0.4 to 0.8°F) and are typically higher after ovulation has occurred. The effectiveness of FAM depends on the consistency of its use and the ability of the woman to correctly identify fertile times of her cycle.

 EMERGENCY CONTRACEPTION

Emergency contraception (EC), or postcoital contraception, is used after a single act of unprotected intercourse regardless of the reason. EC reduces the chance of pregnancy by about 75%. Treatment should be initiated within 72 hours of the unprotected act but can be administered up to 120 hours later. Methods of EC include COCs, progesterone-only pills, or insertion of a copper T IUD. The intended mechanism of action is not that of the abortion pill (RU 486); rather it alters tubal transport of the sperm and egg, inhibits or delays ovulation, and alters the endometrium so it is less receptive to implantation. It will not alter or disrupt an already established pregnancy.

 EC reduces the chance of pregnancy by about 75%. Treatment should be initiated within 72 hours of the unprotected act but can be administered up to 120 hours later.

 EC will not alter or disrupt an already established pregnancy.

Plan B and the Yuzpe method are available in the United States. Plan B is a product containing two 750-µg tablets of levonorgestrel (a progestin). The Yuzpe method uses 200 µg of ethinyl estradiol and 1.0 mg of levonorgestrel, which is achieved by using several pills from a COC pack to equal those doses. There is a higher rate of nausea and vomiting associated with the Yuzpe method. If vomiting occurs within 2 hours of taking the dose, a repeat dose is required for either method used.

Postcoital IUD insertion can be used as EC by preventing fertilization up to 7 days after an act of unprotected intercourse. It may be left in place for future contraception. If a woman does not receive her menses within 2 weeks after the EC, a pregnancy test should be performed.

SECTION II • REVIEW QUESTIONS

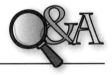

1. The following is true regarding barrier contraception *except*:
   a. They offer protection against STIs
   b. They are coitus related
   c. They sometimes require a prescription
   d. They require use by both partners to be effective

2. The best choice of a contraception for a woman who is newly divorced and dating would be:
   a. Withdrawal method
   b. Barrier contraception, including condoms
   c. IUD
   d. Oral contraceptives

3. Of the following, which is considered the most reliable method?
   a. IUD
   b. Fertility-awareness method
   c. Condoms with foam
   d. Oral contraceptives

4. A woman who uses a diaphragm or cervical cap is more likely to:
   a. Become pregnant than if she used a condom alone
   b. Develop urinary tract infections
   c. Complain of breakthrough bleeding
   d. Have a very light menstrual flow

5. Vaginal discharge or leukorrhea is associated with:
   a. IUDs
   b. Oral contraceptives
   c. Depot medroxyprogesterone acetate
   d. Vaginal ring

6. If a woman weighs 238 pounds she should not use:
   a. an IUD
   b. Today sponge
   c. Ortho Evra patch
   d. Depo-Provera

7. Hormonal methods of contraception include all of the following *except*:

    a. Transdermal patch

    b. Billings method

    c. Vaginal ring

    d. Hormonal implants

8. The mechanism of action for emergency contraception:

    a. Alters the endometrium so it is less receptive to implantation

    b. Causes the basal body temperature to rise slightly

    c. Prevents sperms from traveling through the vas deferens

    d. Suppresses follicle-stimulating hormone and luteinizing hormone production

9. When teaching a patient about barrier contraception, it is important to remind her:

    a. It can be inserted up to 6 hours before intercourse

    b. To use additional spermicide with repeated acts of coitus

    c. Not to use it if she or her partner is allergic to latex

    d. All of the above

10. It is important to consider which of the following when selecting a contraceptive method?

    a. Frequency of intercourse

    b. Cost

    c. Efficacy

    d. All of the above

ANSWERS AND RATIONALES

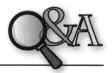

1. **The answer is d.** Rationale: Barrier contraception can be used by just one partner. Contraception methods, such as the cervical cap or diaphragm, need to be fitted by a health care provider and require a prescription.

2. **The answer is b.** Rationale: Barrier contraception protects against pregnancy and sexually transmitted diseases.

3. **The answer is a.** Rationale: IUD is the most reliable of those listed. There are higher failure rates with the other methods if not used correctly.

4. **The answer is b.** Rationale: Women who use diaphragms or cervical caps are at a higher risk for developing urinary tract infections.

5. **The answer is d.** Rationale: Users of the vaginal ring are more likely to complain of leukorrhea.

6. **The answer is c.** Rationale: The patch has decreased effectiveness against birth control if used by women who weigh more than 198 pounds.

7. **The answer is b.** Rationale: The Billings method is one of the fertility-awareness methods, or natural family planning.

8. **The answer is a.** Rationale: EC alters tubal transport of the sperm and egg, inhibits or delays ovulation, and alters the endometrium so it is less receptive to implantation.

9. **The answer is d.** Rationale: All of the above are important teaching aspects with barrier contraception.

10. **The answer is d.** Rationale: All of the answers are important to consider.

III

Antepartum Period

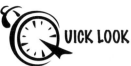

It is very important for women to have and maintain good health practices before pregnancy.

The first visit to the doctor or midwife usually occurs after the first missed menstrual period and continues throughout the pregnancy.

Prenatal care includes laboratory analysis, nutritional guidance, detailed health history, physical examinations, and health education.

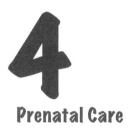

4

Prenatal Care

TERMS
- [ ] **Human chorionic gonadotropin (hCG)**
- [ ] **Medical/surgical history**
- [ ] **Nutritional history**
- [ ] **Obstetric/gynecologic history**
- [ ] **Probable signs of pregnancy**
- [ ] **Psychosocial history**

PRECONCEPTION HEALTH

It is very important for women to have and maintain proper health practices before pregnancy. Preconception counseling, such as premarital and family planning, can be provided as part of routine health examinations. Health promotion involves a healthy diet, maintaining an optimal weight, exercise, rest, safe sex practices, and avoiding substance abuse of tobacco, alcohol, and any recreational drugs. Before becoming pregnant, a routine health examination should be made with a health care provider. At this time a health history, routine physical examination, pelvic exam, Papanicolaou (Pap) test, blood type, Rh factor, and hemoglobin level can be evaluated.

FIRST PRENATAL VISIT

The first visit includes a detailed health history, a complete physical examination (including a pelvic exam), and manual pelvic measurements to determine pelvic adequacy and laboratory tests. The laboratory tests on the initial visit are as follows: blood type and Rh factor, antibody screen, complete blood count, urine analysis and culture, Rubella antibody screen, hepatitis B antigen, human immunodeficiency virus antibody screen, serological test for syphilis, tests for gonorrhea and chlamydia, Pap test, and tuberculosis skin test. Also, a 1-hour glucose tolerance test is done at the initial visit if a woman is at risk for gestational diabetes. However, this test is done routinely at 24 to 28 weeks' gestation for all pregnant women.

Early diagnosis of pregnancy can be done by pregnancy tests. The commonly used laboratory tests for pregnancy are based on detecting the presence of **human chorionic gonadotropin (hCG),** a hormone secreted by the chorionic villi of the placenta, found in urine or blood serum of the pregnant woman. Because all pregnancy tests are only 95% accurate in diagnosing pregnancy, these tests are considered **probable signs of pregnancy** rather than positive signs of pregnancy. In the nonpregnant woman, there are no units that are detectable because there are no trophoblast cells producing hCG. In the pregnant woman trace amounts of hCG appear in the serum as early as 24 to 48 hours after implantation. They reach a measurable level (50 mIU/ml) in 7 to 9 days after conception.

Urine tests are rarely used in the health care setting because blood serum tests give earlier results. Home pregnancy tests based on urine samples are still used by the consumer. The home pregnancy tests are convenient. A woman dips a reagent strip into her stream of urine. A color change on the strip denotes pregnancy.

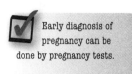 Early diagnosis of pregnancy can be done by pregnancy tests.

 In the pregnant woman trace amounts of hCG appear in the serum as early as 24 to 48 hours after implantation.

NÄGELE'S RULE

An estimated date of delivery (EDD) or estimated date of birth (EDB) is important because it gives the pregnant woman and her family an estimated date in which the birth of the baby may take place. About 10% of pregnant woman deliver on their estimated dates of delivery. However, this date is helpful for the health care provider to monitor and evaluate the progress of gestation.

The method for estimating this date of delivery is called Nägele's rule. To calculate Nägele's rule, count back 3 months from the first day of the last menstrual period and add 7 days:

$$5/12 - 3 \text{ months} = 2/12 + 7 \text{ days} = 2/19, \text{ or February 19}$$

This example shows the first day of the last menstrual period as May 12 minus 3 months, which gives us February 12 plus 7 days equals the expected date of delivery, which is February 19. Nägele's rule assumes a 28-day menstrual cycle with conception occurring on the 14th day. If the menstrual cycle is shorter or longer, the health care provider must take that into consideration when calculating the expected date of delivery.

 To calculate Nägele's rule, count back 3 months from the first day of the last menstrual period (LMP) and add 7 days.

DETAILED HEALTH HISTORY

A detailed health history covers many areas. The **obstetric/gynecologic history** reviews the age of menarche, menstrual history, contraceptive practices, infertility, gynecologic problems, sexually transmitted infections, and all pregnancies as well as their outcomes. Nägele's rule is applied based on the first day of the last menstrual period to determine the EDD.

The **medical/surgical history** is based on any present conditions the pregnant woman may have and their effects on pregnancy. Some examples of medical problems could be hypothyroidism, obesity, diabetes, and hypertension. Any of these conditions may warrant collaboration with specialists in the particular area. A referral for genetic counseling may be appropriate at this time. Any surgery is listed as well as the outcomes. A common surgical operation is an appendectomy, which later can rule out appendicitis.

The **nutritional history** is extremely important based on the fact that the developing embryo/fetus relies on nutrition for proper growth and development. A dietary history can reveal strengths and weaknesses in nutrition. An excellent assessment is one that evaluates a typical diet for 1–2 weeks. This process enables the health care provider to evaluate the overall nutritional habits of the pregnant woman. If a healthy diet including folic acid is not part of the typical diet, then guidance and education can assist the pregnant woman in achieving this goal. Along with nutrition, there needs to be a plan for optimal weight gain, exercise, rest, and avoidance of tobacco, alcohol, caffeine, and any illegal/recreational drugs. Questions need to be asked regarding use of any herbal preparations (e.g., teas), over-the-counter drugs, and prescriptions because some substances pass through the placenta and may harm the developing embryo.

 A dietary history can reveal strengths and weaknesses in nutrition. An excellent assessment is one that evaluates a typical diet for 1–2 weeks.

The **psychosocial history** includes the spouse/partner, family situation, and any history of domestic violence. Family support or other support systems, readiness for pregnancy (age, stress, life goals), and financial resources are part of this process. Another aspect that is very important is the home and workplace (environmental conditions) as well as safety hazards, toxic chemicals, and possible radiation.

 Questions need to be asked regarding use of any herbal preparations (e.g., teas), over-the-counter drugs, and prescriptions because some substances pass through the placenta and may harm the developing embryo.

FIRST, SECOND, AND THIRD TRIMESTER VISITS

A trimester is one of three periods of about 3 months each into which a normal pregnancy is divided. Therefore including the first comprehensive prenatal visit, the follow-up visits are divided into trimesters:

> A trimester is one of three periods of about 3 months each into which a normal pregnancy is divided.

- Every 4 weeks for the first 28 weeks of gestation
- Every 2 weeks to week 36
- After week 36, weekly until birth

 ## SIGNS OF PREGNANCY

Some of the physiological changes that occur in pregnancy are recognized as signs and symptoms of pregnancy.

1. Presumptive (subjective) changes are those symptoms experienced by the pregnant woman. Some conditions other than pregnancy may be the cause.

   - Amenorrhea (4 weeks)
   - Excessive fatigue (12 weeks)
   - Breast changes (3–4 weeks)
   - Nausea/vomiting (4–14 weeks)
   - Urinary frequency (6–12 weeks)
   - Quickening (16–20 weeks) (mother's perception of fetal movement)

2. Probable (objective) changes are those signs observed by the examiner. Some conditions other than pregnancy may be the cause.

   - Goodell's sign (5–6 weeks): Softening of the cervical tip caused by increased vascularity and slight hypertrophy.
   - Hegar's sign (6–12 weeks): Softening of the lower uterine segment and compressibility of the uterine isthmus. The isthmus is the area between the cervix and the body of the uterus.
   - Chadwick's sign (6–8 weeks): Violet-bluish color of vagina and cervix caused by increased vascularity.

- Positive pregnancy test (4–12 weeks): Serum is used.
- Positive pregnancy test (6–12 weeks): Urine is used.
- Braxton-Hicks contractions (16 weeks): Mild, intermittent, painless contractions that occur during pregnancy.
- Ballottement (16–18 weeks): A diagnostic test using palpation. A floating object when tapped or pushed moves away and then returns to touch the examiner's hand. The examiner places his or her hand in the vagina and taps gently upward, causing the fetus to rise. The fetus then sinks and a gentle tap is felt on the finger.
- Uterine souffle: When auscultated over the uterus, a soft blowing sound is made by the blood in the arteries of the pregnant uterus and synchronous with the maternal pulse.

3. Positive signs of pregnancy are those signs attributed only to the presence of the fetus.

- Visualization of the fetus (4 weeks) by transvaginal ultrasonography
- Fetal heart tones (8 weeks) detected by ultrasound examination and electronic Doppler by 10 weeks and fetoscope by 18–20 weeks
- Fetal movement palpated by an experienced examiner (19–22 weeks)

 ## GRAVIDA/PARA CONCEPTS

There are several systems used to describe a woman's pregnancy history. The two most common are the two-digit system and the five-digit system. In the two-digit system a woman pregnant for the first time who has not carried a pregnancy to viability is considered a gravida 1 and para 0 (G1/P0). When the woman delivers she is a gravida 1 and para 1.

In the five-digit system five parameters are considered: gravida, term birth, preterm birth, abortion, and living children (GTPAL). An example of this system would be a woman who is pregnant for the fifth time, has had two term births, one preterm birth (under 37 weeks' gestation), one spontaneous abortion, and three living children. Using the five-digit system she would be considered G5 T2 P1 A1 L3.

Conception takes place when a sperm fertilizes an ovum in the outer one-third of the fallopian tube. After fertilization, the ovum passes through several cell divisions on its journey to the uterus. Once in the uterus, implantation takes place and embryonic layers of cells are formed. The embryonic period is the most critical because all the major organs are forming and are at risk to the influences of the environment.

The fetal period begins at 9 weeks gestation and terminates when the pregnancy ends (usually 40 weeks gestation). During the fetal period, refinement of structure and function take place.

5

Embryology and Fetology

TERMS
- ☐ **Amnion**
- ☐ **Amniotic cavity**
- ☐ **Blastocyst**
- ☐ **Capacitation**
- ☐ **Chorion**
- ☐ **Chorionic villi**
- ☐ **Corona radiata**
- ☐ **Decidua basalis**
- ☐ **Ectoderm**
- ☐ **Endoderm**
- ☐ **Hyaluronidase**
- ☐ **L/S ratio (lecithin/ sphingomyelin)**
- ☐ **Mesoderm**
- ☐ **Morula**
- ☐ **Nuchal cord**
- ☐ **Trophoblasts**
- ☐ **Wharton's jelly**
- ☐ **Zona pellucida**
- ☐ **Zygote**

37

CONCEPTION

Conception takes place when a sperm fertilizes an ovum in the outer one-third of the fallopian tube. This outer one-third is called the ampullar portion. Normally, one ovum matures each month (at the time of ovulation). The ovum needs to be fertilized within the first 24 hours (48 hours at the outermost); if not the ovum disintegrates. The life of a sperm is usually 2 to 3 days; therefore successful fertilization can take place around 48 hours before ovulation or 24 hours after.

 Conception takes place when a sperm fertilizes an ovum in the outer one-third of the fallopian tube.

During the menstrual cycle, when the graafian follicle ruptures and an ovum is ejected from the ovary into the fallopian tube, that ovum is encased by a thick membranous envelope called the **zona pellucida**. This thick membranous envelope along with the **corona radiata** (elongated follicle cells surrounding the zona pellucida of the ovum) are captured by the fimbriated edges of the fallopian tube and propelled into the tube. Once inside the fallopian tube, hairlike structures that line the inside of the fallopian tube move the ovum through the tube along with peristaltic action.

SEXUAL INTERCOURSE

During sexual intercourse the male ejaculates about 200 to 500 million sperm (a teaspoon of semen) into the vagina. The cervical mucus during ovulation is much less viscous and hostile to sperm, thereby aiding spermatozoa greater penetration. Using the flagellar movement of their tails, the sperm can fertilize an ovum in 5 minutes or in 4 to 6 hours, which is usually the average time. Sperm remain viable in the reproductive tract for 2 to 3 days. The great number of sperm ejaculated is necessary because many sperm are lost in the vagina, cervical mucus, and endometrium or enter the wrong fallopian tube, which does not contain an ovum.

A prerequisite for a sperm to fertilize an ovum is called **capacitation,** which is an enzymatic process. Small perforations form in the cap of the sperm (acrosome) which allows **hyaluronidase** (an enzyme) to help the sperm penetrate the protective layers (corona radiata and zona pellucida) around the ovum. Only one sperm can fertilize one ovum in normal circumstances. Once the sperm penetrates the ovum's cell membrane, the cell membrane changes and becomes impenetrable to other spermatozoa, and this process is called the zona reaction.

During the fusion of the ovum and the sperm, cell division begins and the structure is called a zygote. The sex of the embryo is determined at the time of fertilization because the ovum and sperm each carry 23 chromosomes (22 autosomes and 1 sex chromosome); therefore the fertilized ovum has 46 chromosomes. A male child is conceived if a Y-carrying spermatozoon fertilized the ovum. This child will have received an X chromosome from the mother and a Y chromosome from the father, XY. A female child is conceived if an X-carrying spermatozoon fertilized the ovum. This child will have received an X chromosome from the mother and an X chromosome from the father, XX.

 ## PASSAGE THROUGH THE FALLOPIAN TUBE

After fertilization the ovum passes through several cell divisions, during which it is retained in the fallopian tube for about 3 days. Fertilization takes place (day 1), and the fertilized ovum divides and is called a **zygote** (day 2). As cell division continues, a cluster of cells form, called the **morula** (day 3). The morula is still surrounded by the protective cell covering, called the zona pellucida. This cluster of cells continues to travel down the fallopian tube until it enters the upper aspect of the uterus. At this point large cells collect at the periphery of the ball with a fluid space surrounding an inner cell mass; this phase is called the **blastocyst** (day 4). As fluid passes through the zona pellucida, it is eventually shed by the growing structure. The blastocyst is divided into two parts: The inner surface of the blastocyst forms the embryo and amnion and the outer layers of cells surrounding the blastocyst cavity are called the **trophoblasts.** Eventually, the trophoblast develops into one of the embryonic membranes, the chorion, and helps to form the placenta.

As the zona pellucida degenerates, the trophoblast cells burrow into the endometrial lining at the implantation site (usually in the anterior or posterior fundal region). **Chorionic villi** develop out of the trophoblast and manifest "fingerlike projections" and continue to burrow into the blood-filled spaces of the endometrium. These villi obtain oxygen and nutrients from the maternal bloodstream and dispose of carbon dioxide and waste products into the maternal blood. Once implantation has taken place (7–8 days), the endometrium is called the **decidua basalis**.

IMPLANTATION

When implantation has been established the trophoblastic cells secrete human chorionic gonadotropin, which stimulates the corpus luteum in the ovary not to atrophy but to continue secreting estrogen and progesterone until the placenta is fully functioning. Therefore the uterine endometrium (decidua) will not slough off as in a menstrual cycle but will continue to grow in thickness and vascularity.

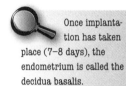

Once implantation has taken place (7–8 days), the endometrium is called the decidua basalis.

Further differentiation of the inner cell mass occurs at the same time with the development of the trophoblast and implantation. Three embryonic layers of cells are formed: the ectoderm, mesoderm, and endoderm. All tissues, organs, and organ systems of the embryo develop from these three primary cell layers:

- The **ectoderm**, the upper layer, forms the central nervous system, special senses, skin, nails, hair, and glands.
- The **mesoderm**, the middle layer, forms the skeletal, urinary, circulatory, spleen, and reproductive organs.
- The **endoderm**, the lower layer, forms the respiratory system, liver, pancreas, and digestive system.

Many women are not aware immediately that a pregnancy has been started. Several weeks may pass before even one of the presumptive signs of pregnancy takes place (e.g., missing the first menstrual period).

DEVELOPMENTAL STAGES OF OVUM, EMBRYO, AND FETUS

The first 2 weeks are considered to be the period of the dividing zygote and implantation (preembryonic development) (Figure 5-1). From day 15 until 8 weeks after conception is considered the embryonic stage (or measurement of the embryo of 3 cm from crown to rump). The embryonic period is the most critical because all the major organs are forming and are at risk to the influences of the environment (e.g., infections, viruses, drugs, and radiation). Intrauterine growth restriction (retardation) can be the result of nutritional deficiencies during pregnancy and can be influenced by

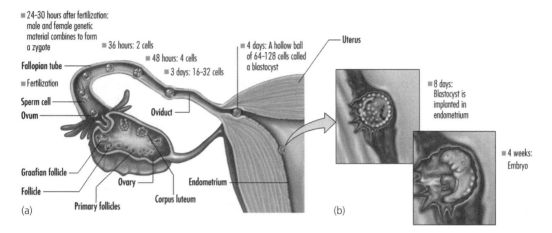

- 24–30 hours after fertilization: male and female genetic material combines to form a zygote
- 36 hours: 2 cells
- 48 hours: 4 cells
- 3 days: 16–32 cells
- 4 days: A hollow ball of 64–128 cells called a blastocyst
- Uterus
- Fertilization
- Fallopian tube
- Sperm cell
- Ovum
- Oviduct
- Graafian follicle
- Ovary
- Endometrium
- Follicle
- Corpus luteum
- Primary follicles

(a)

- 8 days: Blastocyst is implanted in endometrium
- 4 weeks: Embryo

(b)

Figure 5-1 (a) Fertilization and passage through the fallopian tubes. (b) Implantation.

prepregnancy nutritional deficiencies. The fetal period begins at 9 weeks gestation and terminates when the pregnancy ends. During the fetal period, refinement of structure and function take place.

The vulnerability of the fetus to teratogens is less except for the function of the central nervous system, which remains highly sensitive to teratogens until the 32nd week of gestation, when the CNS becomes less sensitive. As far as viability (fetal ability to survive outside the uterus), with modern technology the fetus is viable at 20 weeks' gestation with a fetal weight of 500 grams or more.

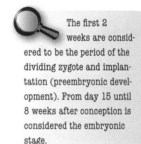

The first 2 weeks are considered to be the period of the dividing zygote and implantation (preembryonic development). From day 15 until 8 weeks after conception is considered the embryonic stage.

The fetal period begins at 9 weeks' gestation and terminates when the pregnancy ends.

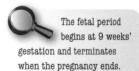

The fetus is viable at 20 weeks' gestation with a fetal weight of 500 grams or more.

PLACENTA

The trophoblastic tissue forms the placenta and becomes a multifunctioning organ. The placenta serves as the fetal lungs, digestive system, kidneys, and an endocrine organ throughout the pregnancy. At term, the placenta covers half the internal surface of the uterus.

There is no direct circulatory connection between the maternal blood and that of the embryo/fetus. The process of exchange is carried out through osmosis. Because there is only one layer (the chorionic villi) of tissue between the maternal blood and fetal capillaries, there is risk of a tissue tear whereby

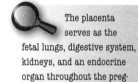

The placenta serves as the fetal lungs, digestive system, kidneys, and an endocrine organ throughout the pregnancy.

fetal blood can enter the maternal circulation. This can cause problems if there is an Rh or ABO incompatibility between mother and fetus. The placenta also produces hormones throughout the pregnancy, such as human chorionic gonadotropin, human placental lactogen, estrogen, progesterone, and relaxin. These hormones are important in maintaining normalcy throughout the pregnancy.

MEMBRANES

Two fetal membranes are formed during implantation and surround the developing embryo; they are the chorion and the amnion. The trophoblast develops into the **chorion,** which covers the fetal side of the placenta. The umbilical blood vessels branch out over

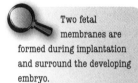

Two fetal membranes are formed during implantation and surround the developing embryo.

the fetal surface of the placenta. The blastocyst develops into the **amnion**, which evolves into the **amniotic cavity,** forming a fluid-filled sac. The amnion covers the umbilical cord and later comes into direct contact with the chorion.

AMNIOTIC FLUID

At term the normal amount of amniotic fluid is between 800 and 1200 ml of clear fluid. There is a constant change in the amniotic fluid volume. The fetus "breathes" the fluid in and out of its lungs, swallows the fluid, and urinates into it. The amniotic fluid has many functions: maintenance of temperature, cushioning the fetus from trauma, oral fluids, waste repository, area for fetal movement and development of the musculoskeletal system, and facilitating symmetrical growth.

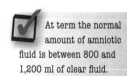

At term the normal amount of amniotic fluid is between 800 and 1,200 ml of clear fluid.

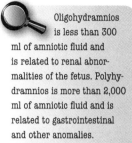

Amniotic fluid volume is used in assessing fetal well-being. Oligohydramnios is less than 300 ml of amniotic fluid and is related to renal abnormalities of the fetus. Polyhydramnios is more than 2,000 ml of amniotic fluid and is related to gastrointestinal and other anomalies.

> Oligohydramnios is less than 300 ml of amniotic fluid and is related to renal abnormalities of the fetus. Polyhydramnios is more than 2,000 ml of amniotic fluid and is related to gastrointestinal and other anomalies.

The volume of amniotic fluid allows for greater information to assess fetal well-being, especially in high risk pregnancies. The **L/S ratio (lecithin/sphingomyelin)** determines the maturity of the fetal lungs, especially useful in preterm labor, as well as other complications. Genetic studies provide information regarding abnormalities of chromosomal structure and number. On a positive note, the sex of the fetus is also determined when amniotic fluid studies are needed.

UMBILICAL CORD

The entire umbilical cord is wrapped in connective tissue, called **Wharton's jelly,** which prevents compression of the blood vessels. At term a usual umbilical cord measures 18–22 inches long (55 cm) and 1 inch wide (2 cm). The cord ensures continued oxygenation and nourishment to the growing embryo/fetus. If the umbilical cord is wrapped around the fetal neck, it is called a **nuchal cord**. Also, any other compression of the cord can occur if the cord lies between the fetal head and the maternal pelvis or is twisted around the fetal body.

There are two arteries and one vein in the umbilical cord. The vessels are so named because of structure, not function. The one umbilical vein brings oxygenated blood from the placenta to the fetus, and the two arteries take away the deoxygenated blood from the fetus to the placenta. The umbilical cord is normally located centrally on the placenta; any other type of insertion is considered abnormal. An example of one type of abnormality is a battledore placenta in which the umbilical cord has a peripheral location.

An example of one type of abnormality is a Battledore placenta in which the umbilical cord has a peripheral location.

SECTION III · REVIEW QUESTIONS

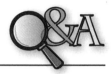

1. The early diagnosis of pregnancy is a test based on detecting the presence of the _____hormone secreted by the chorionic villi found in urine and blood serum of the pregnant woman.
   a. Estrogen
   b. Human chorionic gonadotropin
   c. Progesterone
   d. Luteinizing

2. The ovum needs to be fertilized within a time span of:
   a. 24–48 hours
   b. 72–96 hours
   c. 1 week
   d. 2 weeks

3. This probable sign of pregnancy is a diagnostic test using palpation: a floating object when tapped or pushed moves away and then returns to touch the examiner's hand. This sign is called:
   a. Hegar
   b. Goodell
   c. Chadwick
   d. Ballottement

4. Once the sperm penetrates the ovum's cell membrane, the cell membrane changes and becomes impenetrable to other spermatozoa in a process called:
   a. Corona radiata
   b. Zona reaction
   c. Hyaluronidase
   d. Zona pellucida

5. During prenatal care, a nutritional history is extremely important because the developing embryo relies on nutrition for proper growth and development. The best method to assess the nutrition of the pregnant woman is to:
   a. Ask detailed questions about nutrition
   b. Give the pregnant woman a short quiz based on nutrition
   c. Evaluate the pregnant woman's typical diet for 2 weeks
   d. Give the pregnant woman a book based on nutrition

6. After fertilization cell division takes place. On day 3 a cluster of cells are called morula and are still surrounded by a protective cell covering called the:
    a. Zygote
    b. Blastocyst
    c. Zona pellucida
    d. Trophoblast

7. Prenatal care and doctor visits are divided into:
    a. First, second, and third trimester visits
    b. A visit every 4 weeks throughout the pregnancy
    c. A visit every 2 weeks throughout the pregnancy
    d. A visit every week throughout the pregnancy

8. When implantation has been established the trophoblastic cells secrete _____ hormone, which stimulates the corpus luteum in the ovary not to atrophy but to continue secreting estrogen and progesterone until the placenta is fully functioning.
    a. Relaxin
    b. Human placental lactogen
    c. Estrogen
    d. Human chorionic gonadotropin

9. The visualization of the fetus at 4 weeks of gestation by transvaginal ultrasonography is considered:
    a. A probable sign of pregnancy
    b. A presumptive sign of pregnancy
    c. A positive sign of pregnancy
    d. Both probable and presumptive signs of pregnancy

10. Which period of development during the 40 weeks of gestation is the most critical?
    a. Preembryonic period
    b. Embryonic period
    c. Fetal period
    d. Postfetal period

ANSWERS AND RATIONALES

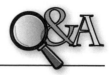

1. **The answer is b.**

2. **The answer is a.** Rationale: If not fertilized within 24–48 hours, the ovum disintegrates.

3. **The answer is d.**

4. **The answer is b.**

5. **The answer is c.**

6. **The answer is c.**

7. **The answer is a.** Rationale: First-trimester visits comprise a visit every 4 weeks for the first 28 weeks of gestation, second trimester a visit every 2 weeks from week 29 through week 36, and third trimester weekly until birth.

8. **The answer is d.**

9. **The answer is c.** Rationale: A positive sign of pregnancy is attributed only to the presence of the fetus.

10. **The answer is b.** Rationale: All the major organs are forming and are at risk to the influences of the environment.

IV

Intrapartum and Postpartum Periods

Labor is a series of processes by which the products of conception are expelled from the mother's body. The cause of labor is unknown.

There are four stages of labor:

- **First stage:** Begins with true labor contractions and results in cervical effacement and dilation and ends with complete effacement and dilation.

- **Second stage:** Begins with complete cervical effacement and dilation and ends with the birth of the baby.

- **Third stage:** Begins with the birth of the baby and ends with the birth/delivery of the placenta.

- **Fourth stage:** Begins with the delivery of the placenta and ends 1–4 hours past the birth process. This stage is also referred to as the recovery phase.

Part of the recovery phase is spent with the mother bonding with the newborn and if she plans on breastfeeding, this is a wonderful time to do so.

6

Labor and Delivery

TERMS
- ☐ **Bloody show**
- ☐ **Labor**
- ☐ **Lightening**

LABOR

Labor is a series of processes by which the products of conception are expelled from the mother's body. However, there are other milestones that need to be addressed. The birth of a newborn results in the expansion of a family. A couple will enter the labor suite and upon discharge a new family emerges.

THEORIES OF LABOR

The cause of labor is unknown; however, there are several theories. One theory states that there is an increased sensitivity of the myometrium to oxytocin, whereas another states that there is a decrease in the progesterone levels. A third theory states that there is an increase in the uterine irritability as a result of stretching from the expanding contents.

The cause of labor is unknown; however, there are several theories.

PREMONITORY SIGNS OF LABOR

During the last few weeks of pregnancy a number of changes may indicate that the time for labor is approaching. Primigravidas have **lightening** occur about 10–14 days before delivery. Lightening means that the fetal presenting part descends into the true pelvis. The woman usually feels pressure on her bladder and reports more frequent urination. However, her breathing is much easier because the fetus is no longer pressing on the diaphragm. A phenomenon called nesting occurs during this time, and some women report a surge of energy before labor. The increased energy level usually occurs in 24 to 48 hours before the onset of labor. It is theorized to be the result of an increase in epinephrine release and a decrease of progesterone.

Lightening means that the fetal presenting part descends into the true pelvis.

A phenomenon called nesting occurs during this time and some women report a surge of energy before labor.

The differences between true labor and false labor are as follows:

- In true labor the contractions occur at regular intervals and increase in frequency, duration, and intensity as the labor progresses. In false labor the contractions occur at irregular intervals and tend to disappear when the patient lies down. The contractions do not increase in frequency or intensity.

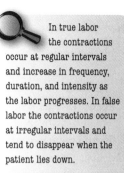 In true labor the contractions occur at regular intervals and increase in frequency, duration, and intensity as the labor progresses. In false labor the contractions occur at irregular intervals and tend to disappear when the patient lies down.

- In true labor the cervix is soft and will admit the examiner's finger easily. In false labor the cervix does not change.

 In true labor the cervix is soft; in false labor the cervix does not change.

- In true labor the discomfort is not relieved by mild sedation. In false labor the discomfort may be relieved by mild sedation.

- In true labor the descent of the presenting part occurs. In false labor the presenting part does not descend.

 In true labor the descent of the presenting part occurs. In false labor the presenting part does not descend.

- In true labor there is a backache due to stretching of the cervix. A **bloody show** appears due to the discharge of the mucous plug that fills the cervical canal during pregnancy. The exposed cervical capillaries release a small amount of blood that mixes with the mucus, resulting in red-tinged secretions. In false labor the discomfort is mainly in the anterior region of the abdomen and pelvis and there is no stretching of the cervix.

 In true labor there is a backache due to stretching of the cervix. In false labor the discomfort is mainly in the anterior region of the abdomen and pelvis and there is no stretching of the cervix.

STAGES OF LABOR

There are four stages of labor (Figure 6-1):

First stage: Begins with true labor contractions and results in cervical effacement and dilation and ends with complete cervical effacement and dilation

Second stage: Begins with complete cervical effacement and dilation and ends with the birth of the baby

Third stage: Begins with the birth of the baby and ends with the birth/delivery of the placenta

Fourth stage: Begins with the delivery of the placenta and ends 1–4 hours past the birth process

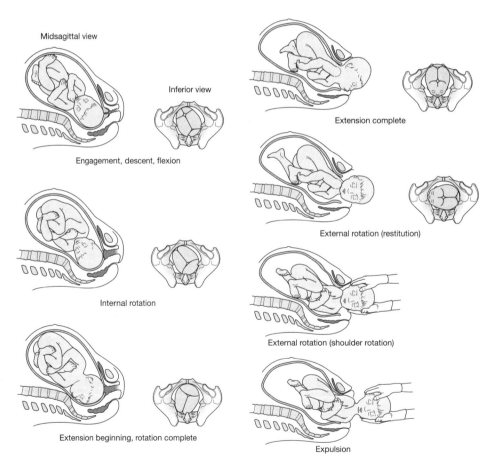

Figure 6-1 Stages of labor.

During the first stage of labor, uterine activity needs to be assessed constantly. This assessment comprises palpation or electronic monitoring, which evaluates the frequency, duration, and intensity of a uterine contraction (a tightening of the uterus).

- Frequency is timed from the beginning of one contraction to the beginning of the next contraction (usually recorded in 1-minute increments).
- Duration is timed from the beginning of a contraction to the end of that same contraction (usually recorded in 30–90 seconds).
- Intensity refers to the strength of a contraction (peak or acme). As a method, evaluation is measured by the indentability of the fundal portion of the uterus at the peak of a contraction. Using this method, the intensity is recorded as mild, moderate, or strong. If using the electronic fetal monitor to measure the intensity, an intrauterine pressure catheter must be in place. This is an accurate measurement of intensity because it is measured in millimeters of mercury.

The first stage of labor and the longest stage are divided into three subgroups: the latent phase, active phase, and transitional phase. Because the first stage of labor is called the dilating stage, the status of progress is determined by the effacement (thinning out of the cervix) and the dilation of the cervix (opening up). The latent phase starts from true labor contractions and ends with the cervix dilated to 4 cm and the effacement of the cervix from 0 to 40%. Usually, the contractions are mild, with the frequency of contractions about every 5 to 10 minutes and a duration of 30 to 45 seconds.

The active phase continues from 5 to 7 cm of cervical dilation, and the cervical effacement is between 40% and 80%. Usually, the contractions are moderate, with a frequency of 2 to 5 minutes and a duration of 45 to 60 seconds.

The transitional phase continues from 8 to 10 cm of cervical dilation, and the cervical effacement is between 80% and 100%. Usually, the contractions are strong, with a frequency of 1 to 2 minutes and a duration of 60 to 90 seconds. The transitional phase is the hardest and most difficult phase to endure. At this stage the laboring mother may manifest nausea and vomiting, apprehension, backache, and feelings of loss of control and of being overwhelmed. At this stage a lot of encouragement is needed. Fortunately, this phase does not last longer than 3 hours for nulliparas (a woman who has not delivered a viable offspring) and 1 hour for multigravidas (a woman who has delivered a viable offspring previously and is pregnant again).

The second stage of labor is the pushing stage and starts when the cervix is completely effaced and dilated (10 cm) and ends with the birth of the baby. This stage basically involves moving the fetus down and out of the birth canal. During this stage the mother is more in control, focused, and less irritable. During this phase the fetal head changes position via internal rotation and presents direct occiput anterior. Active pushing continues, and there is perineal bulging. At this point the fetal head is visible at the vaginal opening (introitus) and may disappear between contractions. Crowning appears when the top of the fetal head no longer disappears between contractions. A burning "ring of fire" is reported by the mother as the head crowns; this is caused by the pressure of the fetal head against the perineum.

The third stage of labor begins with the birth of the baby and ends with the expulsion of the placenta. The signs of placental separation are as follows: the uterus rises up in the abdomen, there is a gush of bright red blood, the umbilical cord descends three or more inches, and the uterus becomes globular in shape. The placenta breaks away from the uterine lining by two different mechanisms. If the central portion of the placenta breaks away first, followed by the edges, the fetal side (shiny membranes) of the placenta presents at the introitus (vaginal opening); this is called the "shiny Schultz" placenta. However, if the edges of the placenta break away from the uterine lining first, followed by the central portion, then the maternal side (red and beefy) of the placenta presents at the introitus; this is called "dirty Duncan." All the maternal cotyledons are visible with this placenta expulsion.

After the placenta is expelled, the uterus is massaged until it is firm. This process promotes the constriction of uterine blood vessels and decreases the possibility of a postpartum hemorrhage. The normal amount of blood volume loss during a vaginal delivery is about 500 ml and, during a cesarean section, 1,000 ml.

The fourth stage of labor begins from the expulsion of the placenta and ends about 1 to 4 hours later. Assessment of mother and baby begin. The fundus should be firm to the touch and contracted. At this point it is usually felt at the umbilicus. If the uterus becomes boggy, it is manually massaged, promptly contracts, and is firm to the touch again. The lochial flow (vaginal discharge) is bright red in color and may have a few small clots, with a moderate amount of lochia. Vital signs are taken every 15 minutes, along with a fundal and lochial flow assessment for the first hour. Temperature is also monitored hourly. If an episiotomy was performed during the second stage of labor, an assessment is also done at this time. The episiotomy should be intact, with the suture line even (well approximated) and no edema or redness visible.

The remainder of the recovery period is spent with the mother bonding with the newborn, and if she plans on breastfeeding this is a wonderful time to do so. During the first hour or so after birth, the sucking reflex in the newborn is the strongest, so this is a perfect time to assist the new mother with proper positioning for breastfeeding.

During the fourth stage of labor both mother and baby are monitored. The newborn's temperature, apical pulse, and respirations are taken every hour for several hours. The baby needs to be kept warm and close to mother. Other parameters that need to be assessed on the mother during this stage are bladder distention, prevention of hemorrhage, and venous thrombosis.

Other parameters that need to be assessed on the mother during the fourth stage of labor are bladder distention, prevention of hemorrhage, and venous thrombosis.

The concept of fetal monitoring is based on the fact that labor is a period of physiologic stress for the fetus. Therefore, frequent monitoring can measure fetal well-being by the response of the fetal heart rate to uterine contractions.

There are two types of electronic fetal monitoring: the external method and the internal method. The external fetal monitor is a noninvasive method and does not require that the membranes be ruptured or that cervical dilation has occurred. The internal fetal monitor is an invasive method and requires the membranes to be ruptured and the cervix to be dilated.

7

Fetal Monitoring

TERMS
- ☐ External method
- ☐ Internal method
- ☐ Intrauterine pressure catheter (IUPC)

The concept of fetal monitoring is based on the fact that labor is a period of physiological stress for the fetus. Therefore frequent monitoring can measure fetal well-being by the response of the fetal heart rate (FHR) to uterine contractions. Fetal oxygen supply must be maintained during labor to prevent fetal compromise and to promote newborn health after birth.

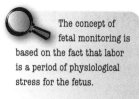

The concept of fetal monitoring is based on the fact that labor is a period of physiological stress for the fetus.

There are normal/reassuring FHR patterns:

- A FHR in the normal range of 110–160 beats per minute is considered to be a baseline FHR provided there are no periodic changes and a moderate baseline variability (fluctuations in the FHR).
- Accelerations with fetal movement (an increase in FHR above the baseline, with a return to baseline within 10 minutes).

There are abnormal/non-reassuring FHR patterns:

- Tachycardia of 160 beats per minute or more.
- Progressive increase or decrease in baseline rate
- Progressive decrease in baseline variability
- Absence of FHR variability
- Severe bradycardia (less than 70 beats per minute)
- Prolonged deceleration (greater than 60–90 seconds)
- Late decelerations that are repetitive and uncorrectable (slowing of the FHR that begins after the onset of a contraction. The FHR returns to baseline after the contraction has ended.)
- Severe variable decelerations (slowing of the FHR due to umbilical cord compression)

 There are abnormal/nonreassuring FHR patterns.

There are two types of electronic fetal monitoring:

1. **External method:** External transducers are placed on the maternal abdomen to assess FHR and uterine activity.

2. **Internal method:** A spiral electrode is applied to the fetal presenting part to assess the fetal electrocardiogram (ECG) and an **intrauterine pressure catheter (IUPC)** assesses uterine activity and pressure.

EXTERNAL FETAL MONITORING

External fetal monitoring is a noninvasive method and does not require that the membranes be ruptured or that cervical dilation has occurred (Figure 7-1). The ultrasound transducer operates by reflecting high-frequency sound waves from a moving object, which is the fetal heart and the fetal heart valves. The external fetal monitor is not as accurate as the internal fetal monitor because it cannot show short-term variability and beat-to-beat changes in the FHR patterns. Another difficulty that exists is that a continuous and precise record of the FHR is sometimes prevented due to artifacts (irregular variations or absence of FHR on the fetal monitor record, resulting from mechanical limitations) introduced by fetal movement and maternal movement.

The tocotransducer measures uterine activity transabdominally. This device is placed over the fundus, above the umbilicus. Uterine contractions depress a pressure-sensitive surface on the side next to the abdomen. The tocotransducer can measure and record the frequency, regularity,

Figure 7-1

Noninvasive fetal monitoring.

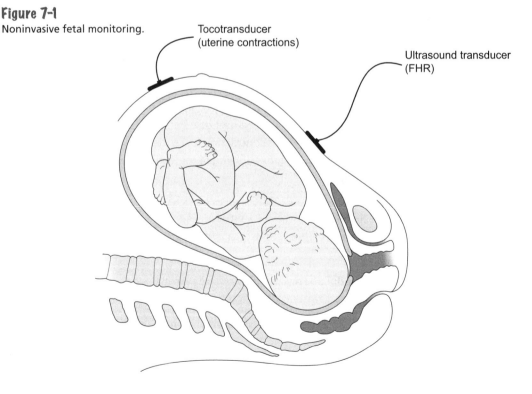

Tocotransducer
(uterine contractions)

Ultrasound transducer
(FHR)

and approximate duration of uterine contractions but not their intensity (mild, moderate, or strong). This type of monitoring is usually beneficial for antepartum testing and first stage of labor in women with intact membranes. However, there are instances when the external monitoring method is used successfully throughout labor.

INTERNAL FETAL MONITORING

Internal fetal monitoring provides an accurate appraisal of fetal well-being during labor. The criteria necessary to use the internal method are that the membranes must be ruptured, the cervix needs to be dilated, and the presenting part needs to be low enough to allow for placement of the electrode. This is an invasive method (Figure 7-2). The spiral electrode shows the FHR and fetal electrocardiogram on the monitor strip.

> ✓ Internal fetal monitoring provides an accurate appraisal of fetal well-being during labor.

Figure 7-2
Invasive fetal monitoring.

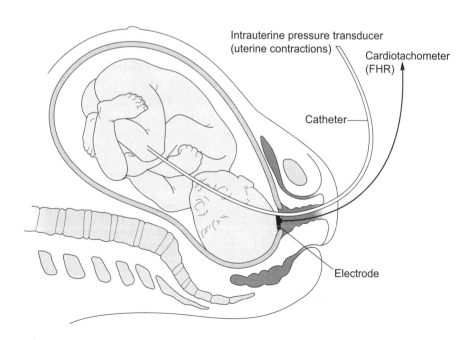

To monitor uterine activity, a solid or fluid-filled intrauterine pressure catheter (IUPC) is introduced into the uterine cavity. The solid catheter has a pressure-sensitive tip that measures changes in intrauterine pressure. A fluid-filled IUPC is a catheter filled with sterile water. As the catheter is compressed during a contraction, pressure is placed on the transducer. This pressure is then converted into a pressure reading in millimeters of mercury (mm Hg). The average pressure during a contraction ranges from 50 to 85 mm Hg. The IUPC can measure frequency, duration, and intensity of uterine contractions.

MONITOR PAPER

The monitor paper has small squares, and each small square stands for 10 seconds. A grouping of six squares comprises a larger box, and this equals 1 minute.

BASELINE FHR

The baseline FHR is observed between contractions during a 10-minute segment. The normal range at a term pregnancy is 110–160 beats per minute. Baseline changes take place during 10-minute periods of time. Therefore changes include tachycardia, bradycardia, and variability of heart rate. Tachycardia is a baseline FHR above 160 beats per minute. Many times this can be considered an early sign of fetal hypoxia from maternal or fetal infection such as prolonged rupture of membranes with amnionitis. Bradycardia is a baseline FHR below 110 beats per minute and is considered a later sign of fetal hypoxia and is known to occur before fetal demise. Also, bradycardia can result from prolonged compression of the umbilical cord or maternal hypotension. Maternal supine hypotensive syndrome is caused by uterine pressure (the weight of the gravid uterus) on the inferior vena cava. When this occurs it decreases the return of blood flow to the maternal heart, which then reduces maternal cardiac output and blood pressure.

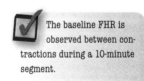

The baseline FHR is observed between contractions during a 10-minute segment.

VARIABILITY

Variability is a normal irregularity of fetal cardiac rhythm. Short-term variability is the beat to beat changes and long-term variability is the rhythmic changes or waves from the baseline value. In clinical practice short-term and long-term variability continue to be used to describe the FHR fluctuations. The absence of or undetected variability is considered a nonreassuring sign. Also, decreased variability can result from fetal hypoxia and drugs that depress the central nervous system, such as analgesics, narcotics, barbiturates, and general anesthetics. Another important point to remember is that a temporary decrease in variability can occur when the fetus is in a sleep state. These sleep states do not usually last longer than 30 minutes.

PERIODIC CHANGES IN FHR

When changes occur from baseline patterns in FHR, they are called periodic changes. These periodic changes occur with uterine contractions.

ACCELERATIONS

Accelerations in the FHR are an abrupt increase in the FHR above the baseline. The acceleration is defined as an increase of 15 beats per minute or greater and lasts 15 seconds or more, with the return to baseline less than 2 minutes from the beginning. The appearance of an acceleration usually denotes fetal movement, which in turn means fetal well-being.

DECELERATIONS

A deceleration is a fall in the FHR from the normal baseline. This is caused by stimulation of the parasympathetic nervous system. There are three types of decelerations: early, late, and variable (Figure 7-3). They are described by their shape and relation to a uterine contraction.

1. Early deceleration is due to pressure on the fetal head as it progresses down the birth canal. The monitor strip resembles an upside down shape of a uterine contraction. It has a uniform shape. The deceleration usually starts at the beginning of the contraction and ends when the contraction is over. The lowest deceleration occurs at the peak of the contraction (it mirrors the appearance of a uterine contraction) and is within the normal FHR range. Early deceleration is a normal and benign finding and is often seen during the active stage of a normal labor, and during the second stage of labor with pushing, crowning, or vacuum extraction. Because this is a benign finding no intervention is needed.

2. Late deceleration is due to uteroplacental insufficiency. As a result there is decreased blood flow and oxygen transfer to the fetus during contractions. The monitor strip resembles a smooth uniform shape that inversely mirrors a contraction. The deceleration begins after the peak of the contraction and lasts past the end of the contraction. Late decelerations usually occur with every contraction and are persistent and consistent, which indicates a pattern. Examples of some conditions that may decrease uteroplacental perfusion are gestational hypertension, placental aging due to postmaturity and diabetes, maternal smoking, maternal hypotension, anemia, conduction anesthetics (producing hypotension), placenta previa, abruptio placenta, and hyperstimulation via oxytocin infusion. Interventions include turning the woman to the left side-lying position or right side-lying position. Findings should be reported to the physician or nurse-midwife. Discontinue oxytocin if it is being administered. Administer oxygen by mask at 7–10 L/min. Monitor maternal blood pressure and pulse for signs of hypotension. And finally, prepare for a cesarean birth if needed.

3. Variable deceleration is due to umbilical cord compression, which decreases the amount of blood flow (including oxygen) to the fetus. This is the most common deceleration pattern and is usually correctable. There is a quick deceleration that occurs abruptly. The shapes of variable decelerations are usually a U, V, or a W. They show an unpredictable (or non-uniform) shape on the FHR baseline and can occur anytime during the uterine contracting phase. This deceleration is a nonreassuring sign, and interventions are needed if the variable decelerations are repetitive or the FHR drops below 90.

Interventions include maternal positional change to one in which the FHR pattern is most improved. Oxygen administered (by face mask) to the woman is sometimes helpful. Findings are reported to the physician or nurse-midwife. Discontinue oxytocin if infusing and there are severe variable decelerations; however, if mild or moderate decelerations, the infusion may be continued. Assist with amnioinfusion (an infusion of normal saline warmed to body temperature through an intrauterine catheter into the uterine cavity in an attempt to increase the fluid around the umbilical cord and prevent compression during uterine contractions), if it is ordered. Try to correct maternal hypotension, and continue to monitor FHR patterns for any further changes. Finally, assist with the preparation for a cesarean section, if needed. When cord compressions are severe or prolonged, variable decelerations cause neonatal depression (i.e., tight nuchal cord, short cord, knot in the cord, or prolapsed cord).

QUICK LOOK AT THE CHAPTER AHEAD

The postpartum period takes place from the birth of the newborn (and placenta) to approximately 6 weeks following the delivery. This time interval is important because it allows all the reproductive organs to return to their prepregnancy state.

The emotional status is equally important. The parenting role is one in which great changes occur for the couple. Caring for the new infant involves both physical and emotional changes for the parents.

8

Physiology of the Postpartum Period

TERMS

☐ Letting-go phase
☐ Lochia alba
☐ Lochia rubra
☐ Lochia serosa
☐ Postpartum period
☐ Taking-in phase
☐ Taking-hold phase

The **postpartum period** takes place from the birth of the newborn (and placenta) to about 6 weeks after delivery (Figure 8-1). This time interval is important because it allows all the reproductive organs to return to their normal prepregnancy state. The postpartum period is also called the puerperium or the fourth trimester.

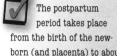

The postpartum period takes place from the birth of the newborn (and placenta) to about 6 weeks after delivery.

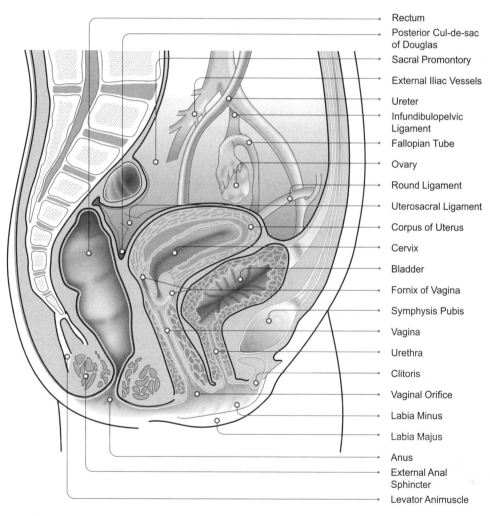

Figure 8-1 The anatomy and physiology of the postpartum period.

UTERUS

Involution is the process whereby the uterus returns to its prepregnancy size. This process starts right after the placenta is delivered and continues for 6 weeks when complete physiological involution is complete. At the end of the third stage of labor (delivery of the placenta) the uterus weighs approximately 2 pounds (1,000 g and about the size of a grapefruit); in its nonpregnant state, the uterus weighs about 1 to 2 ounces (50–100 g).

At the end of the delivery process, the fundus (top portion of the uterus) should be firm upon palpation and be midline and one fingerbreadth (2 cm) below the level of the umbilicus. If the fundus is not firm and feels soft (boggy), it may respond to manual massage and become firm. If it does not respond to manual massage and continues to feel soft or boggy, this may indicate uterine atony and may lead to postpartum hemorrhage. Further monitoring and risk factors need to be considered (e.g., high parity, prolonged labor, and tocolytics).

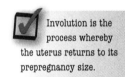
Involution is the process whereby the uterus returns to its prepregnancy size.

Twelve hours after delivery the fundus is 1 cm above the uterus. As the postdelivery hours pass, the uterine fundus involutes 1 to 2 cm (½ to 1 fingerbreadths) every 24 hours. If at any time during uterine assessment of the patient the uterus is deviated above the umbilicus and to the right, this indicates a distended bladder. The postpartum patient should be taught that frequent voiding will alleviate this problem. As the normal fundus continues to involute (by the sixth day), it is located between the umbilicus and the symphysis pubic bone. By the tenth day, the uterus cannot be palpated.

If at any time during uterine assessment of the patient the uterus is deviated above the umbilicus and to the right, this indicates a distended bladder.

LOCHIA

Lochia is a normal uterine discharge of blood, mucus, and tissue after childbirth. There are three different types of lochia, and they are deter-

mined by days (birth through 6 weeks). **Lochia rubra** appears immediately after the delivery of the placenta and is bright red in color and
is composed of blood, decidual and trophoblastic depris, and bacteria.
Lochia rubra continues for the first 3 days after delivery. The amount
is considered moderate for a vaginal delivery, and a small amount for a
cesarean section. There also may be small clots present.

Lochia serosa follows lochia rubra and continues from day 4 to 10
days after delivery. It contains serous fluids, old blood, leukocytes, and
tissue debris. Lochia serosa is pinkish and watery in color or also may be
brown tinged in color. The overall amount is usually lighter than lochia
rubra.

Lochia alba follows lochia serosa and continues for approximately 2
to 6 weeks after delivery. It contains leukocytes, mucus, serum, and decidual cells. Lochia alba is whitish-yellow and creamy in color. Lochia has
a fleshy odor and should never smell or have
an offensive odor; if it does, infection (endometritis) may be indicated. Endometritis is
an infection of the uterine lining, and it usually accompanies a fever, pain, and abdominal tenderness.

 Lochia is a normal
uterine discharge of
blood, mucus, and tissue
after childbirth.

BLADDER

Desensitization of the bladder occurs from
trauma of the birth process, increased bladder capacity after childbirth, and conduction
anesthesia, which together cause a decrease
in the urge to void. Added to this are the
trauma of labor, possible vaginal lacerations,
and an episiotomy, which can decrease the
voiding reflex. Bladder distention can occur
due to decreased voiding combined with
postpartal diuresis. Also, after childbirth if
frequent voiding does not occur, a distended bladder can cause increase
vaginal bleeding by pushing the uterus up and to the right, preventing
proper involution of the uterus.

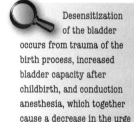 Desensitization
of the bladder
occurs from trauma of the
birth process, increased
bladder capacity after
childbirth, and conduction
anesthesia, which together
cause a decrease in the urge
to void.

BREASTS

Assessment of the breasts after delivery should reveal soft and enlarged breasts (first and second postpartum day) with a small amount of colostrum present, which can be expressed. There should not be any cracked, reddened, tender, or blistered nipples. Assessment of the nipples should also reveal erect nipples; if flattened or inverted, the lactation specialist should be informed so that prompt action can be taken, especially if the mother plans to breastfeed. Usually around the third day postpartum, the breasts start filling and feel firm and warm. By the fourth day postpartum the breasts become engorged (filling of the breasts with milk and secondary to increased vascularity and venous stasis) and are hard and may be reddened. Frequent breastfeeding by the infant every 2 to 3 hours usually relieves the engorgement. If necessary, relief from engorgement can be obtained through pumping of the breasts or manual expression.

 There should not be any cracked, reddened, tender, or blistered nipples.

If the mother chooses to bottle-feed her infant, then methods of milk suppression should be taught to her. Several methods can be used, such as a very tight and supportive fitting bra worn 24 hours daily, applying ice packs to the breasts 15 to 20 minutes every other hour, and avoiding warm/hot showers on the breasts. Analgesics such as acetaminophen (Tylenol) may also be used for breast discomfort. In about 2 to 3 days the engorgement should subside using these measures.

If a firm nodule is detected upon palpation of the breasts, it is usually due to a blocked milk duct. This is a temporary condition and is usually rectified by the infant breast-feeding and sucking. However, if the lump is consistently palpated in the same location, this could be indicative of fibrocystic breast disease or cancer. The physician or nurse-midwife should be notified immediately for further investigation and testing. Remember, a filled milk duct will shift positions from day to day.

If a firm nodule is detected upon palpation of the breasts, it is usually due to a blocked milk duct. However, if the lump is consistently palpated in the same location, this could be indicative of fibrocystic breast disease or cancer.

GASTROINTESTINAL SYSTEM AND BOWELS

In a vaginal delivery without complications, a mother's appetite will return to normal immediately after delivery. The new mother will become hungry about 1 hour after delivery, and regular food may be consumed. Her fluid intake should be increased due to the stresses of labor and the beginning of diaphoresis as well as nourishment with food. If the mother has had heavy blood loss during labor or cesarean section, foods high in protein and iron should be encouraged. Tissue healing and restoration of iron levels are provided by foods that are high in protein and iron. This is necessary because of the normal hemodilution of pregnancy.

Bowel sounds should be active and easily heard during a typical postpartum assessment. However, the passage of stool through the bowel tract may be slow due to the hormone relaxin as well as to pain due to the episiotomy and/or hemorrhoids. Comfort measures and treatments for hemorrhoids are witch hazel and a topical anesthetic spray. A bowel movement should be anticipated within 2 to 3 days after delivery. The mother should be taught to eat foods high in fiber (e.g., fruit, vegetables, and whole grains) and to drink six to eight glasses of water daily. If constipation occurs, a mild laxative may be given such as magnesium hydroxide (Milk of Magnesia), 30 ml/day. Others prefer a stool softener such as docusate (Colace) or bisacodyl (Dulcolax).

HOMANS' SIGN

A very important assessment each day is that of the extremities. This assessment should include examination of deep tendon reflexes, varicosities, tenderness, and any presence of edema on the legs. Some of the risk factors for developing superficial or deep vein thrombosis are traumatic delivery, obesity, vessel damage during birth, immobility, and severe anemia. Local swelling on the legs (and calves), pain, or redness indicate thrombophlebitis. Early ambulation for the new mother reduces the incidence of thrombophlebitis.

Homans' sign is assessed by straightening the mother's leg in the flat position on the bed. The nurse places one hand on the knee to keep the leg straight and with the other hand on the mother's foot gently flexes the foot toward the body. Any calf pain on flexion in either foot indicates a positive Homans' sign (thrombophlebitis).

BLOOD COMPONENTS

During the first 6 weeks after delivery, the blood values usually return to normal. There is marked leukocytosis (a transient increase in the number of leukocytes in the blood) during labor and after labor. This is a protective mechanism in which the leukocyte count increases during and after labor to 25,000–30,000/mm^3. The average leukocyte count is 14,000–16,000/mm^3. If an elevated temperature occurs, a possible infection needs to be ruled out.

Because of blood loss during childbirth, a limited decrease in total blood volume results. However, during pregnancy a normal increase in blood volume from 1,000 to 1,500 ml is seen, but this is reduced after birth and returns to normal values by the sixth postpartum week (hematocrit levels, 37–47%).

EMOTIONAL STATUS

The parenting role is one in which great changes occur for the couple. Caring for the new infant involves both physical and emotional changes for the mother and father. Reva Rubin in the early 1960s described the three phases a mother goes through to adjust to the new parenting role. The **taking-in phase** takes place immediately after delivery and lasts about 2 days. In this phase the mother is more passive and relies on the nurse to help her make decisions. She relives her labor and delivery and openly discusses it with family and friends. The mother is more concerned with her own needs, such as fluids, food, and rest. This also is the time the new mother bonds with her newborn. In the maternity hospital today, discharges occur in relatively short periods of time. Usually, a mother who delivers vaginally and without complications is discharged in 2 days, not counting her delivery day (delivery day, postpartum day 1, and postpartum day 2). Therefore the other stages described by Rubin are not usually observed in the hospital, unless the mother has had a cesarean section, in which discharge takes place on day 4, not counting the operative day.

The **taking-hold phase** starts on the third postpartum day and continues for several weeks. In this stage the mother becomes preoccupied with the present. She is concerned with her health, the infant's, and her ability to care for her newborn. She begins to take charge and wants to care for her infant by herself.

After several weeks the mother moves toward the third phase, called the **letting-go phase.** In this phase the mother reestablishes relationships with others outside the immediate family circle. She is comfortable in the motherhood role and with the care and responsibility of her newborn.

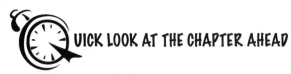

The neonatal period is defined as the first 28 days of life. Immediately after birth (transition period) and throughout the hospital stay, the infant needs to be assessed. The assessments evaluate the infant's adjustment to extra-uterine life. The assessment data covers the respiratory system, cardiac, and temperature regulatory mechanisms. The Apgar score is a procedure that provides immediate assessment for the need of resuscitation of the newborn. The five parameters and the scores of each parameter will determine the physiologic state of the newborn. The five parameters are heart rate, respiratory effort, muscle tone, reflex irritability, and color.

9

Newborn Assessment

TERMS
☐ Apgar score
☐ Neonatal period

The **neonatal period** is defined as the first 28 days of life. Immediately after birth (transition period) and throughout the hospital stay, the infant needs to be assessed. These assessments evaluate the infant's adjustment to extra-uterine life.

> The neonatal period is defined as the first 28 days of life.

Transition of the newborn in most institutions usually takes place between 4 and 6 hours. The assessment data cover the respiratory system, cardiac, and temperature regulatory mechanisms. Immediately after birth the amniotic fluid is dried from the newborn's body. Incorporating this procedure prevents heat loss through evaporation (the dissipation of heat as the energy required to vaporize a liquid). To prevent heat loss and maintain body temperature, the newborn is placed on a radiant warmer for assessment of the Apgar score.

The **Apgar score** is a procedure that provides immediate assessment for the need of resuscitation of the newborn. The five parameters and the scores of each parameter determine the physiological state of the newborn. The five parameters follow:

> The Apgar score is a procedure that provides immediate assessment for the need of resuscitation of the newborn.

1. Heart rate, which is based on auscultation with a stethoscope
2. Respiratory effort, which is based on the observation of the movement of the chest wall
3. Muscle tone, which is based on the degree of flexion and movement of the extremities
4. Reflex irritability, based on the response to gentle taps applied to the soles of the feet
5. Skin color, described as blue and pale, extremities blue only, or total body pink

These parameters are evaluated at 1- and 5- minute intervals after birth. Each parameter with a perfect score is valued at a 2. Therefore if a newborn meets each parameter with a perfect score and there are 5 parameters, then the Apgar score would be a 10. The overall guidelines indicate severe distress (0–3), moderate distress (4–6), and an infant that adjusted to extra-uterine life immediately (7–10).

After the Apgar score has been completed (usually by the nurse attending the delivery), the newborn's temperature needs to be assessed (Table 9-1). At birth, the newborn is placed under a radiant warmer to

Table 9-1. Four Types of Heat Loss in Newborns

1. **Evaporation**: Occurs when heat is lost as water is converted to a vapor.	**Example**: Immediately after birth the amniotic fluid can elicit evaporation heat loss unless the newborn is immediately dried.
2. **Conduction**: Occurs when a warmer object comes in direct contact with a cooler object.	**Example**: A cold scale, a cold examining table, or an unwarmed incubator
3. **Radiation**: Occurs when heat is transferred from the heated body surface (newborn) to cooler surfaces and/or objects not in direct contact with the newborn's body.	**Example**: Placing the newborn's crib against an outside wall, when the inside walls of a home are usually warmer than the outside walls
4. **Convection**: Occurs when heat is lost from a warm body surface to cooler air currents.	**Example**: Placing the newborn in areas such as open doorways or air-conditioning drafts

maintain body temperature. After the temperature (usually axillary, 97–99.5°F), the apical heart rate (120–160 beats per minute), and respiratory rate (40–60 beats per minute) are taken, the infant is weighed (normal range, 5½ to 7½ pounds) and measured (normal length, 18–22 inches). Rectal temperatures are usually not done anymore, due to the risk of damage to the rectal lining.

When these procedures are completed, the newborn may be placed skin-to-skin with the mother. While the mother is holding the infant (skin-to-skin), this is a convenient time to have the newborn breastfeed (if the mother plans on using this method). Because the newborn's sucking reflex is the strongest right after birth, this is the best time to teach the new mother the proper latching-on method and positioning to breastfeed.

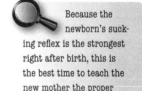

Because the newborn's sucking reflex is the strongest right after birth, this is the best time to teach the new mother the proper latching-on method and positioning to breastfeed.

Usually during transition the vital signs are taken every hour for the first 4–6 hours. Shortly after birth the newborn's head and chest circumference are measured. The normal head circumference for a term newborn at birth is 13–15 inches and chest circumference 12–14 inches. The measurement of the chest circumference is valuable as a comparison with the head circumference but is not necessarily by itself. The chest circumference may be equal to the head but should never be larger than the head; if this occurs, the health care provider needs to be alerted.

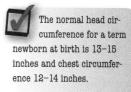
The normal head circumference for a term newborn at birth is 13–15 inches and chest circumference 12–14 inches.

Once the infant's vital signs are stabilized, the newborn needs ophthalmic and vitamin K prophylaxis and an admission (first) bath. To prevent gonococcal and chlamydial infections in the newborn, an ophthalmic ointment is given prophylactically. There are several brands used (depending on the institution), for example, erythromycin ointment 0.5%, tetracycline 1%, or silver nitrate solution 1%. All three medications may cause an irritation to the eyes (chemical conjunctivitis), which ceases in 24 hours. Vitamin K (phytonadione 0.5–1 mg) is also administered prophylactically to stimulate the production of vitamin K by the bacteria in the newborn's intestine. While the newborn is gestating in the uterus and immediately after birth the intestine is sterile, and there is no intestinal flora to produce vitamin K. Soon after birth, when the newborn breastfeeds or ingests infant formula, a bacterial formation stimulates the production of vitamin K to prevent hemorrhagic disorders of the newborn and to promote the formation of clotting factors in the liver. Vitamin K is therefore administered early in the newborn's life (at least 1 hour after birth) and is given as an intramuscular injection into the vastus lateralis muscle (located in the newborn's thigh).

When the umbilical cord is cut immediately after birth, it must be assessed for three vessels. There should be two arteries and one vein. The arteries are easily identified because they protrude out from the umbilical cord, are smaller, and have thicker walls, and the vein is easily identified because it has a larger lumen and thinner walls than the arteries. Having

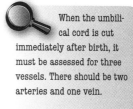
When the umbilical cord is cut immediately after birth, it must be assessed for three vessels. There should be two arteries and one vein.

only one artery indicates a congenital anomaly, and the health care provider should be immediately notified to provide early treatment if needed. Cord care is implemented soon after birth to prevent infection because the cord stump is a medium for bacterial growth. Many institutions use a drying agent to prevent infections and facilitate drying of the cord.

Having only one artery indicates a congenital anomaly, and the health care provider should be immediately notified to provide early treatment if needed.

Once the newborn's temperature has stabilized, a complete physical exam should be implemented. This procedure may be done in a well-lighted room (the parent's room or in the newborn nursery), free of drafts, and if preferred under a radiant warmer (to prevent cold stress). A head to toe examination is usually the easiest and most complete and starts with observation of the overall skin color of the newborn, level of alertness, posture, breathing patterns, and muscle tone.

A head to toe examination is usually the easiest and most complete and starts with observation of the overall skin color of the newborn, level of alertness, posture, breathing patterns, and muscle tone.

- **Head**. Palpate and observe the anterior and posterior fontanelles. The anterior fontanelle is larger and diamond shaped and located on the parietal bone. The posterior fontanelle is triangular in shape and located on the occipital bone. There should not be any bulging of the fontanelles (intracranial pressure) or depressed fontanelles (dehydration). Molding (overriding of the sagittal suture) occurs frequently due to the fetal head passing through the birth canal.

  Caput succedaneum (edema in scalp tissues from trauma) and cephalhematoma (oozing of blood from ruptured vessels between a skull bone and the periosteum) may be present due to a very fast labor (less than 2 hours) or a very long and difficult labor.
- **Eyes**. The eyes should be clear and without drainage and without swelling of the eyelids. The red reflex should be present. Swelling of the eyelids may be from a birth trauma or a reaction to the eye prophylaxis.
- **Ears**. Observe and palpate the outer ear (pinna). The top of the ear should be in alignment with the eyes. The ears should not be too low set. This indicates a congenital anomaly.
- **Nose**. Inspect the nares; they should be open, equal, and clear (without mucus). Newborns are nose breathers; if any stuffiness is noted, the health care provider should be notified. Milia are pinpoint white papules (plugged sebaceous glands) that can be found on the cheeks or across the bridge of the nose. There should be no nasal flaring, retractions, or grunting. Assess respirations immediately and note skin color.
- **Mouth**. Inspect the inside of the mouth. Both the hard and soft palate should be intact (easier to see when the newborn cries).

If an opening is found, this indicates a cleft palate (notify health care provider). If any white patches are found on the mucous membranes and cannot be wiped off with a gauze pad, *Candida albicans* (thrush) may be suspected (alert the health care provider).

- **Chest**. The chest should be symmetrical with the breasts slightly enlarged due to the mother's estrogen levels during pregnancy. Assess respiratory rate for 1 full minute. Observe the movement of the chest and abdomen. Observe for sternal and intercostal retractions; if present give oxygen as needed (alert health care provider).

- **Abdomen**. Inspect, palpate, and auscultate the abdomen. It should be soft and slightly rounded, and bowel sounds should be heard in all four quadrants. There should be no distention in the abdomen, and the umbilical cord stump should be drying without any redness, discharge, or bleeding present (alert health care provider).

- **Genitals**. Inspect the genitals. The female infant's labia majora and minora will be slightly swollen, along with clear mucous drainage from the vagina. If a small amount of vaginal bleeding (pseudomenstruation) occurs in the female newborn, this is due to the exposure of maternal estrogen while in utero.

  The male newborn's genitals should be clearly visible. Palpation of the scrotum should find both testicles descended. The urinary meatus should be centered on the end shaft of the penis; if not and it is on top (epispadias) or underside (hypospadias), the health care provider should be notified (omit circumcision; foreskin needed for reconstruction of the urinary meatus).

- **Hips**. Inspect the newborn's hips. The legs should be equal in length, and the skinfolds on both the right and left posterior thighs should be symmetrical (equal). Perform Ortolani's maneuver to rule out hip dislocation. If a crepitus sound (clunk) is heard, notify the health care provider.

- **Extremities**. All four extremities should be symmetrical and display equal movement. Ten fingers and ten toes should be found. If any extra digits are found or clubfoot or webbing (syndactyly) noted, the health care provider should be notified. Note the amount of creases on the palms of the hands and the soles of the feet (preterm infants have less and areas appear smooth).

> Note the amount of creases on the palms of the hands and the soles of the feet (preterm infants have less and areas appear smooth).

SECTION IV · REVIEW QUESTIONS

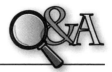

1. Primigravidas experience lightening 10–14 days before delivery. Lightening is:
   a. The descent of the fetal presenting part into the true pelvis
   b. A surge of energy before labor begins
   c. A decrease in the progesterone levels
   d. An increase in uterine irritability

2. At what period of time during a labor contraction is the baseline fetal heart rate observed?
   a. At the beginning of a uterine contraction
   b. At the end of a uterine contraction
   c. At the acme of a uterine contraction
   d. Between contractions

3. This process starts right after the placenta is delivered and continues for 6 weeks when the process is complete. This process is called:
   a. Involution of the fundus
   b. Involution of the uterus
   c. Involution of the puerperium
   d. Involution of the endometrium

4. The Apgar score is a procedure that provides immediate assessment for the need of resuscitation of the newborn. The five parameters are:
   a. Temperature, heart rate, respiratory effort, muscle tone, and color
   b. Heart rate, respiratory effort, muscle tone, reflex irritability, and color
   c. Temperature, heart rate, respiratory effort, reflex irritability, and color
   d. Temperature, heart rate, respiratory effort, reflex irritability, and muscle tone

5. There are many differences between true labor and false labor. In true labor:
   a. The discomfort is mainly in the anterior portion of the pelvis.
   b. Discomfort may be relieved by mild sedation.
   c. There is a backache due to stretching of the cervix.
   d. The cervix does not change.

6. A late deceleration is due to:
  a. Head compression
  b. Umbilical cord compression
  c. Uteroplacental insufficiency
  d. Beat to beat variability

7. What position of the uterine fundus during uterine assessment indicates a distended bladder?
  a. Above the umbilicus and to the right
  b. At the umbilicus and centered
  c. One fingerbreadth (2 cm) below the umbilicus
  d. Two fingerbreadths (4 cm) below the umbilicus

8. Immediately after birth the amniotic fluid is dried from the newborn's body. This procedure prevents heat loss through:
  a. Conduction
  b. Convection
  c. Evaporation
  d. Radiation

9. The second stage of labor begins:
  a. With true labor contractions
  b. With complete cervical effacement and dilation
  c. With the birth of the baby
  d. With the delivery of the placenta

10. A variable deceleration is due to:
  a. Head compression
  b. Umbilical cord compression
  c. Uteroplacental insufficiency
  d. Beat to beat variability

11. During the postpartum assessment, what causes desensitization of the bladder?
  a. Natural childbirth
  b. Trauma of the birth process
  c. Breast-feeding immediately after delivery
  d. Ice to the perineum

12. The neonatal period is defined as:
  a. The first 28 days of life
  b. The first 2 months of life
  c. The first 3 months of life
  d. The first 6 months of life

13. The third stage of labor ends:
- a. With the birth of the baby
- b. With the delivery of the placenta
- c. With complete cervical effacement and dilation
- d. One to 4 hours after the birth process

14. Using the external fetal monitoring method, the tocotransducer can measure and record:
- a. Frequency, regularity, and approximate duration of uterine contractions
- b. Frequency, intensity, and regularity
- c. Intensity, regularity, and approximate duration of uterine contractions
- d. Frequency, intensity, and approximate duration of uterine contractions

15. This lochia appears immediately after birth and continues for the first 3 days after delivery. What is this lochia called?
- a. Lochia alba
- b. Lochia serosa
- c. Lochia negra
- d. Lochia rubra

16. The normal apical heart rate of a newborn for 1 full minute is usually:
- a. 60–80 beats per minute
- b. 80–100 beats per minute
- c. 120–160 beats per minute
- d. 180–200 beats per minute

17. During the first stage of labor, uterine contractions are assessed. The term frequency means:
- a. The strength of a contraction (peak or acme)
- b. The time from the beginning of one contraction to the beginning of the next contraction
- c. The time from the beginning of one contraction to the end of that same contraction
- d. The sensitivity of the myometrium to oxytocin

18. The fetal monitor paper has small squares, and each square stands for:
  a.   10 seconds
  b.   20 seconds
  c.   40 seconds
  d.   60 seconds

19. During breast-feeding, around the fourth day postpartum the breasts become engorged and are hard and may be reddened. What advice or treatment can relieve engorgement?
  a.   Alternate breast-feeding with bottle feeding
  b.   Omit breast-feeding at night
  c.   Frequent breast-feeding every 2 to 3 hours
  d.   Limit breast-feeding to every 4 hours

20. Ortolani's maneuver is part of the physical assessment. It is used to rule out:
  a.   Clavicular dislocation
  b.   Femoral dislocation
  c.   Hip dislocation
  d.   Ankle dislocation

ANSWERS AND RATIONALES

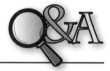

1. The answer is a.

2. The answer is d.

3. The answer is b.

4. The answer is b.

5. The answer is c.

6. The answer is c.

7. The answer is a.

8. The answer is c.

9. The answer is b.

10. The answer is b.

11. The answer is b.

12. The answer is a.

13. The answer is b.

14. **The answer is a.** Rationale: The intensity of a uterine contraction can only be measured by the internal fetal monitor method, using the intrauterine pressure catheter.

15. **The answer is d.**

16. **The answer is c.** Rationale: The other parameters are too low, reflecting bradycardia, or too high, reflecting tachycardia.

17. The answer is b.

18. The answer is a.

19. The answer is c.

20. The answer is c.

V

Complications of Pregnancy

Ectopic pregnancies can occur within the fallopian tube or anywhere outside of the uterus. Because the fertilized embryo is implanted into an inhospitable environment, it can cause rupture of the structure it is in, causing hemorrhage and death.

Women who have had pelvic surgeries, IUDs, or pelvic infections are at the greatest risk for developing an ectopic pregnancy.

Signs and symptoms are often subtle, such as mild to moderate menstrual cramping progressing to localized and extreme pain. Women do not know they have an ectopic pregnancy until the pain is so severe that they seek treatment.

10
Ectopic Pregnancy

TERMS
- ☐ **Culdocentesis**
- ☐ **Ectopic pregnancy**

An **ectopic pregnancy** is the implantation of a fertilized ovum outside of the endometrial cavity. Approximately 95% of ectopic pregnancies occur within the fallopian tube, but implantation can also occur on the ovary and within the cervix or abdominal cavity (Figure 10-1). As the embryo grows, rupture of the structure is inevitable. It is the leading cause of pregnancy-related deaths in the first trimester secondary to hemorrhage.

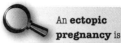 An **ectopic pregnancy** is the implantation of a fertilized ovum outside of the endometrial cavity. Approximately 95% of ectopic pregnancies occur within the fallopian tube, but implantation can also occur on the ovary and within the cervix or abdominal cavity.

 ## CONTRIBUTING FACTORS

Any woman with a history of pelvic inflammatory disease, a history of abdominal or pelvic surgery, or who uses an intrauterine device has an increased risk of an ectopic pregnancy. Tubal scarring decreases the ability of the fertilized ovum to move through the fallopian tube, causing it to become implanted into the wall of the tube itself. As the pregnancy progresses, serum human chorionic gonadotropin levels continue to rise while the fetus continues to grow.

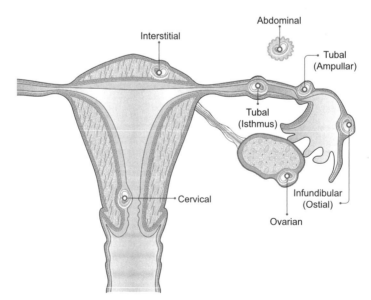

Figure 10-1 Sites of ectopic pregnancy.

Any woman with a history of pelvic inflammatory disease, a history of abdominal or pelvic surgery, or who uses an intrauterine device has an increased risk of an ectopic pregnancy.

 ## SIGNS AND SYMPTOMS

It is difficult to diagnose an ectopic pregnancy until the patient experiences consequences of an impending rupture. Unilateral lower quadrant pain is generally the first symptom of an ectopic pregnancy. The pain may be dull to constant or colicky in nature and progressively worsens. Symptoms are not apparent until the tube ruptures when the embryo becomes too large.

There may be a palpable adnexal mass or unilateral tenderness on bimanual examination. Other signs and symptoms include positive pregnancy test, missed menses, and dark red or brown vaginal bleeding. Once the rupture occurs, the patient complains of referred shoulder pain due to diaphragmatic irritation from bleeding into the peritoneal cavity. It is important to note that these signs and symptoms may also be caused by other pelvic disorders such as appendicitis, ruptured corpus luteum cysts, ovarian torsion, pelvic inflammatory disease, or bowel disorders. The patient may also exhibit syncopal symptoms due to hypovolemia. It is critical to obtain quick diagnosis and treatment for symptomatic patients.

Ask patients about positive pregnancy tests, missed menses, and dark red or brown vaginal bleeding. It is critical to obtain quick diagnosis and treatment for symptomatic patients.

 The patient may also exhibit syncopal symptoms due to hypovolemia.

 ## DIAGNOSIS AND TREATMENT

β-Human chorionic gonadotropin tests will be elevated if there is a pregnancy. Those levels double every few days in a normal intrauterine pregnancy. Low β-human chorionic gonadotropin levels are indicative of impending pregnancy loss. Hemoglobin and hematocrit levels determine blood loss. Pelvic ultrasound tests confirm the presence of a tubal pregnancy.

A procedure called a **culdocentesis** may be performed to determine intraperitoneal bleeding. This is done by insertion of a needle through the vaginal wall into the cul-de-sac. Nonclotted blood is indicative of hemorrhage. If it is confirmed that the patient has an ectopic pregnancy, surgical intervention, such as a laparoscopy or laparotomy, is indicated if the patient has life-threatening symptoms. Nonsurgical management includes the use of methotrexate intramuscularly, prostaglandins, or misoprostol in stable patients who prefer not to undergo surgery and whose mass is less than 4 cm and is unruptured.

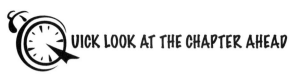

Spontaneous abortions are commonly referred to as miscarriages and can occur anytime during the first half of pregnancy. There are many reasons why spontaneous abortions occur, including genetic deficiencies (such as fetal anomalies), infections, or metabolic and endocrine abnormalities.

The first sign of an impending abortion is vaginal bleeding. Bleeding at any time during the pregnancy is cause for concern. An ultrasound will confirm or deny the presence of fetal heart tones.

11

Spontaneous Abortion

TERMS
☐ Spontaneous abortion

The most common causes of bleeding during the first half of pregnancy are spontaneous abortion and hydatidiform mole. Bleeding anytime during pregnancy is cause for concern because it can be life-threatening. **Spontaneous abortions**, commonly referred to as miscarriages, are defined as the loss or termination of a pregnancy before 20 weeks' gestation. There are several types of spontaneous abortions (Table 11-1).

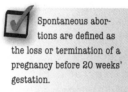

Spontaneous abortions are defined as the loss or termination of a pregnancy before 20 weeks' gestation.

Bleeding anytime during pregnancy is cause for concern because it can be life-threatening.

PATHOPHYSIOLOGY

The causes for spontaneous abortions vary from genetic abnormalities, maternal infections, endocrine or metabolic disorders, to fetal abnormalities. Premature dilation of the cervix or other abnormalities of the reproductive tract also contribute to the incidence of spontaneous abor-

Table 11-1 Types of Spontaneous Abortions

	Description
Threatened abortion	Potential for miscarriage; pregnancy may continue but prognosis is unpredictable
Inevitable abortion	Moderate bleeding, ruptured membranes with dilated cervical os; expulsion of products of conception
Incomplete abortion	Moderate to severe cramping and bleeding; a portion of the products of conception passed; cervical os is dilated; poor prognosis
Missed abortion	Uterine growth ceases; uterine size decreases; fetus is nonviable
Habitual abortion or recurrent spontaneous	Spontaneous loss of three or more consecutive pregnancies
Complete abortion	All products of conception passed; uterus is normal prepregnancy size

tions. At least 50% of all documented pregnancy losses are due to chromosomal abnormalities. Advanced maternal age increases the risk for spontaneous abortion.

SIGNS AND SYMPTOMS

The most common recognizable signs of a spontaneous abortion are light bleeding or cramping. Women who are unaware of a pregnancy may report heavier than normal menstrual flow with moderate cramping once the spontaneous abortion progresses. Vaginal bleeding is generally bright red. She may also notice the products of conception, which are commonly mistaken for increased clotting.

DIAGNOSIS AND TREATMENT

Elevated β-human chorionic gonadotropin levels confirm pregnancy. A pelvic ultrasound confirms or denies the presence of a fetal heart rate as well as an embryonic sac. Uterine size is less than the expected gestational size. Because blood loss is rarely excessive with a spontaneous abortion, there should be no change in the hemoglobin or hematocrit levels. A pelvic exam determines whether or not the cervical os is dilated.

Depending on the gestational age and the type of spontaneous abortion, the patient may be instructed to be on strict bed rest. Although commonly prescribed, no data exist to support any increased outcome of the pregnancy. Pelvic rest is indicated, and the patient should be instructed to avoid any sexual activity that may increase uterine contractions.

This chapter describes molar pregnancy and its clinical manifestations and treatment. Molar pregnancies are rare but occur as a result of an overproduction of placental cells which produce a mass but not a pregnancy.

Patients will have positive pregnancy signs such as a missed menses, a positive pregnancy test, breast tenderness, and nausea. The patient will also have a larger than gestational age-sized uterus.

12

Hydatidiform Mole

TERMS
☐ Hydatidiform mole

Hydatidiform moles are also known as a molar pregnancy. The incidence is 1 in every 1,000 pregnancies and increases with advanced maternal age. The etiology is unknown. It is a form of gestational trophoblastic disease and is a result of a higher than normal production of the cells that originate in the placenta. This overproduction of cells produces a mass instead of a viable pregnancy.

There are two types of hydatidiform moles: complete (or classic) and partial mole. Approximately 10–15% of hydatidiform moles may develop into invasive moles or, more rarely, choriocarcinoma, a malignant form of cancer.

 ## SIGNS AND SYMPTOMS

Signs and symptoms are similar to that of an early pregnancy: amenorrhea, breast tenderness, and nausea as well as a positive pregnancy test. Vaginal bleeding may occur at about the 12th week in 95% of all cases. The client may believe she is experiencing a spontaneous abortion. Examination of the client may reveal an abnormal growth in the size of the uterus for gestational size. The client may also have symptoms similar to preeclampsia: hypertension, edema, and proteinuria.

 The client may also have symptoms similar to preeclampsia: hypertension, edema, and proteinuria.

 ## DIAGNOSIS AND TREATMENT

A pelvic ultrasound confirms the absence of fetal heart tones or gestational sac. β-Human chorionic gonadotropin levels will be high due to the placental cells that comprise the tumor. Upon confirmation that there is no fetus, a dilation and curettage is performed. Tissue is sent to pathology for further examination and confirmation of diagnosis. Serum β-human chorionic gonadotropin levels are monitored until they return to nonpregnant levels.

SECTION V · REVIEW QUESTIONS

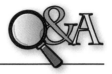

1. An ectopic pregnancy can occur:
   a. In the fallopian tubes
   b. On the ovary
   c. In the cervix
   d. All of the above

2. Abnormal vaginal bleeding in the second half of pregnancy is common.
   a. True
   b. False

3. Moderate vaginal bleeding with expulsion of the products of conception occurs with:
   a. Threatened abortion
   b. Ectopic pregnancy
   c. Missed abortion
   d. Inevitable abortion

4. Which of the following tests is appropriate for a hydatidiform mole?
   a. Pelvic ultrasound
   b. Culdocentesis
   c. Hemoglobin and hematocrit
   d. Pelvic exam

5. Spontaneous abortions are defined as:
   a. Missed menses
   b. Loss of pregnancy before 20 weeks' gestation
   c. Loss of pregnancy at 20–25 weeks' gestation
   d. Any time during the pregnancy

6. Which of the following is a common symptom of an ectopic pregnancy?
   a. Heavy vaginal bleeding
   b. Normal β-human chorionic gonadotropin
   c. Rectal pressure
   d. Shoulder pain

7. Treatment options for an ectopic pregnancy include:
   a. Surgery for removal of ectopic
   b. Methotrexate
   c. Misoprostol
   d. All of the above

8. Of the following tests, which one is the most diagnostic for a missed abortion?
   a. Pelvic ultrasound
   b. β-Human chorionic gonadotropin
   c. Abdominal x-ray
   d. Culdocentesis

9. Which of the following is considered a risk factor for ectopic pregnancy?
   a. Pelvic inflammatory disease
   b. Use of IUD
   c. Prior history of pelvic surgery
   d. All of the above

10. An abortion in which the fetus dies but is retained in the placenta is known as:
    a. Inevitable abortion
    b. Missed abortion
    c. Incomplete abortion
    d. Threatened abortion

ANSWERS AND RATIONALES

1. **The answer is d.** Rationale: Ectopic pregnancies can occur in the fallopian tube, on the ovary, in the cervix, or the abdominal cavity.

2. **The answer is b.** Rationale: Vaginal bleeding anytime during pregnancy is cause for concern but is not common during the second half of pregnancy.

3. **The answer is d.** Rationale: Inevitable abortions cause moderate bleeding, ruptured membranes with dilated cervical os, and expulsion of the products of conception.

4. **The answer is a.** Rationale: Pelvic ultrasound confirms or denies the presence of fetal heart tones and gestational sac.

5. **The answer is b.** Rationale: Pregnancies are considered viable after week 2.

6. **The answer is d.** Rationale: Shoulder pain is referred pain due to diaphragmatic irritation from intraabdominal bleeding.

7. **The answer is d.** Rationale: All of the above are considered options for an ectopic pregnancy.

8. **The answer is a.** Rationale: A pelvic ultrasound confirms or denies the presence of fetal heart tones.

9. **The answer is d.** Rationale: All of the options increase the risk of an ectopic pregnancy.

10. **The answer is b.** Rationale: A missed abortion occurs when uterine growth ceases, uterine size decreases, and the fetus is nonviable.

VI

High-Risk Conditions of Pregnancy

Placenta previa is an abnormally implanted placenta. Instead of the placenta being implanted in the upper uterine segment, it is implanted in the lower uterine segment. Placenta previa is usually diagnosed after the onset of sudden, painless vaginal bleeding during the second or third trimester of pregnancy. The diagnosis of placenta previa is obtained through the use of a transabdominal ultrasound or a transvaginal ultrasound examination.

Abruptio placenta is the premature separation of a normally implanted placenta. The detachment from the implantation site occurs before the delivery of the fetus. This can occur after the 20th week of gestation. It is one of the causes of third trimester bleeding, and is attributable to a high mortality rate. One of the main clinical manifestations of abruptio placenta is pain which can range from mild to severe. There is also mild to severe uterine hypertonicity which can be localized in one area or manifest as a hard "boardlike" abdomen. Ultrasounds (sonograms) are not as effective in the diagnosis of abruption as in placenta previa. The success rate using ultrasounds for diagnosing the abruption placenta is only 25%.

13

Placenta Previa and Abruptio Placentae

TERMS
☐ Abruptio placentae
☐ Placenta previa

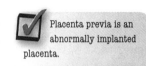

PLACENTA PREVIA

Placenta previa is an abnormally implanted placenta (Figure 13-1). Instead of the placenta being implanted in the upper uterine segment, it is implanted in the lower uterine segment. Placenta previa occurs in 1 in 200 pregnancies.

> ✓ Placenta previa is an abnormally implanted placenta.

There are three different types of placenta previa:

1. Complete, total, or central: This occurs when the placenta completely covers the internal cervical os.
2. Partial or incomplete: This occurs when there is incomplete coverage of the internal cervical os.
3. Low lying or marginal: This occurs when the placenta is located in the lower uterine segment but away from the internal cervical os.

When a complete placenta previa is diagnosed in the second trimester, only 1–12 complete placentae previae are a previa at term. This occurs because as the pregnancy continues, the lower uterine segment elongates and the uterine muscle enlarges, placing the placenta in the upper uterine segment.

Risk Factors

The cause of placenta previa is not known; however, certain risk factors seem to increase the incidence of this occurring. Scarring from uterine surgery reduces the vascularity of the upper uterine segment (induced abortion, previous cesarean sections, past molar pregnancy, and fibroid tumors). Factors that increase risk include previous placenta previa, multiple fetal gestation (because multiple fetal gestation requires a larger surface area for placental implantation), maternal age (over 35 years), smoking, cocaine use, closely spaced pregnancies, and multiparity.

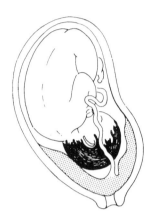

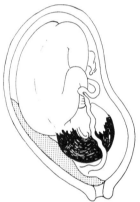

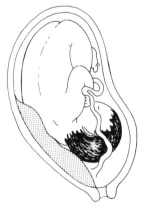

Figure 13-1 Placenta previa.

Clinical Presentation and Treatment

Placenta previa is usually diagnosed after the onset of sudden painless vaginal bleeding during the second or third trimester of pregnancy. Also, bleeding can occur when there is stretching and thinning of the lower uterine segment during the third trimester. It could start when a woman is resting or during any activity. The bleeding is bright

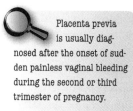

Placenta previa is usually diagnosed after the onset of sudden painless vaginal bleeding during the second or third trimester of pregnancy.

red and can be intermittent, occur in gushes, or, less commonly, be continuous. Because a pregnant woman can lose up to 40% of blood volume without showing signs of shock (heavy blood loss included) and her vital signs can be normal, the most accurate assessment of this problem is decreasing urinary output. Vigorous fetal heart rate assessment is necessary to ensure the integrity of fetal health status. Vaginal examinations or other methods to stimulate uterine contractions should be omitted until the physician further assesses the pregnant woman.

The diagnosis of placenta previa is obtained through the use of a transabdominal ultrasound or a transvaginal ultrasound examination; the accuracy rate is very high (95%). Treatment is based on the placement of the previa, gestational age of the fetus, and degree and amount of vaginal bleeding. In patients who have a marginal placenta previa, it may be permissible to labor and deliver vaginally provided that, if the emergency arises, a cesarean section can be accomplished immediately. If hemorrhage occurs, immediate delivery takes place (via cesarean section), regardless of the gestational age of the fetus. However, if the woman is preterm, not in labor, and bleeding has stopped or is minimal, the delivery can be delayed until the pregnancy is closer to term. Some physicians prefer their patients to remain in the hospital until delivery time, whereas in other circumstances their patients remain at home. Those women who remain at home need to be instructed to call their physician and return to the hospital immediately if vaginal bleeding, uterine contractions, or decrease in fetal movement occurs.

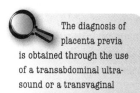

The diagnosis of placenta previa is obtained through the use of a transabdominal ultrasound or a transvaginal ultrasound examination.

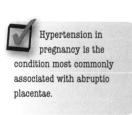 ## ABRUPTIO PLACENTAE

Abruptio placentae is defined as the premature separation of a normally implanted placenta (Figure 13-2). The detachment from the implantation site occurs before the delivery of the fetus. This can occur after the 20th week of gestation. Abruptio placentae

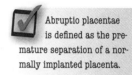

occurs in 1 in 150 deliveries. It is one of the causes of third-trimester bleeding and is attributable to a high mortality rate. The fetal mortality rate for abruptio placentae is 20–40% based on the type of abruption.

There are three different types of abruptio placentae:

1. Partial separation: There is a central separation (abruption) with concealed hemorrhage.
2. Partial (marginal) separation: There is a marginal detachment with external hemorrhage.
3. Complete (total) separation: There is a complete abruption with concealed hemorrhage (could also be external).

Risk Factors

Hypertension in pregnancy is the condition most commonly associated with abruptio placentae. Other situations are trauma (possible car accidents), cocaine use (during pregnancy), cigarette smoking, preterm premature rupture of membranes (causes sudden uterine decompression), women with a gravida of five or more, prior history of abruptio placentae, and history of reproductive loss.

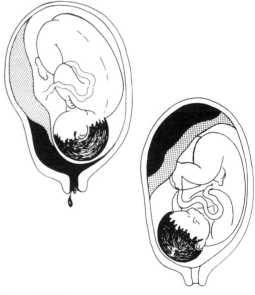

Hypertension in pregnancy is the condition most commonly associated with abruptio placentae.

Figure 13-2 Abruptio placentae.

Clinical Presentation and Treatment

One of the main clinical manifestations of abruptio placentae is pain, which can range from mild to severe. There is also mild to severe uterine hypertonicity that can be localized in one area or manifest as a hard "board-like" abdomen. Other classical symptoms may include vaginal bleeding (80% of cases), uterine tenderness, and contractions. Ultrasounds (sonograms) are not as effective in the diagnosis of abruptio placentae as in placenta previa. The success rate, using sonograms, for diagnosing the abruptio placentae is only 25%.

One of the main clinical manifestations of abruptio placentae is pain, which can range from mild to severe.

The uterine muscle can be damaged by extensive myometrial bleeding. If this occurs, it can lead to a Couvelaire uterus (a reddish or purplish uterus that is ecchymotic and contractility is lost) when blood accumulates between the separated placenta and the uterine wall. Shock ensues, and laboratory findings show blood in the amniotic fluid (a positive Apt test), a drop in hemoglobin and hematocrit levels (or hemoglobin and hematocrit levels will later drop), and a drop in coagulation factor levels, which could lead to disseminated intravascular coagulation. If the mother is Rh negative, a Kleihauer-Betke test detects fetal red blood cells in the maternal circulation. This test determines the degree of fetal–maternal hemorrhage and assists in calculating the correct dosage of RhoGAM for Rh-negative women.

Abruptio placentae is one of the leading causes of maternal death. Several factors affect the mother's prognosis: the overall blood loss, placental detachment (marginal or complete), and the time between the placental detachment and the birth. Massive blood loss results in decreased kidney perfusion and may cause oliguria. The treatment for decreased kidney perfusion is volume resuscitation with intravenous fluids and blood. However, if ischemia occurs, it can result in renal failure and pituitary necrosis.

Preterm birth, respiratory distress syndrome, and anemia are the neonatal complications of abruptio placentae. Third-trimester fetal deaths due to abruptio placentae are about 35%.

Preterm birth, respiratory distress syndrome, and anemia are the neonatal complications of abruptio placentae.

The overall treatment for abruptio placentae is to assess, monitor, and replace the amount of blood lost to enable the mother to deliver a healthy baby. Vigilant observation is needed to prevent coagulation disorders. Close monitoring is needed to avoid hypovolemia; if it occurs, intravenous infusions of lactated Ringer's or normal saline can be used to restore blood volume. Blood specimens should be obtained for evaluation of the hemodynamic status and for typing and crossmatching if blood replacement is needed. Cesarean birth is done immediately, once the mother has been stabilized and the abruption diagnosed.

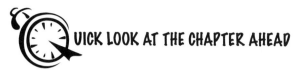

In the United States the population with Rh-negative type blood [missing the Rh (D) factor] is 15% in white couples and 10% in African-American couples; it is rarely found in Asian couples. This hemolytic disease is caused by the excessive destruction of red blood cells in the newborn and is caused by maternal antigens responding to Rh or ABO blood incompatibilities. Hemolytic disorders occur when the blood groups of the mother and the fetus differ. The most common of these are Rh factor and ABO incompatibilities.

14

Rh Incompatibility and ABO Incompatibility

TERMS
☐ ABO incompatibility
☐ Amniocentesis
☐ Direct Coombs test
☐ Hemolysis
☐ Percutaneous umbilical blood sampling
☐ Phototherapy
☐ Rh incompatibility

Maternal antibodies are present naturally (blood groups O, A, B, and AB) or form in response to an antigen from the fetal blood (Rh-positive factor) crossing the placenta and entering the maternal circulation. The maternal antibodies cross the placenta, causing **hemolysis** (destruction) of the fetal red blood cells, resulting in hyperbilirubinemia and jaundice. This disease can have severe effects on the fetus, whereas there are little or no risks to the mother. As early as the 1900s, severe fetal hemolytic disease was described in the literature, but the exact problem or cause was not known until the discovery of the Rh factor in 1940. This disease has been decreasing in the United States for the last 30 years due to the availability of Rh antibody prevention. In 1969 Rh (anti-D) globulin became commercially available (RhoGAM), and the ability to prevent Rh sensitization occurred. RhoGAM prevents sensitization by clearing the fetal cells from the maternal circulation and depressing the mothers' immune response.

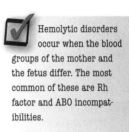 Hemolytic disorders occur when the blood groups of the mother and the fetus differ. The most common of these are Rh factor and ABO incompatibilities.

 RhoGAM prevents sensitization by clearing the fetal cells from the maternal circulation and depressing the mothers' immune response.

PATHOPHYSIOLOGY OF RH INCOMPATIBILITY

Rh incompatibility is defined as a sensitization that occurs when an Rh-negative (blood type) mother delivers an Rh-positive (blood type) baby. This sensitization occurs when fetal blood (Rh positive) enters the maternal circulation (Rh negative) and stimulates the formation of antibodies in the mother's blood (Figure 14-1). Once the formation of antibodies occurs (in the mother's blood), these antibodies have the capability to cross the placental barrier into the fetal circulation and attack (destroy) fetal red blood cells. Rh-negative blood lacks the Rh (D) antigen as compared with Rh-positive blood. Because this antigen only exists in someone who is Rh positive, problems arise during pregnancy when a woman with Rh-negative blood is pregnant with a fetus with Rh-positive blood.

 Rh incompatibility is defined as a sensitization that occurs when an Rh-negative (blood type) mother delivers an Rh-positive (blood type) baby.

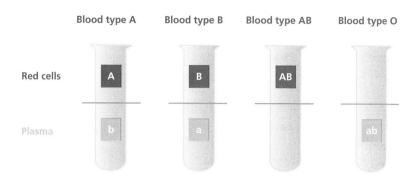

Capital letters represent antigens
Lowercase letters represent naturally occurring antibodies

Figure 14-1 How Rh disease develops.

Although there is no direct connection between maternal blood and fetal blood in the placenta, this blood is separated by a single cell membrane. Anytime during pregnancy there is the possibility that a (small leak) tear in this membrane could occur. It only takes a very small amount of Rh-positive fetal blood to enter the maternal bloodstream and actively stimulate maternal antibodies to form against the Rh-positive blood. Usually, the mixing of fetal blood cells and maternal blood cells takes place at the time of placental separation (third stage of labor). However, the danger exists during pregnancy as well as after delivery (28 weeks' gestation and 3 days after delivery).

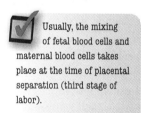

Usually, the mixing of fetal blood cells and maternal blood cells takes place at the time of placental separation (third stage of labor).

Other situations can lead to sensitization: after an abortion (antepartal period), after an invasive procedure (amniocentesis), or during pregnancy (placenta previa, abruptio placentae, or trauma). Remember, once active immunity takes place (antibodies actively formed), future pregnancies are at risk for hemolytic disease of the fetus and newborn.

Remember, once active immunity takes place (antibodies actively formed), future pregnancies are at risk for hemolytic disease of the fetus and newborn.

PATHOPHYSIOLOGY FOR ABO INCOMPATIBILITY

Since the advent of RhoGAM and its use for Rh-negative women who have not been sensitized to the Rh-positive blood of their newborns, ABO incompatibility is more common. **ABO incompatibility** is a less serious problem for newborns as compared with Rh incompatibility. This problem usually occurs when a mother is blood type O and her infant is either blood type A, B, or AB. Because in blood groups there are naturally occurring anti-A and anti-B antibodies, these naturally occurring antibodies may cross the placental barrier. This situation can occur because of a tear in the membrane of the placenta separating the maternal blood from the fetal blood as well as placenta previa, abruptio placentae, trauma (a physical blow to the abdomen), and amniocentesis.

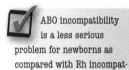

ABO incompatibility is a less serious problem for newborns as compared with Rh incompatibility.

One of the main distinctions between Rh incompatibility and ABO incompatibility is that ABO incompatibility may affect first-born infants. This occurs because mothers with type O blood already have antibodies (anti-A and anti-B antibodies) in their blood because that blood type is genetically determined at the time of conception. Blood is drawn at birth from the umbilical cord, and a **direct Coombs test** is performed. A direct Coombs test determines whether there are maternal antibodies in fetal cord blood. Positive test results indicate the presence of antibodies, and phototherapy treatment for hyperbilirubinemia is implemented.

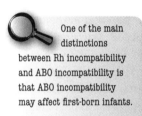

One of the main distinctions between Rh incompatibility and ABO incompatibility is that ABO incompatibility may affect first-born infants.

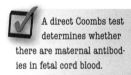

A direct Coombs test determines whether there are maternal antibodies in fetal cord blood.

MANAGEMENT

During the initial prenatal visit blood work is always ordered. The blood type and Rh factor and antibody titer tests (indirect Coombs test) are part of this workup. If the pregnant woman is Rh negative, an in-depth history needs to be taken to determine whether there are any high-risk events that would cause a potential Rh incompatibility problem. If high-risk events are present, it should then be determined whether she received RhoGAM [Rho (D) immune globulin] to prevent Rh sensitization development. The high-risk events are a previous pregnancy resulting in an Rh-positive baby, any blood transfusion with Rh-positive blood, any spontaneous or elective abortion (usually after 8 weeks' gestation) or ectopic pregnancy, any invasive procedures done during past pregnancies (chorionic villus sampling, amniocentesis), placenta previa, abruptio placentae, and trauma.

A pregnant woman who has had a negative indirect antibody test (indirect Coombs test) result during the initial prenatal visit is tested again at 28 weeks' gestation. An intramuscular injection of RhoGAM [Rho (D) immune globulin] is given prophylactically if her test results are negative for sensitization. However, a titer count of 1:8 or higher (tests results positive) indicates that sensitization has occurred. Further monitoring of her sensitization needs to be done, so a schedule of tests at 4-week intervals is performed to evaluate her antibody titer count. If the titer count keeps increasing, several tests need to be done.

Ultrasonography evaluates fetal growth, and an amniocentesis evaluates the condition of the fetus. **Amniocentesis** is used to withdraw amniotic fluid (using a needle) from the uterus to detect and evaluate the amount of bilirubin (hemolysis taking place). Using ultrasonography as a guide, **percutaneous umbilical blood sampling** directly takes a sample of fetal blood from the umbilical cord to determine whether the fetus is severely compromised.

For the severely compromised fetus, a transfusion of blood (intrauterine fetal transfusion) is given via the umbilical vein or into the fetal peritoneal cavity. As soon as the fetus is stabilized (adequate lecithin-to-sphingomyelin ratio), a preterm birth is inevitable. At delivery, the newborn is assessed and evaluated for the degree of hemolytic disease. Depending on the severity of hemolytic disease of the newborn, phototherapy or exchange transfusion may be used.

If sensitization does not occur during pregnancy or at the time of delivery in a woman who is Rh negative and her baby is Rh positive (Coombs test negative), then an injection of RhoGAM is needed. RhoGAM must be given within 72 hours after birth to prevent Rh sensitization.

With ABO incompatibility a positive result in the direct Coombs test (at birth, greater than 4 mg/dl) can be treated with early feedings, phototherapy, and exchange transfusions. Hyperbilirubinemia (excessive amounts of bilirubin in the blood) commonly occurs with ABO incompatibility. Immediate treatment is of utmost importance. Starting early feedings (at delivery, breast-feeding or formula feeding very soon after birth) assists in the removal of bilirubin from the body through newborn stools (early feeding stimulates bowel peristalsis). **Phototherapy** exposes the newborn to high-intensity light (bulbs in the blue-light spectrum) and decreases serum bilirubin levels in the skin. This therapy assists biliary excretion of unconjugated bilirubin. Through phototherapy, bilirubin is also excreted through the urine. Also, fiberoptic blankets may be used in conjunction with phototherapy and when the newborn is taken out of the isolette and brought to the mother for feedings.

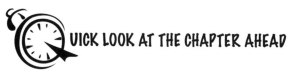

QUICK LOOK AT THE CHAPTER AHEAD

Pregnancy-induced hypertension is the leading cause of maternal death in the United States. It is a multi-system failure that occurs only during pregnancy and regresses after delivery. It is thought to be caused by an imbalance in thromboxane A2 (a vasoconstrictor) and placental prostacyclin (a platelet inhibitor).

Early signs of PIH include high blood pressure, sudden weight gain, edema, and proteinuria. Late signs of PIH manifest as visual acuity changes, headaches, and abdominal pain due to the impact on multiple organ systems.

Treatment is aimed at prevention of complications and convulsions due to eclampsia.

15

Pregnancy-Induced Hypertension

TERMS
☐ Eclampsia
☐ Hydralazine (Apresoline)
☐ Magnesium sulfate (MgSO$_4$)

Pregnancy-induced hypertension (PIH), once known as "toxemia of pregnancy" (this term is no longer acceptable or used), is the most common medical complication of pregnancy reported and is the leading cause of maternal death in the United States, accounting for approximately 15–18% of deaths. It occurs in approximately 6–8% of pregnancies. PIH is a multiorgan disease process and develops as a consequence of pregnancy. It progresses rapidly and regresses in the postpartum period. Delivery is the only definitive treatment for this condition.

PREDISPOSING FACTORS AND CAUSES

Although there are no known causes for PIH, several factors contribute to its development. This disease usually occurs if a woman is a primipara, carrying multiple gestations, of advanced maternal age, diabetic, or obese. The incidence rate is higher among African-American women, those with an Rh incompatibility, and those with a prior history of lupus or renal disease.

PIH is thought to be caused by an imbalance of the placental prostacyclin, a vasodilator that inhibits platelet aggregation, and thromboxane A_2, a vasoconstrictor that stimulates platelet aggregation, resulting in vasospasm, which in turn increases peripheral vascular resistance.

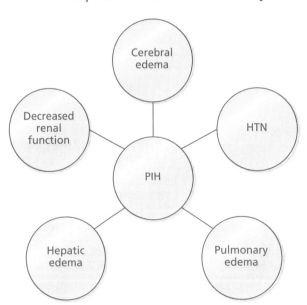

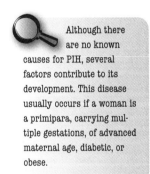

Although there are no known causes for PIH, several factors contribute to its development. This disease usually occurs if a woman is a primipara, carrying multiple gestations, of advanced maternal age, diabetic, or obese.

Figure 15-1 Types of PIH.

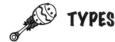

TYPES

Figure 15-1 presents the different types of PIH. Table 15-1 outlines signs and symptoms of PIH, and clinical presentations and descriptions are also defined.

Mild preeclampsia occurs when blood pressure readings after gestational week 20 are higher than 140/90 mm Hg on two occasions or when mean arterial pressure is greater than 105 mm Hg. The presence of proteinuria greater than 1+ on urine dipstick or more than 3g per 24-hour urine is also part of the diagnostic criteria. There may be generalized edema in the face, hands, or abdomen that does not resolve after 12 hours of bed rest. Although edema is common, it is no longer considered part of the diagnostic criteria. The patient generally reports a rapid weight gain of approximately 4–5 pounds in 1 week.

Severe preeclampsia is defined as blood pressure exceeding 160/110 mm Hg, proteinuria greater than 5 g/24 hours, oliguria less than 400 ml/24 hours, and hyperactive deep tendon reflexes. Visual acuity changes, severe headache, mental status changes, or vascular disturbances occur as a result of

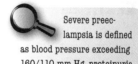 Severe preeclampsia is defined as blood pressure exceeding 160/110 mm Hg, proteinuria greater than 5 g/24 hours, oliguria less than 400 ml/24 hours, and hyperactive deep tendon reflexes. Visual acuity changes, severe headache, mental status changes, or vascular disturbances occur as a result of cerebral edema and central nervous system irritability.

Table 15-1 Signs and Symptoms of PIH and How Each Affects the Relationship to Other Organs

Type	Clinical Presentation	Description
Preeclampsia	Occurs after week 20; blood pressure 140/90 on two occasions; + proteinuria trace to 1+ or 0.3 g/24-hr urine; edema slight, generalized; rapid weight gain	Mild or severe nonconvulsive form of PIH occurring after week 20; determined by the presence of proteinuria
Eclampsia	Occurrence of seizures in absence of other causes	Convulsive form of PIH
Gestational Hypertension	Blood pressure 140/90 on two occasions; no proteinuria	Elevation of blood pressure without proteinuria; usually resolves by 12 weeks postpartum

cerebral edema and central nervous system irritability. Decreased glomerular filtration rates cause oliguria but rarely cause permanent damage to the kidneys. Hepatic irritability due to ischemia and necrosis causes generalized abdominal pain or, more specifically, pain localized to the right upper quadrant. Pulmonary edema, cyanosis, and jaundice are late stages of advancing disease.

Eclampsia is the occurrence of seizures in a pregnant woman who has no other metabolic or physiological reason for seizure activity, such as epilepsy or a brain mass.

TREATMENT

The goal of treatment is to prevent complications of PIH and convulsions until it is safe to deliver. If the patient has mild PIH, the gestational age determines whether or not to deliver. Ultrasound and nonstress tests evaluate fetal status. Monitoring of laboratory tests, especially complete blood count with differential, platelets, renal and liver function, coagulation studies, and urinalysis with a specific gravity, contributes to the patient's status. The patient is on bed rest with little to no stimulation.

Magnesium sulfate (MgSO$_4$) is a Pregnancy Category A anticonvulsant medication used to prevent or control seizures and acts as a smooth muscle relaxant to decrease vasoconstriction. MgSO$_4$ blocks acetylcholine and has a transient hypotensive effect. Serum magnesium levels must be monitored to determine therapeutic levels (4–6 mEq/l). The patient needs to be monitored for signs and symptoms of MgSO$_4$ toxicity defined as loss of patellar reflexes or a blood level of 10 mEq/l. Supplemental oxygen may also be administered.

> The patient needs to be monitored for signs and symptoms of MgSO$_4$ toxicity defined as loss of patellar reflexes or a blood level of 10 mEq/l.

Hydralazine (Apresoline) is a Pregnancy Category A vasodilator used to control high blood pressure. It decreases arteriolar spasms, produces vasodilation, and decreases blood pressure.

QUICK LOOK AT THE CHAPTER AHEAD

Gestational Diabetes occurs in less than 10% of all pregnancies in the United States today but a woman with a previous history of GDM has a 60–70% risk of developing it with subsequent pregnancies. All women should be screened during their 24th to 28th week of pregnancy and again 6 weeks postpartum.

Strict adherence to dietary restriction and monitoring of blood glucose is key to successful management of this disease during pregnancy. Complications that occur as a result of GDM include large for gestational age (LGA) infants, ketoacidosis which can be life-threatening, Polyhydramnios, and respiratory distress syndrome.

16

Gestational Diabetes Mellitus

TERMS
- ☐ Diabetic ketoacidosis
- ☐ Gestational diabetes mellitus (GDM)
- ☐ Human placental lactogen
- ☐ Hyperglycemia
- ☐ Macrosomia
- ☐ Polyhydramnios

Gestational diabetes mellitus (GDM) is the onset of impaired glucose or carbohydrate metabolism that is diagnosed during pregnancy. In the past GDM had a high maternal mortality rate. Approximately 30% of pregnant women died due to diabetic ketoacidosis, and the perinatal mortality rate was between 60% and 70%. Today, complications due to GDM have dramatically declined because of advances in research and successful management of blood glucose levels during pregnancy.

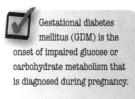

Gestational diabetes mellitus (GDM) is the onset of impaired glucose or carbohydrate metabolism that is diagnosed during pregnancy.

Impaired glucose metabolism is influenced by the hormones of pregnancy but may have been present before pregnancy. Gestational diabetes is diagnosed during the 24th to 28th week of pregnancy, and values generally return to normal after delivery. GDM is the most common medical complication in pregnancy and affects approximately 3–8% of all pregnancies in the United

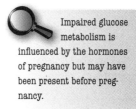

Impaired glucose metabolism is influenced by the hormones of pregnancy but may have been present before pregnancy.

States. Any woman who has had GDM in a previous pregnancy has a 60–70% risk for developing it with subsequent pregnancies or to develop adult-onset diabetes in the future.

GDM carries certain risks to both the woman and her fetus. Those risks increase if the woman does not have adequate blood sugar control during the perinatal period. The American Diabetes Association recommends that all pregnant women be screened for GDM by gestational weeks 24–28 by using a 50-g glucose tolerance test. It is also recommended that women with GDM undergo reclassification of the disease 6 weeks postpartum.

The American Diabetes Association recommends that all pregnant women be screened for GDM by gestational weeks 24–28 by using a 50-g glucose tolerance test. It is also recommended that women with GDM undergo reclassification of the disease 6 weeks postpartum.

PATHOPHYSIOLOGY

GDM is primarily caused by the inability of the beta cells of the pancreas to partially or completely secrete insulin needed to transport glucose across cell membranes. When glucose is unable to enter the cell, it remains in the bloodstream, resulting in high blood sugar levels, or **hyperglycemia.**

The basal metabolic rate of a pregnant woman increases in response to fetal growth, resulting in higher utilization of glucose, which crosses the placental membrane by diffusion. Insulin does not cross the placental membrane. The fetal pancreas secretes insulin as early as week 10 in response to glucose from maternal circulation. There is a direct correlation between high maternal glucose levels and high fetal glucose levels. Increased levels of glucose from maternal circulation cause increased fetal growth. **Human placental lactogen** is maternally produced by the placenta to assist with appropriate regulation of glucose. Human placental lactogen decreases the sensitivity of maternal cells to insulin.

 MATERNAL EFFECTS

Table 16-1 lists maternal complications of GDM. Women with good diabetic control during pregnancy have significantly less risks than those with poor diabetic control. **Diabetic ketoacidosis** is diagnosed when a woman's blood sugar exceeds 200 mg/dl. She may experience polyuria and polydipsia as well as headache, malaise, nausea, and vomiting. It is imperative that those with diabetic ketoacidosis receive prompt treatment because this can be life-threatening.

Hypertensive disorders of pregnancy occur more commonly with women diagnosed with diabetes prepregnancy. Established vascular disease increases the risk of preeclampsia and pregnancy-induced hypertension.

Infection, especially urinary tract infections, is greater when blood glucose levels are elevated. Glomerular filtration rates are increased, and the presence of glycosuria increases the risk of urinary infections. If urinary tract infections are not treated promptly, bacteria ascend into the kidneys, causing pyelonephritis. Elevated glucose levels also increase the risk of development of vaginal or oral candidiasis.

The incidence of **macrosomia** is approximately 20–50% among women with GDM. Typically, these large-for-gestational-age infants weigh about

Table 16-1 Maternal Complications and Fetal and Infant Risks

Maternal Complications
Diabetic ketoacidosis
Pregnancy-induced hypertension or preeclampsia
Urinary tract infections and pyelonephritis
Difficult labor, vaginal trauma, or cesarean birth
Polyhydramnios, which may lead to preterm labor
Progression of chronic systemic complications
Fetal and Infant Risks
Macrosomia
Intrauterine growth retardation
Respiratory distress syndrome
Birth trauma or shoulder dystocia due to large for gestational age
Hypoglycemia caused by withdrawal of maternal glucose

4,000 g and can cause vaginal trauma if not delivered via cesarean birth. These women are more likely to experience failure to progress, resulting in an assisted delivery (forceps, episiotomy, cesarean).

Polyhydramnios occurs when there is more than 200 ml of amniotic fluid. This is 10 times more likely to occur in women with diabetes; these women are also more likely to suffer from preterm labor as a result of premature rupture of membranes.

 FETAL OR INFANT EFFECTS

Intrauterine growth retardation causes small-for-gestational-age infants who are less than the 10th percentile for height and weight. This is a result of decreased uteroplacental perfusion due to the effects of diabetes on the vascular system and is more common among type 1 diabetic patients.

Respiratory distress syndrome occurs four to six times more often in infants born to women who are diabetic or have GDM. Elevated levels of maternal glucose inhibit the production of surfactant necessary for lung maturity. Fetal oxygen saturation rates are monitored after delivery, as are routine respiratory assessments.

> Respiratory distress syndrome occurs four to six times more often in infants born to women who are diabetic or have GDM.

Insulin acts as a growth hormone, increasing placental and fetal growth. Infants exposed to high levels of glucose in utero suffer from hypoglycemia after the birth. Macrosomia or large-for-gestational-age infants are at a higher risk for developing birth traumas such as shoulder dystocia, cephalohematoma, clavicular fractures, brachial plexus injuries, or perinatal hypoxia. These injuries happen when the fetus is too large for the maternal pelvis or occur as the fetus is descending through the vaginal canal. The neonate is monitored for hyperbilirubinemia as the cephalohematoma resolves. Fractures and brachial plexus injuries are treated by immobilization and proper positioning.

Hypoglycemia in the neonate occurs when there is withdrawal of maternal glucose and is a common effect of GDM on the newborn. Blood sugar levels are high at birth, causing the fetal pancreas to increase secretion of insulin. These blood sugar levels then decrease to less than 40 mg/dl within the early hours after birth. A heel stick performed on the infant determines blood sugar levels, which are frequently monitored during the first 24 hour of the neonate's life. Signs and symptoms of hypoglycemia in the neonate are lethargy, tachypnea, and tremors. Treatment is aimed at frequent feedings or intravenous glucose.

TREATMENT

Monitoring of blood sugar levels is the cornerstone in diabetic therapy and requires daily self-monitoring of blood glucose (Table 16-2). This self-monitoring enables patients to determine their response to dietary influences on their blood glucose levels and to make adjustments accordingly. During pregnancy, insulin levels vary widely due to hormonal fluctuations and may require multiple self-monitorings in the course of the day. Typically, patients obtain a fasting blood glucose level upon rising in the morning, a 2-hour postprandial level, and a bedtime level. For those with fluctuating blood glucose levels, monitoring before and after each meal, at bedtime, and a 3 AM glucose reading are recommended. A random glucose reading is also advised at any time the patient is symptomatic.

Dietary therapy and education, including a nutritional assessment by a registered dietitian or nutritionist, are equally important components of diabetic therapy. It is imperative that the patient is motivated and committed to making dietary changes to achieve tight glycemic control.

Subcutaneous insulin injections are used for patients with type 1 diabetes and GDM because it mimics the body's natural glycemic cycle and is achieved by using bolus doses of insulin. If the patient is not using an insulin pump, both short-acting and long-acting insulin are prescribed. For patients who are on insulin therapy, a sliding scale is often used depending on the blood glucose reading.

The newest technology includes the use of a continuous glucose monitoring system. It is a sensor that is implanted under the skin and connected to an external monitor that is attached by a plastic cannula. The monitor continuously records blood glucose levels every 5 minutes. An alternative to a continuous glucose monitoring system is the continuous subcutaneous insulin infusion pump. A small amount of insulin is delivered continuously throughout the day and allows for bolus injections to be administered if indicated.

Oral hypoglycemic agents are currently contraindicated during pregnancy because of their ability to cross the placental barrier. Ongoing studies regarding the safety of oral agents are being performed. Currently, the only agent that has been evaluated and does not appear to cross the placental barrier is glyburide. However, larger studies need to take place before this is widely accepted for use.

Table 16-2 Self-Monitoring Blood Glucose Levels

Time of Monitoring	Levels
Fasting blood glucose	≤ 95 mg/dl
1-hour postprandial blood glucose	≤ 55 mg/dl
2-hour postprandial blood glucose	≤ 120 mg/dl

HELLP syndrome is an acronym for a severe variant of preeclampsia. It is believed to occur as a result of fragmented red blood cells passing though damaged vessels that contain fibrin. These fibrin deposits cause a series of events leading to obstruction of vessels and consequent impaired blood flow to the liver. Monitoring of CBC and LFTs is imperative in early diagnosis of this syndrome.

17

HELLP Syndrome

TERMS
☐ **HELLP syndrome**

HELLP syndrome is an acronym for *hemolysis* (H), *elevated liver enzymes* (EL), and *low platelets* (LP). It is a severe variant of preeclampsia. The incidence of HELLP syndrome is highest among whites, multiparous women, and those diagnosed with preeclampsia. It occurs in only 2–16% of all pregnancies, compared with 5–7% for preeclampsia.

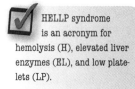
HELLP syndrome is an acronym for hemolysis (H), elevated liver enzymes (EL), and low platelets (LP).

PATHOPHYSIOLOGY

HELLP syndrome is believed to occur when fragmented red blood cells pass through vessels that have endothelial damage and deposits of fibrin. These fibrin deposits obstruct blood flow to the liver, causing impaired liver function and possible necrosis or intrahepatic hemorrhage. Thrombocytopenia may occur as a result of platelet aggregation at the site of vascular damage from vasospasm, leading to tissue hypoxia.

SIGNS AND SYMPTOMS

Approximately 90% of all patients with HELLP syndrome present with a complaint of malaise for several days. Most may also experience epigastric or right upper quadrant pain or tenderness, thought to be related to hepatic ischemia, nausea, and/or vomiting, as well as some influenza type symptoms. The patient may also have symptoms of preeclampsia such as severe hypertension, edema, and weight gain.

LABORATORY VALUES AND TREATMENT

It is important to monitor the patient's liver function and complete blood count with differential. It is typical to find decreased hemoglobin, hematocrit, and platelets (< 100,000/mm³) and elevated liver function tests, most specifically alanine and aspartate aminotransferases. Prothrombin time and partial thromboplastin time are normal unless the patient is developing disseminated intravascular coagulation, a potentially life-threatening defect of coagulation. Because of the high risk of rupture, it is important avoid palpation of the liver until further diagnostic tests are performed.

 It is important to monitor the patient's liver function and complete blood count with differential.

"TORCH" is an acronym for a collection of infections that can cross and enter the placenta causing fetal anomalies or death. The mother may experience mild flu-type symptoms but the infection can have devastating consequences on the developing fetus and may cause spontaneous abortion.

Each infection carries its own signs and symptoms as well as transmission of the individual infectious agent.

18

TORCH

TERMS

☐ **Cytomegalovirus (CMV)**
☐ **Group B streptococcus (GBS)**
☐ **Herpes simplex virus**
☐ **Rubella**
☐ **TORCH**
☐ **Toxoplasmosis**
☐ **Varicella**

"**TORCH**" is an acronym for a collection of infections that are capable of crossing the placenta, causing adverse effects on the developing fetus. The infections include *T*oxoplasmosis, *O*ther infections, *R*ubella, *C*ytomegalovirus, and *H*erpes simplex virus. The maternal symptoms experienced are flu-like and can cause miscarriage or severe fetal anomalies.

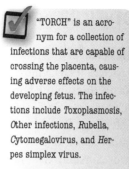

"TORCH" is an acronym for a collection of infections that are capable of crossing the placenta, causing adverse effects on the developing fetus. The infections include *T*oxoplasmosis, *O*ther infections, *R*ubella, *C*ytomegalovirus, and *H*erpes simplex virus.

TOXOPLASMOSIS

Toxoplasmosis is a disease caused by the protozoan parasite *Toxoplasma gondii* and is associated with eating raw or undercooked meat and through handling of infected cat feces and infected mice or farm animals. It can also be transmitted through eating unwashed fruits or vegetables whose surfaces have become contaminated with the parasite.

Acute infection produces symptoms such as rash, fever, malaise, lymphadenopathy, headaches, and/or sore throat. Changes in vision or eye pain may also be present. Symptoms are frequently mistaken for influenza or mononucleosis and can occur 1–2 weeks after exposure. Previous maternal infection provides immunity.

Infections during pregnancy are associated with spontaneous abortion, preterm delivery, fetal demise, or congenital infection with symptoms appearing at birth. Toxoplasmosis titers are performed to determine infection. Approximately 10% of infected infants exposed to the disease develop chorioretinitis, pneumonia, jaundice, and thrombocytopenia purpura. This rate increases to approximately 60% if exposed during the third trimester. They may also suffer permanent neurological deficits.

The drugs of choice for this infection include spiramycin, sulfadine, pyrimethamine, and folinic acid. Pyrimethamine is not recommended during the first trimester because of the potential for teratogenicity. If the patient is allergic to sulfonamides, an alternative is to treat with clindamycin or azithromycin.

OTHER INFECTIONS

This category includes infections such as group B streptococcus (GBS), varicella (chickenpox), hepatitis, and human immunodeficiency virus. **Varicella** is in the family of all herpes viruses. Once exposed to it, varicella can remain dormant in the dorsal root of the ganglia for many years before reactivating. It is transmitted through direct contact with respiratory secretions from an infected individual. The incubation period is approximately 10–14 days.

Signs and symptoms include fever, malaise, and a generalized pruritic vesicular rash on the body. The vesicles evolve to pustules that crust over before resolving. Individuals are considered contagious 24 hours before the onset of the rash and until all the lesions have completely crusted over. Treatment is aimed at prevention by individuals becoming immunized preconceptually. Symptomatic relief includes acetaminophen for fevers and cool or tepid baths to relieve itching. In severe infections, intravenous acyclovir may be safely used in all trimesters of pregnancy.

Once an individual has had varicella zoster, they usually have lifetime immunity. However, in pregnant women who have not had the disease or vaccination, an infection during the first trimester carries an approximate 10–20% risk for congenital defects, such as mental retardation, growth retardation, limb and digit hypoplasia, and eye anomalies. These signs usually develop within the first 10 days of the neonates' life.

Group B streptococcus (GBS) is a gram-positive bacterium that is normally found in the vaginas of nonpregnant women and in approximately 9–23% of healthy pregnant women. It causes vertical transmission (from mother to infant) during birth and is the leading cause of neonatal infections in the United States.

Women with GBS are generally asymptomatic; however, once the infection has progressed, patients may initially complain of fever. Late signs and symptoms include uterine tenderness (amnionitis), foul-smelling amniotic fluid, and tachycardia.

The current recommendations are to screen all pregnant women at 35–37 weeks' gestation for GBS by obtaining vaginal and anorectal cultures. All positive results are treated with antibiotics such as penicillin G or ampicillin. Monitoring of the newborn for respiratory distress or signs of infection should be performed.

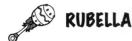

RUBELLA

Rubella, also known as German measles, is caused by the rubella virus. The infection is transmitted by respiratory contact with an infected individual. Patients commonly report fever, myalgias, arthralgias, lymphadenopathy, and a nonpruritic rash. It is vertically transmitted. Rubella is diagnosed based on signs and symptoms and a hemagglutination inhibition antigen test.

Fetal complications are much more serious than maternal complications and can cause miscarriage, congenital anomalies known as congenital rubella syndrome, and death. The incidence of such anomalies is 50–90% if infection occurs during the first trimester. Malformations of the fetal heart and brain occur if exposure happens during the first 2 months. If infection occurs after the fourth month, hearing loss, mental retardation, intrauterine growth retardation, and systemic infections can occur in the fetus.

Vaccination against rubella is widely available, but women are recommended to be screened during the initial prenatal visit to determine immunity. Otherwise, vaccination should take place a minimum of 3 months before conception or in the immediate postpartum period. It is contraindicated in pregnant women. It is not contraindicated in breast-feeding women.

CYTOMEGALOVIRUS

Cytomegalovirus (CMV) is a DNA virus in the herpes family that is transmitted maternally through sexual contact, blood transfusions, or respiratory contact. Women are at risk for contracting CMV if they work or have children in day care or in institutions for the mentally retarded.

Infected women are primarily asymptomatic but may present with flulike symptoms and elevated liver function tests. A positive CMV-specific antigen IgM test confirms the presence of an infection. Women with a positive infection need to decide on elective termination of the pregnancy due to the high rate of fetal anomalies associated with CMV. Reactivation of a previous infection can also occur because there is no immunity once the disease has been contracted.

Currently, there is no therapy to treat CMV. Proper hand-washing techniques, good hygiene, and safe sex help to prevent spreading the virus to others.

HERPES SIMPLEX VIRUS

Approximately 20% of the adult population has been diagnosed with **herpes simplex virus** type 2 (HSV-2). Genital herpes is a recurrent life-long viral infection that can reoccur at any time. The virus can be shed at any time without symptoms.

Approximately 2% of women acquire HSV-2 during pregnancy. It is associated with a high rate of infant mortality (40–60%) if primary infection occurs during either the first trimester or near the time of delivery.

Signs and symptoms include painful vesicular lesions on or around the inner and outer labia, fever, malaise, and dysuria. Diagnosis is based on clinical symptoms, viral cultures of the lesions, and type-specific serological testing for HSV. Oral antiviral medications are used to decrease the severity of the outbreak along with topical antibiotic ointments or creams to prevent secondary bacterial infections. If the outbreak occurs near or at the time of delivery, a cesarean section is recommended to prevent complications and transmission to the newborn.

SECTION 6 • REVIEW QUESTIONS

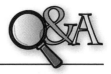

1. Placenta previa is a (an) _____ implanted placenta.
   a. Normally
   b. Abnormally
   c. Centrally
   d. Laterally

2. What medication prevents sensitization by clearing the fetal cells from the maternal circulation and depressing the mothers' immune response?
   a. Tetracycline
   b. RhoGAM
   c. Vitamin K
   d. Erythromycin

3. Which of the following symptoms indicates increasing severity of PIH?
   a. 2+ edema in hands and feet
   b. Fatigue and headache
   c. Epigastric pain and oliguria
   d. Three-pound weight gain over 2 months and shortness of breath

4. Which of the following are the three different types of placenta previa?
   a. Complete, partial, and low lying
   b. Complete, normal, and marginal
   c. Partial, incomplete, and low lying
   d. Total, central, and marginal

5. When will a primigravida who is Rh negative and pregnant with an Rh-positive fetus most likely to become sensitized to the Rh-positive blood?
   a. At the time of placental separation
   b. During the birth of the baby
   c. As soon as labor begins
   d. At the time of fertilization

6. A patient is being treated for PIH with bed rest and intravenous $MgSO_4$. The classification of this drug is a:
   a. Prostaglandin inhibitor
   b. Anticonvulsant
   c. Antihypertensive
   d. Diuretic

7. The diagnosis of placenta previa is obtained through a(an):
   a. X-ray
   b. Ultrasound
   c. Fetal monitor
   d. Cesarean section

8. When a woman is Rh negative, what other situations can lead to sensitization?
   a. When she is pregnant with Rh-negative twins
   b. When the father is Rh negative
   c. After an abortion
   d. If she develops gestational diabetes

9. What is the only known cure for preeclampsia?
   a. $MgSO_4$
   b. Antihypertensive medications
   c. Delivery of the fetus
   d. Administration of ASA (aspirin) every day for the remainder of the pregnancy

10. When reviewing risk factors, what condition is most commonly associated with abruptio placenta?
    a. Large term infant
    b. Preterm infant
    c. Hypertension
    d. Hypothyroid

11. ABO incompatibility usually occurs when:
    a. The mother and infant are A blood type
    b. The mother and infant are AB blood type
    c. The mother and infant are B blood type
    d. The mother is O blood type and the infant is A blood type

12. Which of the following clinical signs is not included in the classic symptoms of preeclampsia?
    a. Hypertension
    b. Edema
    c. Proteinuria
    d. Glucosuria

13. One of the main clinical manifestations of abruptio placentae is:
    a. Hypertension
    b. Hypotension
    c. Mild to severe pain
    d. Mild uterine relaxation

14. One of the main distinctions between Rh incompatibility and ABO incompatibility is that ABO incompatibility may affect:
    a. First-born infants
    b. Only male infants
    c. Only female infants
    d. No first-born infants

15. Which of the following assessment findings would encourage the nurse to hold the next dose of $MgSO_4$?
    a. Absence of DTRs (deep tendon reflexes)
    b. U/O (urine output) of 100 cc for the past 2 hours
    c. RR (respiratory rate) 14/min
    d. Decrease in blood pressure from 160/100 to 140/85

16. When caring for a patient with HELLP syndrome, which of the following assessments should be avoided?
    a. Auscultation of the heart and lungs
    b. Palpation of the abdomen
    c. Checking DTRs every 4 hours
    d. Daily phlebotomy for laboratory values

17. Signs and symptoms for HELLP syndrome include all of the following *except:*
    a. Epigastric pain
    b. Elevated fasting blood sugar
    c. Malaise
    d. Nausea and vomiting

18. In teaching patients about TORCH, all of the following are true *except:*
   a.   Wash all foods well
   b.   Avoid handling cat litter boxes
   c.   Avoid eating sushi
   d.   Wear sunglasses when outside

19. A woman in labor has tested positive for group B streptococcus. Which of the following is *true?*
   a.   Monitor the newborn for signs and symptoms of respiratory distress
   b.   Avoid anyone who has not had the chickenpox
   c.   Avoid working in day care or other institutions
   d.   Practice safe sex

20. Rubella, if contracted during the first trimester of pregnancy, can cause:
   a.   Amnionitis
   b.   Malformation of the fetal heart and brain
   c.   Painful generalized rash on one side of the body
   d.   Maternal blindness

21. Maternal complications for GDM include all of the following *except:*
   a.   Diabetic ketoacidosis
   b.   Pyelonephritis
   c.   Intrauterine growth retardation
   d.   Pregnancy-induced hypertension

22. Diabetic ketoacidosis occurs when:
   a.   Fasting blood sugar is no more than 95 mg/dl
   b.   One-hour postprandial blood glucose is no more than 155 mg/dl
   c.   Two hour postprandial blood glucose is no more than 120 mg/dl
   d.   Blood glucose exceeds 200 mg/dl

23. All pregnant women should undergo a glucose tolerance test by:
   a.   Weeks 15–17
   b.   Weeks 18–20
   c.   Weeks 22–24
   d.   Weeks 24–28

24. Insulin crosses the placental membrane.
    a. True
    b. False

25. Large-for-gestational-age infants are typically born to women who have:
    a. Gestational diabetes mellitus
    b. Type 1 diabetes mellitus
    c. Type 2 diabetes mellitus
    d. Any type of diabetes

26. Macrosomic infants are at higher risk for developing:
    a. Shoulder dystocia and cephalohematoma
    b. Postdelivery hyperglycemia
    c. Vaginal trauma
    d. Polyhydramnios

27. A large-for-gestational-age infant who has a cephalohematoma should be monitored for:
    a. Respiratory distress syndrome
    b. Polyhydramnios
    c. Hyperbilirubinemia
    d. Excitability

28. Treatment for diabetes in pregnancy includes all of the following *except:*
    a. Insulin
    b. Continuous glucose monitoring system
    c. Oral hypoglycemic agents
    d. Diet therapy

29. _____ diabetes generally resolves after delivery.
    a. Type 1
    b. Type 2
    c. Gestational
    d. None of the above

30. There is a direct correlation between:
    a. High maternal glucose levels and high fetal glucose levels
    b. Low maternal glucose levels and low fetal glucose levels
    c. High maternal glucose levels and low fetal glucose levels
    d. Low maternal glucose levels and high fetal glucose levels

ANSWERS AND RATIONALES

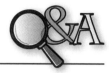

1. The answer is b.

2. The answer is b.

3. **The answer is c.** Rationale: Epigastric pain and oliguria indicate worsening of PIH. Mild edema is not uncommon in late pregnancy as well as fatigue. Women with worsening PIH notice a rapid weight gain of 4–5 pounds in 1 week.

4. The answer is a.

5. **The answer is a.** Rationale: Usually, the mixing of fetal blood cells and maternal blood cells take place during the third stage of labor. There is also a danger at 28 weeks of gestation and 3 days after delivery.

6. **The answer is b.** Rational: Magnesium sulfate is a Category A anticonvulsant medication with some transient hypotensive effects as it decreases vasoconstriction.

7. The answer is b.

8. **The answer is c.** Rationale: If the embryo/fetus is Rh positive and if RhoGAM is not given, she will then become sensitized.

9. **The answer is c.** Rationale: Delivery is the only known cure for preeclampsia. $MgSO_4$ and antihypertensive medications are used to control symptoms, not cure them.

10. The answer is c.

11. **The answer is d.** Rationale: Because blood groups have naturally occurring anti-A and anti-B antibodies, there is the opportunity that these naturally occurring antibodies can cross the placental barrier. This problem can also occur if the infant has blood type B or AB and the mother is O blood type.

12. **The answer is d.** Rationale: Glucosuria is not considered diagnostic criteria for preeclampsia. The others are.

13. The answer is c.

14. **The answer is a.**

15. **The answer is a.** Rationale: $MgSO_4$ toxicity causes loss of patellar reflexes.

16. **The answer is b.** Rationale: Palpation of the abdomen in a patient with HELLP syndrome is contraindicated due to the high risk of liver rupture.

17. **The answer is b.** Rationale: An elevated fasting blood sugar is not considered part of the diagnostic criteria for HELLP syndrome.

18. **The answer is d.** Rationale: All of the choices are important to teach patients about TORCH.

19. **The answer is a.** Rationale: Infants born to women with GBS are at risk for developing respiratory distress syndrome.

20. **The answer is b.** Rationale: Rubella, or German measles, can cause severe fetal anomalies if contracted or exposed during the first trimester of pregnancy.

21. **The answer is c.** Rationale: Intrauterine growth retardation is a fetal risk.

22. **The answer is d.** Rationale: Diabetic ketoacidosis occurs when blood glucose exceeds 200 mg/dl.

23. **The answer is d.** Rationale: The American Diabetes Association recommends that all pregnant women be screened by weeks 24–28.

24. **The answer is b.** Rationale: Insulin does not cross the placental membrane. The fetal pancreas secretes insulin as early as week 10.

25. **The answer is a.** Rationale: Insulin acts as a growth hormone and increases fetal growth.

26. **The answer is a.** Rationale: Infants with macrosomia are at higher risk for developing birth traumas such as shoulder dystocia and cephalohematoma due to the infant being too large for the maternal pelvis.

27. **The answer is c.** Rationale: Infants with a cephalohematoma are monitored for hyperbilirubinemia due to the breakdown of the cephalohematoma.

28. **The answer is c.** Rationale: Oral hypoglycemic agents are contraindicated in pregnancy.

29. **The answer is c.** Rationale: Gestational diabetics have impaired glucose metabolism that is influenced by the hormones of pregnancy. Values generally return to normal after delivery.

30. **The answer is a.** Rationale: High levels of maternal glucose directly influence fetal glucose levels.

VII

Menopause

Menopause is defined as the cessation of menses for 12 consecutive months. The age at which menopause occurs is predetermined genetically. There are several possible stages of menopause: perimenopause, menopause, induced menopause, premature menopause, and postmenopause. Currently, diagnosing menopause is based solely on the patient's symptomatology. Traditionally, measuring a serum estradiol, follicle-stimulating hormone (FSH), and luteinizing hormone (LH) were enough to determine whether a woman was in menopause.

Consequences of menopause include increased risk of cardiovascular disease, hypertension, hyperlipidemia, and osteoporosis or osteopenia.

Treatment options for menopause include hormone therapy (HT), which continues to be controversial, and complementary or alternative therapies. Life-style changes are also recommended to help reduce menopausal symptoms.

19

Menopause

TERMS
☐ **Menopause**

Menopause is defined as the cessation of menses for 12 consecutive months. It is also referred to as the climacteric phase of a woman's life. The average age of menopause in the United States is 51 years of age. Women today can expect more than one-third of their lives to be ahead of them when they reach menopause and have a mean life expectancy of 84 years. The age at which menopause occurs is predetermined genetically as is the onset of menarche in young women. A woman can expect menopause at about the same age that her mother or older sisters experienced it. Cigarette smoking can increase the onset of menopause by about 2 years. Table 19-1 describes the different stages of menopause.

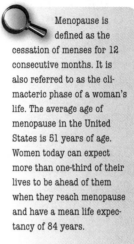

Menopause is defined as the cessation of menses for 12 consecutive months. It is also referred to as the climacteric phase of a woman's life. The average age of menopause in the United States is 51 years of age. Women today can expect more than one-third of their lives to be ahead of them when they reach menopause and have a mean life expectancy of 84 years.

Table 19-1 Stages of Menopause

Stage	Characteristics
Perimenopause	Two to 8 years before the last menstrual period when changes occur *plus* 1 year after menopause Begins in mid-40s with subtle changes in menstrual cycle characteristics Occurs when incidence of pelvic disorders are statistically high Cessation of menses could be due to endometrial polyps, cancer, or precancerous condition
Menopause	No menses for 12 consecutive months or when ovaries are surgically removed or damaged

Induced menopause	Immediate menopause caused by medical intervention such as
	  Surgery
	  Chemotherapy
	  Radiation
	  Certain drugs, such as immunosuppressive therapy

Premature menopause (also known as physiological menopause)	Naturally occurring menopause before the age of 40 Only found in one in four women Caused by autoimmune disorders, endocrine disorders, childhood illnesses (i.e., mumps, viral infections), reproductive tract tumors, or malnourishment
Postmenopause	All the years beyond menopause Greatest risk for developing complications due to lack of estrogen

PATHOPHYSIOLOGY

Ovaries are responsible for the production of estrogen and progesterone as well as small amounts of androgens, including testosterone, which are responsible for a woman's libido. The other function of the ovaries is to produce eggs. At birth, the ovaries contain approximately a half million follicles, which decrease with age. When puberty occurs, the follicles mature to become eggs. As the number of follicles or eggs decrease, estrogen levels begin to decrease. Approximately 90% of all circulating estrogen is produced by the ovaries; however, androgens produced by the adrenal glands convert the adipose cells into estrogen.

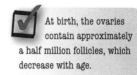

At birth, the ovaries contain approximately a half million follicles, which decrease with age.

The pituitary gland produces follicle-stimulating hormone (FSH) and luteinizing hormone (LH). FSH causes stimulation of the follicles to develop, whereas LH causes the release of the egg from the ovary. The biofeedback between the ovaries, the hypothalamus, and the pituitary gland must be well regulated for menstruation to occur. As the ovary produces less estrogen and progesterone, FSH and LH levels rise and irregular menses occur. Ultimately, the production of ovarian follicles ceases, leading to decreased estrogen and progesterone levels while FSH and LH levels remain high. This causes menstruation to stop.

Vaginal dryness and thinning of the vagina from low levels of estrogen and low levels of androgen all contribute to dyspareunia. The elasticity, length, and width of the vagina all change as a result of estrogen withdrawal. Hot flashes result when there is a burst of hormonal activity, creating instability within the vessels and causing dilation and increased blood flow to the skin. Profuse sweating and redness in the face, neck, and ears can last for several minutes. These episodes typically occur in the middle of the night, disrupting sleep, and women may experience them for 5 to 7 years (Table 19-2).

LABORATORY TESTS

Traditionally, measuring a serum estradiol, FSH, and LH were enough to determine whether a woman was in menopause. Estradiol levels fluctuate widely, and recent research and review of the literature no longer

Table 19-2 Signs and Symptoms of Menopause

Change in characteristics of menstrual cycle: lighter, shorter, longer, or heavier, irregular bleeding patterns
Decreased libido
Mood swings or irritability
Hot flashes or flushes, night sweats
Vaginal dryness, pain and atrophy of vaginal tissue
Thinning and/or graying of hair
Sleep disruption or insomnia
Signs/symptoms of clinical depression
Changes in skin: dryness, acne, increased facial hair
Urinary frequency or increased number of urinary tract infections

recommend these tests due to the inaccuracies of these levels at any given time during a woman's cycle. However, many practitioners still order these tests as a baseline. Currently, diagnosing menopause is based solely on the patient's symptomatology. If a woman has not had menses for 12 consecutive months and suddenly has a period, an endometrial biopsy is recommended to rule out any pathological process that may be developing.

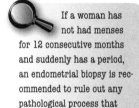 If a woman has not had menses for 12 consecutive months and suddenly has a period, an endometrial biopsy is recommended to rule out any pathological process that may be developing.

 ## CONSEQUENCES OF MENOPAUSE

Cardiovascular disease poses the greatest health risk to women and increases after the age of 50 due to the lack of estrogen. Women in this age group are also at increased risk of developing hypertension, hyperlipidemia, and osteoporosis or osteopenia.

Osteoporosis or osteopenia, caused by the lack of influence of estrogen and calcium absorption on bone, occurs when the body loses bone more quickly than it can produce bone cells, leading to thinning of the bone. An estimated 10 million women have osteoporosis, and 34 million women have osteopenia. The greatest bone loss occurs during the first year after menopause.

 ## TREATMENT OPTIONS FOR MENOPAUSE

Much controversy exists for hormone therapy (HT) since the cessation of the Women's Health Initiative Study in 2002 when it was discovered that the risk of invasive breast cancer in the participants was statistically significant and outweighed the benefits of using HT. The current recommendations are to limit HT to short-term therapy (1–4 years) for those women seeking relief of acute menopausal symptoms. Currently, several major studies are ongoing to further determine those at risk from using HT.

Uses for HT therapy include estrogen *plus* progesterone for women with an intact uterus and estrogen only for hysterectomy patients. Forms of HT available include oral, transdermal patches, silicone rings, or topical creams.

Benefits of HT are as follows:

- Increases high-density lipoproteins
- Increases bone density
- Decreases vasomotor symptoms
- Enhances collagen and improves skin elasticity

There also several risks of HT:

- Increased risk for thromboembolic events
- Vaginal bleeding
- Potential increased risk for Alzheimer's disease

Few studies exist to support the use of complementary or alternative therapies. They are not regulated by the U.S. Food and Drug Administration, and there are no studies to prove their safety or efficacy. There are many interactions with herbal therapy and prescription medication.

Life-style changes are recommended to help reduce menopausal symptoms. These changes include increased exercise to improve circulation and to help boost metabolism and dietary changes such as avoidance of hot spicy foods, caffeine, and alcoholic beverages. To prevent any further bone loss, intake of calcium should be between 1,000 and 1,500 mg daily. If a woman is lactose intolerant or does not consume enough dietary calcium, dietary supplements are an acceptable alternative, as are the use of bisphosphonates and selective estrogen receptor modulators to help reduce the risk of fractures. If a woman has been diagnosed with osteopenia or osteoporosis, there are alternative prescription medications that prevent further bone loss. Vaginal lubricants are recommended to help relieve vaginal dryness. Smoking increases instability of vessels; therefore smoking cessation is recommended.

SECTION VII · REVIEW QUESTIONS

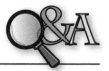

1. Endocrine or autoimmune disorders can cause:
    a. Induced menopause
    b. Perimenopause
    c. Premature menopause
    d. Postmenopause

2. Irregular menstrual cycles occur during perimenopause due to:
    a. Increased FSH and LH levels
    b. Decreased FSH and LH levels
    c. Overgrowth of the endometrial lining
    d. Increased production of estrogen

3. Which of the following tests can predict the stage of menopause that a woman is in?
    a. Estradiol, FSH, and LH levels
    b. Estradiol levels only
    c. FSH and LH levels only
    d. None of the above

4. A patient who has had a complete hysterectomy but still has her ovaries would benefit from which type of hormone therapy?
    a. Combination estrogen and progesterone
    b. Estrogen only
    c. Progesterone only
    d. None of the above

5. Some of the consequences of menopause include:
    a. Osteoporosis
    b. Hypertension
    c. Hyperlipidemia
    d. All of the above

6. The use of bisphosphonates are recommended for:
    a. Women with a family history of breast cancer
    b. Women with a personal history of breast cancer
    c. Women who smoke cigarettes
    d. All women who are perimenopausal or lactose intolerant

7. Women who decide to take HT can do so safely:
a. Indefinitely
b. For 1–4 years
c. Only if they are having acute symptoms
d. None of the above

8. A woman is considered postmenopausal when:
a. Her menses are shorter, lighter, and longer between cycles
b. There is an increase in hot flashes or sleep disruption
c. She complains of loss of libido or vaginal dryness
d. When she has not had a menses in 12 consecutive months

9. Factors that influence the onset of menopause include all of the following *except:*
a. Cigarette smoking
b. Familial history of onset of menopause
c. Any surgical intervention to the ovaries or uterus
d. History of a fracture

10. Which of the following are considered signs and symptoms of menopause?
a. Decreased libido, excessive sleep, dysphagia
b. Dyspareunia, night sweats, insomnia
c. Excessive fatigue, dysphagia, mood swings, oily skin
d. Hot flashes, increased libido, increased hunger

ANSWERS AND RATIONALES

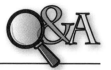

1. **The answer is c.** Rationale: Premature menopause can be caused by autoimmune disorders, endocrine disorders, childhood illnesses, reproductive tract tumors, or malnourishment.

2. **The answer is a.** Rationale: As the ovary produces less estrogen and progesterone, FSH and LH levels rise, causing irregular menses to occur.

3. **The answer is d.** Rationale: Currently, diagnosing menopause is based solely on the patient's symptomatology, although practitioners may order these tests as a baseline.

4. **The answer is b.** Rationale: Women who no longer have a uterus should receive estrogen only. Progesterone is needed to shed or decrease the uterine lining.

5. **The answer is d.** Rationale: Postmenopausal women are at risk for all of the above due to the lack of influence of estrogen on those body systems.

6. **The answer is d.** Rationale: To prevent further bone loss, the use of bisphosphonates and selective estrogen receptor modulators are used to reduce the risk of fractures in any woman who cannot tolerate dietary calcium or who is lactose intolerant.

7. **The answer is b.** Rationale: The current recommendations are to limit HT to short-term therapy of 1–4 years until further studies determine longer use safety.

8. **The answer is d.** Rationale: A woman is considered postmenopausal when she has not had a menses in 12 consecutive months.

9. **The answer is d.** Rationale: History of fracture is important in determining a patient's risk for osteoporosis but does not influence the onset of menopause.

10. **The answer is b.** Low levels of estrogen and androgen cause vaginal dryness, sleep disruption, and instability of blood vessels that cause flushing of skin.

VIII

Sexually Transmitted Infections

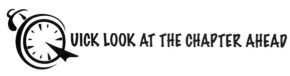

Viral sexually transmitted infections can occur as a result of direct intimate contact, such as kissing, with an infected individual. Viruses are highly transmissible during the shedding period. It is impossible to know when the virus is shedding but it is important to know that transmission is highest when there is a visible lesion.

HSV-1 occurs generally in the mouth but can be transmitted to the genital area during oral sex. HSV-2 can also be transmitted to other areas of the body during intimate contact.

HPV has over 80 strains, some which have onogenic potential. There is now a vaccine available to prevent two known types of HPV which cause cervical cancer.

20

Viral Sexually Transmitted Infections

TERMS
- ☐ Hepatitis B and C
- ☐ Human immunodeficiency virus (HIV)
- ☐ Human papilloma virus (HPV)
- ☐ Sexually transmitted infections (STIs)
- ☐ Viral STIs

Sexually transmitted infections (STIs), also known as sexually transmitted diseases, are transmitted through direct intimate contact with an infected person. The causative organisms are viral, bacterial, or protozoan and can coexist. Approximately 15 million new cases are diagnosed annually, with the incidence of STIs peaking during adolescence. The prevalence of viral STIs exceeds that of bacterial STIs. Some STIs are uncomplicated, such as with *Trichomonas* infection, but others, such as chlamydia and gonorrhea, if left untreated, can lead to long-term health problems such as pelvic inflammatory disease, infertility, chronic pelvic pain, and ectopic pregnancy.

RISK FACTORS

Those who are sexually active (anal, oral, or vaginal) with multiple sexual partners with or without barrier contraception, substance abuse, gay or bisexual males, those not in a mutually monogamous relationship, those who exchange sex for money or drugs, and those who have been previously infected with an STI are at increased risk for contracting an STI.

> Those who are sexually active (anal, oral, or vaginal) with multiple sexual partners with or without barrier contraception, substance abuse, gay or bisexual males, those not in a mutually monogamous relationship, those who exchange sex for money or drugs, and those who have been previously infected with an STI are at increased risk for contracting an STI.

VIRAL STIs

Viral STIs are incurable infections that can cause recurrent episodes and remain in the patient's body for life (Table 20-1). There are no known cures for viral STIs. There are two types of herpes viruses: HSV-1 and HSV-2. HSV-1 is generally oral in nature but can be transmitted to other places on the body, such as the genital region. HSV-2 primarily causes lesions in the genital area but can also occur anywhere on or in the body. Other viral STIs include human papilloma virus (HPV), hepatitis, and human immunodeficiency virus (HIV). Both hepatitis and HIV are covered in greater detail in other chapters of this text.

Table 20-1 Types of Viral STIs

	Causative Organism	Signs and Symptoms	Diagnosis	Management and Treatment
Herpes	Herpes simplex virus (HSV)	Prodrome: pain, burning, itching at site; tiny vesicles or ulcerations; flulike or urinary tract infection symptoms	By clinical exam: HSV culture (Tzanck smear) or Herpes Select (serum)	Valacyclovir, acyclovir, famciclovir, prevention of secondary bacterial infections
Human papilloma virus (HPV)	Over 80 strains identified	Perineal itching; visible warty growths anywhere in perineum, vagina, cervix, or rectal area	Clinical exam, viral DNA testing	Patient applied: imiquimod 5% cream or podofilox 0.5% Provider applied: podophyllin resin, trichloroacetic acid (TCA), or bichloracetic acid (BCA); cryotherapy; laser surgery if severe
Hepatitis B and C	Hepatitis B virus	Flulike symptoms, rash, abdominal pain, dark urine, scleral icterus, jaundice	Hepatitis antibodies and surface antigens, liver function tests, liver ultrasound	Symptomatic, universal precautions, hepatitis C treated with interferon-alpha-2b
Human immunodeficiency virus (HIV)	Retrovirus	Persistent flulike symptoms	Complete blood count with differential, erythrocyte sedimentation rate, CD4 levels, HIV antibodies (must have informed consent)	Antiretrovirals

HERPES SIMPLEX VIRUSES

Herpes simplex viruses are transmitted by direct intimate contact with someone who is shedding the virus. The virus enters through microscopic breaks in the skin and resides in the dorsal root of the ganglia where it may remain latent for many years. Viral replication begins at the portal of entry. The patient generally complains of burning, itching, or tingling at the site and then develops multiple painful vesicles, flulike symptoms, and dysuria. Primary outbreaks also cause bilateral inguinal lymphadenopathy. Symptoms may last up to 2–3 weeks. The vesicles then ulcerate, crust over, and disappear without scarring. Recurrent episodes are generally less painful and shorter and can occur at any time, especially during times of physical or emotional stress. The patient is considered contagious until the lesions have crusted over and healed. The virus can be transmitted to another person anytime the virus is shedding even if the person is without symptoms.

Management

Herpes is diagnosed based on clinical exam and a viral or Tzanck culture. The vesicle is swabbed with cotton or Dacron-tipped swab and placed in the culture tube that contains the appropriate medium to prevent drying of the specimen. Antiviral therapy is used for both primary and recurrent infections and includes acyclovir, famciclovir, or valacyclovir. Comfort measures include sitz baths and topical antibiotic cream or ointment to prevent secondary infections. Abstinence is highly recommended during the prodrome and when lesions are present.

HUMAN PAPILLOMA VIRUS

Human papilloma virus (HPV), or condylomata acuminata, is also known as genital or venereal warts. It is estimated that approximately 1 million new cases are diagnosed annually; HPV is thought to be the most common viral STI in the United States but is not a reportable disease.

HPV is a slow-growing papovavirus and is most commonly spread by sexual or intimate contact. It enters through breaks in the skin or mucous membranes, infecting the basal cells of the epithelium. Those cells multiply and form fleshy lesions that may appear singularly or may coalesce into a cauliflower-like mass. The growths are generally painless but can cause itching or bleeding after intercourse. Incubation of the virus is 1 to 6 months or longer but can remain dormant for decades. There are more than 80 known strains of the virus, some of which cause genital warts and others with known oncogenic potential.

Management

There are several ways to treat condylomata acuminata: Patient-applied or provider-applied therapies are equally as efficacious. Patient-applied therapy includes imiquimod 5% cream or podofilox 0.5% solution gel. Provider-applied therapy requires treatment in the office setting with trichloracetic acid, bichloracetic acid, and podophyllin resin 10–25% in compound tincture of benzoin or cryotherapy with liquid nitrogen or cryoprobe. Severe cases can be treated with laser surgery or intralesional interferon. Clinical trials of a vaccine have shown 100% effectiveness in preventing cervical cancer caused by HPV strains numbers 16 and 18. The U.S. Food and Drug Administration recently approved this vaccine.

 ## HEPATITIS B AND C

Hepatitis B and C are considered STIs due to their transmission during intimate sexual activity. Those at risk for developing hepatitis B and C include intravenous drug abusers, those with multiple sexual partners, and contact of hepatitis B and C virus carriers.

 ## HIV

Human immunodeficiency virus (HIV) infection can result in acquired immunodeficiency syndrome (AIDS), which can be transmitted sexually, through sharing of needles and through vertical transmission from mother to fetus. High-risk behaviors for developing HIV/AIDS include anal, vaginal, or oral intercourse with an infected person; sharing needles during intravenous drug use; multiple sexual partners; and unprotected sex with an infected individual. Individuals who are HIV positive may be without symptoms for 10 years or longer.

Bacterial sexually transmitted infections often co-exist and many times do not have outward symptoms of infection. If left untreated, these infections can impact on a woman's ability to bear children due to scarring from untreated infections. If a woman does not know she is infected, she can unknowingly pass the infection to someone else. It is important that every partner is treated before engaging in sexual activity again.

Bacterial infections are diagnosed using amplified nucleic acid tests, cultures, or blood tests.

21

Bacterial Sexually Transmitted Infections

TERMS
☐ Chlamydia
☐ Gonorrhea
☐ Syphilis

There are three main types of bacterial sexually transmitted infections (STIs). Table 21-1 gives an overview of gonorrhea, chlamydia, and syphilis.

Table 21-1 Types of Bacterial STIs

	Causative Organism	Signs and Symptoms	Diagnosis	Management and Treatment
Chlamydia	*Chlamydia trachomatis*	Usually asymptomatic; irregular menses, postcoital spotting, purulent cervical discharge, dysuria	Culture, DNA probe, enzyme immunoassay, nucleic acid amplification	Azithromycin single dose; doxycycline; erythromycin or amoxicillin if pregnant
Gonorrhea	*Neisseria gonorrhoeae*	Usually asymptomatic; purulent cervical discharge, menstrual irregularities, pelvic pain	Thayer-Martin cultures	Cefixime, ceftriaxone, ciprofloxacin, ofloxacin, levofloxacin, treat presumptively for chlamydia
Syphilis	*Treponema pallidum*	Periods of active symptoms and latency. Primary: chancre. Secondary: maculopapular rash on palms and soles. Tertiary: central nervous system, cardiovascular changes; gumma lesions.	Venereal Disease Research Laboratory or rapid plasma reagent. To confirm: fluorescent treponemal antibody absorbed and microhemagglutination assays for antibody to *T. pallidum*	Penicillin G; if penicillin allergic, doxycycline or tetracycline

GONORRHEA

Gonorrhea is caused by the bacteria *Neisseria gonorrhoeae*, a gram-negative intracellular diplococcus. Approximately 600,000 new infections are reported annually, and it often coexists with chlamydia. It is transmitted by direct contact of the mucous membranes with an infected individual, across amniotic membranes, or during passage through the birth canal. The bacteria attach to the walls of the epithelium in mucous membranes and cause damage to the mucosal cells, leading to an inflammatory response.

Incubation is 3–10 days, and in most cases women are asymptomatic until the organism causes recognizable symptoms such as pelvic pain, fever, and purulent cervical discharge. Other symptoms include pharyngitis or conjunctivitis. Rectal pain and anal discharge can occur after anal intercourse with an infected individual. Gonorrhea can cause pelvic inflammatory disease and tubal scarring, resulting in infertility. Common manifestations of the disease for men include mucopurulent penile discharge and dysuria.

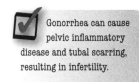

Gonorrhea can cause pelvic inflammatory disease and tubal scarring, resulting in infertility.

Management

Culture and sensitivity specimens should be obtained for definitive diagnosis and to rule out coexisting chlamydia infections. All partners must be treated to prevent reinfection. Medications include cefixime or ceftriaxone. Ciprofloxacin is also recommended; however, there is now a quinolone-resistant *N. gonorrhoeae* (QRNG) strain that is common in parts of Asia and the Pacific. Because of this, quinolone therapy is not recommended for treatment of gonorrhea in the State of Hawaii or for infections thought to have been acquired in Asia or the Pacific. There is an increased prevalence for QRNG found in California, and the use of fluoroquinolones is not advisable in that state.

CHLAMYDIA

The most common reportable bacterial STI in the United States, **chlamydia** infections are more common among adolescents than older women, with most infections causing no symptoms. The causative organism, *Chlamydia trachomatis,* is classified a bacteria but has properties of both bacteria and viruses. They can only reproduce within a host cell and therefore do not live on inanimate objects. Transmission occurs through direct intimate contact or vertical transmission from mother to fetus and is associated with high fetal morbidity. Untreated infections can cause pelvic inflammatory disease, acute salpingitis, ectopic pregnancy, and infertility.

The incubation period for *C. trachomatis* is approximately 10 days to 2 weeks after exposure. Most women are asymptomatic, but symptoms can include abnormal vaginal discharge, postcoital bleeding, pelvic pain, or dysuria. Manifestations of the infection in men include epididymitis, prostatitis, or urethral discharge. Newborns exposed to *C. trachomatis* may be afflicted with conjunctivitis or pneumonia.

Management

Asymptomatic infections can continue for months or years without treatment. All women under age 25 who are sexually active or those with other high-risk factors should be screened.

Cultures, once considered the gold standard, are no longer used today. The nucleic acid amplification test of the endocervical sample or a urine sample is used for definitive diagnosis because each provides the highest sensitivity of any screening method used today. It is also recommended that screening for *N. gonorrhoeae* is performed due to the high rate of coexistence with chlamydia. Azithromycin is the most frequently prescribed antibiotic due to compliance with single dosing and may also be used to treat a pregnant person who is infected. Alternatives include doxycycline, erythromycin, or ofloxacin.

 SYPHILIS

Syphilis, a chronic and systemic disease, is one of the oldest known STIs. It is characterized by periods of active symptoms and latency. It has four stages: primary, secondary, latent, and tertiary. Since 1991 the rates of syphilis have declined overall but are rising among men having sex with men.

Syphilis is caused by *Treponema pallidum,* a motile spirochete. It is transmitted through microscopic abrasions in the skin and mucous membranes and can be transmitted in utero.

Primary syphilis is characterized by a single painless chancre at the site of infection. The chancre ulcerates and erodes. It is the site of the spirochetes that allows transmission of the infection to others. Secondary syphilis occurs approximately 6 weeks after the initial infection. The patient may experience flulike symptoms or develop a widespread maculopapular rash on the palms and soles of the feet. The patient may also complain of generalized lymphadenopathy. In latent infection stage the patient is completely asymptomatic and is detected only by serologic testing. Tertiary syphilis involves widespread systemic disease characterized by central nervous system changes, cardiovascular changes, and the presence of "gumma" lesions that destroy tissue and bone.

Management

Syphilis is diagnosed by nontreponemal antibody tests such as Venereal Disease Research Laboratory or rapid plasma reagent screening tests. A high titer is indicative of active disease and should be followed up with treponemal tests such as fluorescent treponemal antibody absorbed and microhemagglutination assays for antibody to *T. pallidum*. Initial testing may result in a false-negative result; therefore it is important to retest the patient approximately 6 weeks later when seroconversion has most likely occurred. Patients should also be screened for other STIs.

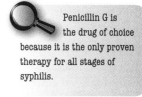
Penicillin G is the drug of choice because it is the only proven therapy for all stages of syphilis.

Penicillin G is the drug of choice because it is the only proven therapy for all stages of syphilis. If a patient is allergic to penicillin, alternative treatment with doxycycline or tetracycline is indicated.

If a patient is allergic to penicillin, alternative treatment with doxycycline or tetracycline is indicated.

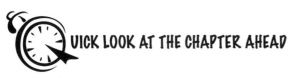

Trichomonas vaginalis is an organism that lives in the female genitalia and is a sexually transmitted infection. It has a characteristic green or yellow frothy vaginal discharge and most women are unaware they have been infected until they become symptomatic. There is no incubation period for it. Easily treated with a single dose antibiotic, it is important that both or all partners are treated before having sexual intercourse again.

22

Protozoan Sexually Transmitted Infections

TERMS
☐ Trichomoniasis

Trichomoniasis is a disease cause by infection with a species of anaerobic one-celled protozoan with flagellate, *Trichomonas vaginalis* (Table 22-1). Approximately 5 million cases occur annually and are transmitted during penile–vaginal intercourse and can facilitate HIV transmission. The organism lives in the urethra and vagina of women and in the urethra and prostate gland of men. There is no incubation period. It is not a reportable disease.

Signs and symptoms include a characteristic frothy yellow or green vaginal discharge that is malodorous and worsens after menstruation. Women frequently complain of dyspareunia or dysuria, although men are generally asymptomatic with rare reports of urethritis or prostatitis. On examination, a woman's cervix may be friable and have hallmark "strawberry spots" or petechiae. The pH of the vagina will be high.

Diagnosis is made based on a wet mount, but there is also a culture available that has the highest sensitivity and specificity. Pap smears or Thin preps are not reliable diagnostic tests for trichomoniasis.

 Pap smears or Thin preps are not reliable diagnostic tests for trichomoniasis.

Metronidazole 2 g single dose is the most commonly recommended antiprotozoal and antibacterial agent. Intravaginal preparations are not recommended. Both partners need to be treated and should be advised to avoid alcohol during treatment and for 24 hours after due to the interaction of alcohol with the medication.

 Both partners need to be treated and should be advised to avoid alcohol during treatment and for 24 hours after due to the interaction of alcohol with the medication.

Table 22-1 Types of Protozoan STIs

	Causative Organism	Signs and Symptoms	Diagnosis	Management and Treatment
Trichomoniasis	*Trichomonas vaginalis*	Asymptomatic in 50% of women; yellow/green frothy malodorous vaginal discharge, dysuria, dyspareunia	Wet mount culture	Metronidazole single dose; treat all partners

SECTION VIII • REVIEW QUESTIONS

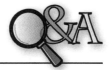

1. Which of the following statements is *true* regarding HPV?
   a. All women with HPV will go on to develop cervical cancer.
   b. All women with HPV will develop genital warts.
   c. Only a few strains of HPV are considered oncogenic.
   d. Only men with HPV can pass the virus onto their partners.

2. Risk factors for acquiring a sexually transmitted infection include all of the following *except:*
   a. Hormonal imbalances
   b. Substance abuse
   c. Multiple sex partners
   d. Lack of contraception

3. The most common bacterial STI is:
   a. Herpes simplex
   b. Human papilloma virus
   c. Chlamydia
   d. Hepatitis

4. The most common reportable STI in the United States is:
   a. Gonorrhea
   b. Chlamydia
   c. Herpes simplex virus
   d. Syphilis

5. A patient complains of abnormal menses, pelvic pain, and urinary tract infection symptoms. She reports her last sexual contact as 14 days ago. She most likely is infected with:
   a. Gonorrhea
   b. Herpes simplex virus
   c. Human papilloma virus
   d. Chlamydia

6. A painless chancre anywhere in the genital area is a symptom of:
   a. Syphilis
   b. Herpes simplex virus
   c. Gonorrhea
   d. Human papilloma virus

7. Appropriate treatment for gonorrhea includes:
a.   Penicillin G
b.   Azithromycin
c.   Ceftriaxone
d.   Ciprofloxacin

8. A frothy green vaginal discharge is indicative of:
a.   HPV
b.   Syphilis
c.   Trichomoniasis
d.   Chlamydia

9. In treating a woman and her partner for trichomoniasis, it is important to instruct the patient to:
a.   Avoid all sexual or intimate contact until both or all partners have been treated
b.   Avoid any alcoholic beverages for 24 hours after treatment
c.   Take the medication all at once
d.   All of the above

10. Prodromal symptoms and flulike or urinary tract infection symptoms are characteristic of:
a.   Herpes simplex virus
b.   Human papilloma virus
c.   Hepatitis
d.   Syphilis

ANSWERS AND RATIONALES

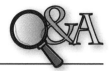

1. **The answer is c.** Rationale: Only a few strains are considered oncogenic. Not all women who are infected with HPV will develop cervical cancer and only certain strains of HPV cause genital warts.

2. **The answer is a.** Rationale: Hormonal imbalances do not contribute to acquiring an STI.

3. **The answer is c.** Rationale: Chlamydia is the most common bacterial STI in the United States. All the others are viral STIs.

4. **The answer is b.** Rationale: Chlamydia is the most common reportable STI in the United States. Gonorrhea and herpes simplex virus are not considered reportable.

5. **The answer is d.** Rationale: The incubation period for chlamydia is 10–14 days.

6. **The answer is a.** Rationale: A syphilitic chancre is painless.

7. **The answer is c.** Rationale: Ceftriaxone is the medication of choice for gonorrhea infections. There is a quinolone-resistant strain of *N. gonorrhea*; therefore quinolones are no longer used.

8. **The answer is c.** Rationale: Malodorous yellow or green frothy vaginal discharge is characteristic of trichomoniasis.

9. **The answer is d.** Rationale: All of the choices should be reviewed with the patient.

10. **The answer is a.** Rationale: Herpes simplex virus symptoms include pain, burning, or itching at the site of vesicles before they appear as well as flulike or urinary tract infection symptoms.

IX

Cancer

Cancer in children differs from adult cancer in many ways. In adult cancer, there is often a strong environmental relationship. Children have not lived long enough for exposure to carcinogens and may not present for diagnosis until symptoms appear. By the time of diagnosis, 80% of cancers are metastatic. Cancer in children is treated aggressively with periods of exacerbations and remissions causing psychological distress for parents and families.

In children under 15 years of age, cancer is the second leading cause of death. However, cure rates have improved over the years and greater than 70% of children diagnosed with cancer will survive. As the number of survivors increases, so too does the late effects of cancer therapy, as well as secondary malignant neoplasms.

Cancer refers to a group of diseases in which there is abnormal cell growth. The neoplasm may be benign or malignant. Leukemia is the most common form of cancer in children, followed by brain tumors.

23

Cancer

TERMS
- ☐ **Cell differentiation**
- ☐ **Ewing's sarcoma**
- ☐ **Hodgkin's disease**
- ☐ **Leukemia**
- ☐ **Lymphoblast**
- ☐ **Malignant brain tumors**
- ☐ **Non-Hodgkin's lymphoma**
- ☐ **Osteogenic sarcoma (osteosarcoma)**
- ☐ **Remission**
- ☐ **Wilms' tumor**

Childhood cancer is the second leading cause of death in children ages 1 to 14. Although survival rates and prognosis have improved over the years, it still continues to be a devastating illness. Leukemia continues to be the most frequent type of cancer, followed by brain tumors.

Cancer results when the body is unable to regulate cell production, causing altered cell differentiation and growth. **Cell differentiation** is defined as the process when dividing cells become more specialized, acquiring the structure and function of the cells they replace. Cell proliferation is defined as the process by which cells divide and reproduce. Cancer cells grow rapidly, spread widely, and do not follow the normal process of cell differentiation and cell proliferation. As a result, malignant cells do not look like the normal cells of the tissue from which they arose, and they do not grow at the rate they should.

> Cell differentiation is defined as the process when dividing cells become more specialized, acquiring the structure and function of the cells they replace. Cell proliferation is defined as the process by which cells divide and reproduce.

An understanding of the cell cycle assists in understanding the process of malignancy as well as treatment options. Chemotherapeutic agents disrupt the cell cycle of proliferating malignant cells with as little damage to normal cells as possible. They are classified as noncell cycle specific or cell cycle specific.

Once diagnosed, many of the cancers are classified according to staging. Staging depends on the size of the main tumor, the presence or absence of metastasis, and the extent or spread to nearby lymph nodes. As the staging number increases, the prognosis becomes worse.

 ## LEUKEMIA

Leukemia is the most common malignancy in children under the age of 15. It is a broad classification of malignant neoplasms of cells that arise from the hematopoietic stem cell. The two most common forms in children are acute lymphocytic leukemia (ALL) and acute myelogenous leukemia (AML). ALL accounts for 75% of all childhood leukemias. The peak incidence occurs in children at 4 years of age. Viruses, radiation, chemical and drug exposure, familial predisposition, and a variety of chromosomal aberrations have been cited as precipitating factors.

AML accounts for 15–20% of childhood leukemia and can be seen at any age. It is often associated with Down syndrome, exposure to radiation and chemotherapy from previous cancer, and exposure to toxins.

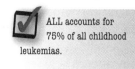
ALL accounts for 75% of all childhood leukemias.

Pathophysiology

A leukemic cell is a type of immature white blood cell that accumulates in the marrow, blood, and tissue. Because they are immature and poorly differentiated, they have a prolonged life span and rapid rate of proliferation. Production of normal red cells, white cells, and platelets is inhibited. A **lymphoblast** is an immature white cell that crowds out normal cells, resulting in pancytopenia and immunosuppression. In a child with ALL, the bone marrow may be replaced by 80–100% blast cells.

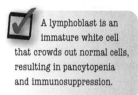
A lymphoblast is an immature white cell that crowds out normal cells, resulting in pancytopenia and immunosuppression.

Leukemic cells can cross the blood–brain barrier, causing involvement of the central nervous system (CNS). Because of this, presenting symptoms in ALL include fever, pallor, bruising, and bone pain. Lymphadenopathy, splenomegaly, and hepatomegaly caused by infiltration of lymphoblasts are common in ALL. In AML, children may present with vague flulike symptoms, or symptoms may be severe and life-threatening with bleeding and severe hemorrhage. There is a higher incidence of CNS involvement at the time of diagnosis.

A bone marrow aspiration and blood work confirm the diagnosis. In ALL, the white blood count and age of the child at diagnosis are prognostic indicators. Children between the ages of 3 and 5 and those with a white blood cell count less than 50,000/mm³ have the best prognosis. Children who are younger than 2 years or older than 10 years of age at diagnosis and those with a white blood cell count over 50,000/mm³ have a poorer prognosis.

Treatment

Chemotherapy is the treatment of choice and is started shortly after confirmation of diagnosis. The goal of the first phase is **remission,** meaning that there is no detectable sign of leukemia on physical exam or lab results. This usually occurs within 4 weeks. CNS prophylaxis is also administered intrathecally into the cerebrospinal fluid space.

Consolidation is the next phase of treatment and starts after remission has been attained to further decrease the number of leukemic cells in the body. Chemotherapy is again given in high doses to eradicate any residual leukemic cells. This phase is intense and lasts several months.

The goal of maintenance therapy is to prolong remission with monthly blood counts to evaluate the marrow's response to the drugs. Almost 80% of children achieve a long-term disease-free life. The maintenance phase lasts for 2–3 years after diagnosis.

HODGKIN'S DISEASE

Hodgkin's disease in one of two types of malignant lymphomas found in young adults. Its peak incidence occurs in the early twenties with a second peak incidence found in adults over the age of 50. In individuals diagnosed in their twenties, the incidence of men and women are equal, whereas for those individuals diagnosed in their fifties, there are more men than women diagnosed. While no known single agent has been reported as responsible for Hodgkin's disease, several studies have identified possible inflammatory reaction to a viral infectious agent, possibly the Epstein-Barr virus.

Pathophysiology

Hodgkin's disease most often originates in the cervical lymph node regions, and a definitive cure is possible depending on staging, histology, and time of diagnosis. In 60–90% of cases individuals present with nontender enlarged lymph nodes. In children, anorexia, malaise, and weight loss may also be accompanying symptoms. Hodgkin's disease is classified as either "A" or "B" depending on

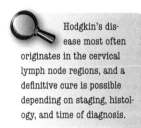

Hodgkin's disease most often originates in the cervical lymph node regions, and a definitive cure is possible depending on staging, histology, and time of diagnosis.

whether or not significant weight loss, fever, or night sweats are present ("A," not present; "B," present). As the disease progresses metastasis to the liver, lungs, digestive tract, and spleen may occur.

A complete workup includes a complete blood count, platelet count, erythrocyte sedimentation rate, and serum copper and iron levels. Biopsy of the lymph nodes confirms diagnosis and determines staging.

Treatment

Irradiation and chemotherapy are the treatments of choice for Hodgkin's disease. In localized disease, radiation alone may be used. Those with more advanced disease are treated with both. Long-term survival rates have greatly increased over the years. Individuals with Hodgkin's disease are living longer lives but continue to be monitored for secondary neoplasms, especially leukemia, and for cardiac disease and fertility issues.

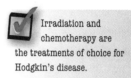 Irradiation and chemotherapy are the treatments of choice for Hodgkin's disease.

NON-HODGKIN'S LYMPHOMA

Non-Hodgkin's lymphoma differs significantly from Hodgkin's disease in several ways. It is a malignant tumor that may originate in any lymphatic tissue in the body, has rapid onset, and presents with widespread involvement at the time of diagnosis. Non-Hodgkin's lymphoma occurs three times more frequently than Hodgkin's and increases steadily with age.

Pathophysiology

Over the years studies have indicated viruses, radiation, genetics, and immune deficiencies as possible factors that play a role in the onset of non-Hodgkin's lymphoma. There is a strong correlation with Epstein-Barr virus and African Burkitt lymphoma. Determination of a primary site is difficult but is often considered as the site with the largest degree of involvement. The most common primary site is intraabdominal, with mediastinal and peripheral nodal involvement following next.

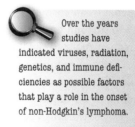 Over the years studies have indicated viruses, radiation, genetics, and immune deficiencies as possible factors that play a role in the onset of non-Hodgkin's lymphoma.

The child usually presents with pain, fever, anemia, malaise, and other gastrointestinal symptoms such as vomiting, diarrhea, constipation, and menstrual irregularity. With mediastinal disease symptoms include cough, dyspnea, chest pain, and compromised respiratory status.

Treatment

Diagnosis is confirmed by lymph node biopsy, and treatment is started as soon as possible. Aggressive multiagent chemotherapy is started as soon as possible. Prognosis is very good, with the possibility of a cure depending on the type of lymphoma. Children with advanced intraabdominal lymphoma have the poorest prognosis.

 # OSTEOGENIC SARCOMA

Osteogenic sarcoma, also known as osteosarcoma, is one of two common malignant bone tumors in children. It accounts for 60% of all malignant bone tumors, affects children primarily in early adolescence, and incidence follows growth pattern progression. It usually occurs in the growth metaphysis or end of the long bones, most commonly the distal femur, proximal tibia, and proximal humerus.

Pathophysiology

Osteogenic sarcoma is a primary bone tumor that arises from the mesenchymal matrix-forming cells of the bone, causing bone destruction and osteoid tissue formation. It is an aggressive tumor with frequent spreading to surrounding soft tissue. Osteosarcoma travels through the bloodstream, usually to the lungs.

Common symptoms are localized pain associated with swelling or a palpable mass. Although a sports injury does not cause osteosarcoma, the child may be diagnosed when brought in for a sports-related injury. Metastasis to the lungs occurs in 25% of patients at the time of diagnosis.

Treatment

Treatment has changed over the years; initially, amputation above the lesion was the treatment of choice. Today, various limb-saving procedures are preferred over amputation depending on presentation of the bone at the time of diagnosis. This cancer is radiation resistant, but multiagent chemotherapy is used both before and after surgery. Long-term prognosis depends on the presence of metastatic lesions at the time of diagnosis.

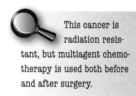

This cancer is radiation resistant, but multiagent chemotherapy is used both before and after surgery.

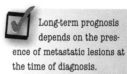

Long-term prognosis depends on the presence of metastatic lesions at the time of diagnosis.

EWING'S SARCOMA

Ewing's sarcoma is the second type of malignant bone tumors found in children and young adults. It is highly malignant and can be found in any bone of the body but is most often found in the pelvis, tibia, fibula, and femur. It is seen most often in young adults less than 25 years of age and more frequently in males.

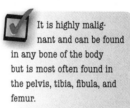

It is highly malignant and can be found in any bone of the body but is most often found in the pelvis, tibia, fibula, and femur.

Pathophysiology

Ewing's sarcoma is a primary bone tumor that arises from immature cells within the bone marrow space, causing bone destruction within. It is usually seen in the midshaft of long or flat bones and may break through the cortex of the bone to form a soft tissue mass.

Individuals often present with pain, limitation of movement, and tenderness over the involved bone. Unlike osteosarcoma, presentation of systemic symptoms such as fever, weight loss, and an increased sedimentation rate may also be noted. Metastasis to the lungs, bone, or other bone marrow at the time of diagnosis is also possible.

Treatment

Diagnosis is determined by biopsy with confirmation of metastasis to other organs. Treatment depends on the location of the bone mass. Surgical resection may be possible, but radiation therapy is the treatment of choice. Chemotherapy is used to control metastasis to other organs. As with other cancers, long-term follow-up is important to monitor for secondary malignancies and other complications.

WILMS' TUMOR

Wilms' tumor (nephroblastoma) occurs primarily in infants and young children. It is a tumor of the kidney that is the most common malignant kidney tumor in children. It represents 6% of childhood cancer, and peak incidence is between 1 and 3 years of age. Eighteen percent of children with Wilms' tumor also have other congenital anomalies. It occurs more often in black children and is very rare in the Asian population.

Pathophysiology

Wilms' tumors are rapidly growing large lesions that may reach a considerable size before being diagnosed. They are an encapsulated tumor with a thin membrane that easily ruptures. Rupture of the capsule may cause spread of malignant cells; if Wilms' is suspected, manipulation of the abdomen and liver should be avoided. A sign is usually placed over the child's head of the bed as a warning.

> Rupture of the capsule may cause spread of malignant cells; if Wilms' is suspected, manipulation of the abdomen and liver should be avoided. A sign is usually placed over the child's head of the bed as a warning.

In 1899 Dr. Wilms was the first to suggest that the tumor is derived from undifferentiated embryonic tissue. Lesions are made up of mesenchymal and epithelial elements in a variety of ratios and stages of maturity. Prognosis is determined by histology type and stage of tumor at diagnosis. Metastasis to the lungs, liver, and uninvolved kidney occurs early.

Diagnosis is confirmed by abdominal ultrasound, lab work, and often a chest x-ray and liver ultrasound to determine any metastasis. Monitoring for hypertension is also an important assessment.

Treatment

The usual treatment for Wilms' tumor is surgery, usually followed by chemotherapy and radiation. A treatment regimen is determined by the staging of the disease. A stage I tumor is limited to the kidney and can be excised with careful attention to not rupturing the capsule. In stage II, the tumor extends

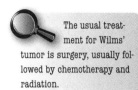

The usual treatment for Wilms' tumor is surgery, usually followed by chemotherapy and radiation.

beyond the kidney but can be completely excised. In stage III, the tumor is confined to the abdomen, and treatment depends on existence of several variables. In stage IV there is metastasis, and in stage V there is bilateral kidney involvement. The prognosis for children with Wilms' tumor continues to improve depending on level of staging at diagnosis. Various treatment protocols have extended the overall survival rate to 92%. Long-term care to the surviving kidney is important as well as monitoring for scoliosis and second neoplasms in children who have had radiation.

MALIGNANT BRAIN TUMORS

In children **malignant brain tumors** are the second leading cause of cancer after leukemia. There are 3.9 cases per 100,000 children diagnosed each year, with the greatest frequency seen in children between 5 to 10 years of age, with boys affected slightly more than girls. Although no known cause of brain tumors exists, there are suggestions that environmental and hereditary factors may play a role.

Pathophysiology

Brain tumors can be classified according to their location and histopathology. In the pediatric patient 60% of primary tumors occur in the infratentorial area. These include the cerebellum, brainstem, and below the tentorium. The other locations where tumors may be found are the supratentorial region, which includes the cerebrum and the tentorium, and the dura mater located between the cerebrum and

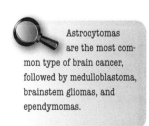

Astrocytomas are the most common type of brain cancer, followed by medulloblastoma, brainstem gliomas, and ependymomas.

cerebellum. Astrocytomas are the most common type of brain cancer, followed by medulloblastoma, brainstem gliomas, and ependymomas.

Early signs of a growing lesion may be difficult to detect. These include irritability, changes in personality, and learning difficulties. Vomiting and anorexia may mimic the flu and so may not be seen as important. Headaches begin as intermittent but increase in duration and intensity as the tumor increases. Increased intracranial pressure and other neurological symptoms should alert the health care professional to seek a specialized diagnostic workup. Diagnosis is confirmed by computed tomography, magnetic resonance imaging, cerebral angiography, and presence of specific neurological symptoms.

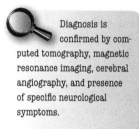

Diagnosis is confirmed by computed tomography, magnetic resonance imaging, cerebral angiography, and presence of specific neurological symptoms.

Treatment

The location and pathology of the tumor determine whether or not surgery, chemotherapy, and radiation are used. All of them carry risks to the young child who is developing and growing. New treatment options continue to be researched to lessen the complications that may occur.

SECTION IX • REVIEW QUESTIONS

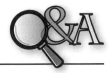

1. Leukemia occurs when stem cells in the bone marrow produce:
    a. Lymphoblasts
    b. Platelets
    c. Retroviruses
    d. Leukocytes

2. Osteogenic sarcoma is a common bone cancer in children. Where is a primary tumor site?
    a. Humerus
    b. Femur
    c. Tibia
    d. Shoulder

3. A 16-year-old is recently admitted for Hodgkin's lymphoma. You would expect to see:
    a. Lymphadenopathy with abdominal involvement
    b. Fever and painless adenopathy
    c. Pallor, bleeding, and fatigue
    d. Sore throat and ear ache

4. Which of the following diagnostic studies is most useful for assessing Wilms' tumor?
    a. Bone marrow aspiration
    b. Spinal tap
    c. Abdominal ultrasound and biopsy
    d. Magnetic resonance imaging

5. The primary treatment modality(ies) for Hodgkin's disease is (are):
    a. Chemotherapy
    b. Surgery and chemotherapy
    c. Surgery and radiation
    d. Irradiation and chemotherapy

6. A 4-year-old is recently admitted to your unit for ALL. You would expect to see which of the following signs and symptoms?
    a. Fever, pallor, bruising, bone pain
    b. Sensitive lymph nodes
    c. Abdominal distention and mass
    d. Sore throat and ear ache

7. The lymphomas have been found to occur more often in people who have a history of:
   a. Living near high tension wires
   b. Epstein-Barr virus
   c. Parasites
   d. Yeast infections

8. Treatment for Ewing's sarcoma usually involves:
   a. Chemotherapy and radiation
   b. Limb-saving procedure and chemotherapy
   c. Amputation and chemotherapy
   d. Radiation and limb-saving procedure

9. The most common form of brain tumors are:
   a. Medulloblastomas
   b. Ependymomas
   c. Gliomas
   d. Astrocytomas

10. Anemia in a child with ALL is due to:
    a. Low platelet count
    b. Low white blood cell count
    c. Loss of blood
    d. Low red blood cell count

11. Mrs. Jones asks why her daughter who has just been diagnosed with ALL has bruises on her body. You respond based on the fact that bruising is caused by:
    a. Low platelet count
    b. Low white blood cell count
    c. Loss of blood
    d. Low red blood cell count

12. Which of the following symptoms should warrant further investigation in an otherwise healthy child?
    a. Vomiting in the morning
    b. Morning headache
    c. Frequent napping
    d. Change in appetite

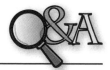

ANSWERS AND RATIONALES

1. **The answer is a.** Rationale: A lymphoblast is an immature white cell that crowds out normal cells that result in pancytopenia and immunosuppression.

2. **The answer is b.** Rationale: The greatest majority of osteosarcomas are found in the end of long bones, especially the distal femur.

3. **The answer is b.** Rationale: In most cases of Hodgkin's lymphoma, children present with nontender enlarged lymph nodes.

4. **The answer is c.** Rationale: An abdominal ultrasound and biopsy confirm Wilms' tumor.

5. **The answer is d.** Rationale: Irradiation and chemotherapy are the treatments of choice for Hodgkin's disease.

6. **The answer is a.** Rationale: Characteristic symptoms of ALL include fever, pallor, bruising, and bone pain.

7. **The answer is b.** Rationale: A strong correlation exists between the lymphomas and Epstein-Barr virus.

8. **The answer is a.** Rationale: Radiation therapy is the treatment of choice along with chemotherapy to control metastasis to other organs. Surgical resection may be done but is not the first line of treatment.

9. **The answer is d.** Rationale: Astrocytomas account for most brain tumors in children.

10. **The answer is d.** Rationale: Anemia in children with ALL is due to decreased red blood cells.

11. **The answer is a.** Rationale: Children with ALL have a decreased platelet count that causes bruising, bleeding, and, at its worst, hemorrhage.

12. **The answer is b.** Rationale: A brain tumor may be suspected in a child who complains of repeated and worsening headaches in the morning that improve as the day progresses.

X

Cardiovascular Disorders

The heart is a complex organ with pumping and endocrine functions. The heart keeps blood moving in a clockwise direction through two connected circulatory pathways and secrets neurohormonal substances (peptides) that stimulate the excretion of sodium and water by the kidneys, thereby helping to regulate blood pressure and blood volume. The circulatory pathway originating from the left side of the heart (systemic circulation) carries oxygenated blood to all parts of the body except the lungs, whereas the pathway originating from the right side of the heart (pulmonary circulation) carries deoxygenated blood to the lungs via the pulmonary artery and returns oxygenated blood to the left atria via the pulmonary veins. Arteries carry blood away from the heart, whereas veins carry blood back to the heart. The smallest arteries are called capillaries, whereas the smallest veins are called venules.

24

Cardiac Anatomy and Physiology

The heart chambers and blood vessels secrete **natriuretic peptides**, which promote diuresis. These peptides are classified as A-type natriuretic peptide, produced mainly by the atrial myocardium; B-type natriuretic peptide, produced by the ventricular myocardium; and C-type natriuretic peptide, produced by both endothelial cells that line the blood vessels and by the kidneys. These peptide hormones, which are antagonists to the renin-aldosterone-angiotensin system, limit aldosterone secretion and promote salt and water loss. They also lower blood pressure by promoting vasodilation by inhibiting the sympathetic nervous system and reducing circulating blood volume.

 The heart chambers and blood vessels secrete natriuretic peptides, which promote diuresis.

TERMS

- ☐ Afterload
- ☐ Bicuspid valve or mitral valve
- ☐ Cardiac output
- ☐ Chordae tendineae
- ☐ Depolarization
- ☐ Diastole
- ☐ End-diastolic volume
- ☐ Endocardium
- ☐ Fibrous pericardium
- ☐ Myocardial contractility
- ☐ Myocardium
- ☐ Natriuretic peptides
- ☐ Negatively inotropic
- ☐ Parietal pericardium
- ☐ Pericardial sac
- ☐ Positively inotropic
- ☐ Preload
- ☐ Semilunar valves
- ☐ Stroke volume
- ☐ Systole
- ☐ Tricuspid valve
- ☐ Visceral pericardium

185

HEART STRUCTURE

Pericardium

The heart wall is composed of the pericardium, myocardium, and endocardium. The pericardium has a tough outer layer and two serous membranes. The outermost layer, the **fibrous pericardium**, is composed of fibrous connective tissue. This layer holds the heart in place. Next is one of the serous membranes, the **parietal pericardium**, which lines the inner surface of the fibrous pericardium. The fibrous pericardium and parietal pericardium are called the **pericardial sac**. The other serous membrane, the **visceral pericardium** (epicardium), covers the heart's surface. The serous membranes secrete a thin pericardial fluid that fills the space between them. This fluid (15–50 mL) reduces friction during the pumping cycle.

The **myocardium** is the muscle that forms the chambers of the heart (atria and ventricles). The muscle fibers between the atria and ventricles are arranged in a loop and circle pattern, not a parallel pattern. When these fibers contract they create a very efficient wringing motion that constricts the ventricular lumen. The **endocardium** is the internal lining of the myocardium and is continuous with the endothelium that lines all blood vessels, creating one continuous circuit.

Heart Chambers

The heart has four chambers that act as piston pumps. The upper chambers are composed of a right and left atria, which have thin walls, and the two lower chambers, the right and left ventricles, which have thicker walls. The two atria are separated by a thin septum, and the ventricles are separated by a thicker muscular septum.

The atria act as storage basins and conduits for blood returning to the heart from the systemic and pulmonary circulations. During diastole, blood trickles from the atria to the ventricles through the atrioventricular (AV) valves. Before ventricular contraction the atria contract (known as the atrial kick) to push the final 20–30% of blood into the waiting ventricles.

The right side of the heart (right atrium and right ventricle) functions as a volume pump by receiving blood from the inferior vena cava, the superior vena cava, and the coronary sinus and then pumping it into the low-pressure pulmonary circulation. Deoxygenated blood then becomes oxygenated in the lungs. The left side of the heart (left atrium and left ventricle) functions as a pressure pump, receiving oxygenated blood from the four pulmonary veins and then pumping it out into the high-pressure systemic circulation. The ventricles account for 60% of the heart's mass and receive most of the coronary artery blood flow. Because the left ventricle pumps blood to the high-pressure aorta it is three times thicker than the right ventricle, which pumps blood to the low-pressure pulmonary artery.

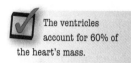

The ventricles account for 60% of the heart's mass.

Cardiac Valves

There are four passive cardiac valves that are responsible for keeping blood flowing through the heart chambers in a forward motion. These delicate valves are composed of leaflets (cusps) lined by endothelium. The valves move passively in response to pressure. The cusps either move out of the way to promote forward blood flow or make contact with each other and impede backward flow.

The AV valves control blood flow between the atria and corresponding ventricles. The right AV valve has three cusps, or leaflets, and is called the **tricuspid valve**. The left AV valve has two cusps, or leaflets, and is called the **bicuspid valve** or **mitral valve** because when it is closed it resembles a bishop's hat (miter). When the ventricles contract they create pressure that closes the AV valves. Because the pressure created is high, the AV valves need help staying closed. The **chordae tendineae** are strong, inelastic, tendon-like cords that are attached on one end to the ventricular surface of an AV cusp and on the other end to a small protrusion on the ventricular myocardium (papillary muscle) to hold the closed AV valves in place.

The **semilunar valves** prevent back flow of blood from the aorta and pulmonary artery to the right and left ventricles. Each semilunar valve has three cusps. The pulmonary semilunar valve separates the right ventricle from the pulmonary artery, whereas the aortic semilunar valve separates the left ventricle from the aorta.

THE CARDIAC CYCLE

The rhythmic repeating pumping action of the heart is called the cardiac cycle. Ventricular contraction is termed **systole,** and ventricular relaxation is called **diastole.** Each ventricular contraction ejects 65–70% of this volume (ejection fraction). **Stroke volume** is the amount of blood pumped from the ventricle during one contraction. Because only 65–70% of the blood in the ventricle is pumped during each contraction, some blood always remains in the ventricle. **End-diastolic volume** is the amount of blood each ventricle contains at the end of its filling period. The amount of blood pumped to the general circulation from the left ventricle each minute is called the **cardiac output.** Cardiac output depends on how fast the heart is beating and the stroke volume.

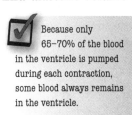

Because only 65–70% of the blood in the ventricle is pumped during each contraction, some blood always remains in the ventricle.

CONTROL OF HEART RATE

Each cell in the heart can trigger an electrical impulse, resulting in a contraction. In a healthy heart this initial triggering mechanism is the responsibility of the sinoatrial node, also called the pacemaker. The electrical pathway follows a prescribed route: the sinoatrial node to the atrioventricular node (pauses briefly to allow the atrial kick), to the bundle of His, to the right and left bundle branches, to the Purkinje fibers, and finally to the cells of the myocardium. As the electrical impulse travels through the myocardial cells, calcium, the contraction regulator, is released from the cardiac cells and binds to troponin. Sodium then flows into the cells and potassium moves out of the cells. This process is called **depolarization,** and it shortens muscle fibers, resulting in a wringing contraction of the ventricles. Any disruption in the electrical pathway or triggering mechanism results in either an abnormal rate, rhythm, or both. This disruption can affect cardiac output and therefore perfusion to the lungs and systemic circulation.

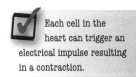

Each cell in the heart can trigger an electrical impulse resulting in a contraction.

STROKE VOLUME CONTROL

Stroke volume, the amount of blood pumped from one systolic contraction, is determined by the amount of blood in the ventricle at the end of diastole (end-diastolic volume, also called **preload**), the vascular resistance to receiving the blood pumped by the ventricle (**afterload**), and how forcefully the ventricle contracts (**myocardial contractility**). Any factor that weakens the contraction force of the ventricles, such as hypoxia, is considered to be **negatively inotropic**, whereas any factor that strengthens the force of a ventricular contraction, such as digoxin, sympathetic nervous stimulation, and epinephrine, is considered to be **positively inotropic**.

This chapter begins with a brief description of fetal circulation and then discusses common structural cardiac defects in the newborn. The etiology of the defect and resulting impact on cardiac function is discussed.

25

Cardiac Structural Defects

TERMS
- Arial septal defect (ASD)
- Coarctation of the aorta
- Foramen ovale
- Patent ductus arteriosus (PDA)
- Pulmonary stenosis
- Subvalvular aortic stenosis
- Supravalvular aortic stenosis
- Tetralogy of Fallot (ToF)
- Transposition of the great arteries (TGA)
- Valvular aortic stenosis
- Ventricular septal defect (VSD)

PERINATAL AND NEONATAL CIRCULATION

Labor benefits the fetus' impending transition to life by moving fluid present in the alveoli during fetal development into the interstitial space and speeding up its absorption. In addition, by 34 weeks of gestation surfactant is produced, which prevents the alveoli from collapsing with expiration.

The first breath is taken in response to hypoxia at birth, reexpansion of the chest when vaginal delivery is complete, and changes in skin temperature when the neonate emerges from the womb. This initial breath causes the pulmonary artery blood flow to increase and the pulmonary vascular resistance to decrease. As the pulmonary vascular resistance falls below that of the systemic circulation, blood flow across the ductus arteriosus shifts from left to right. This initiates the functional closure of the ductus arteriosus. By the time the neonate is 8 hours old, right-to-left shunting has stopped, and the vessel closes completely by the time the infant is 1 to 3 weeks old.

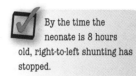
By the time the neonate is 8 hours old, right-to-left shunting has stopped.

During fetal life a one-way valve, the **foramen ovale,** permits shunting of blood from the inferior vena cava through the right atrium to the left atrium. At birth, left atrial pressure rises above right atrium pressure and closes the foramen ovale flap.

By 2 months of age the infant's pulmonary artery has reverted from a thick-walled vessel to a thin-walled vessel and pulmonary artery pressure drops. If the infant continues to have left-to-right shunting, causing pulmonary overload, the signs and symptoms become apparent by 2 months of age.

Table 25-1 lists assessments and their significance for cardiac structural defects in the newborn.

CONGENITAL HEART DISEASE

Approximately 1% of neonates have congenital heart disease, the most common structural malformation observed. Maternal diabetes, alcohol use, excessive smoking, teratogen exposure, progesterone use, and maternal viral infections (rubella) are some of the causes of congenital heart disease.

Table 25-1 Assessments and Significance for Cardiac Structural Defects in the Newborn

Assessment	Significance
Left precordial bulge	Cardiomyopathy
Thrills	Murmur
Palpable fourth heart sound	Hypertrophic cardiomyopathy
Bounding pulse	Patent ductus arteriosus Aortic regurgitation Arteriovenous malformation Fever Anemia Shock
Thready pulse	Reduced cardiac output Severe aortic stenosis
Absent, weak, delayed femoral pulse	Coarctation of the aorta
Cyanosis (Assess lips, nail beds, and mucous membranes)	Low cardiac output Hypothermia Systemic venous congestion Pulmonary obstruction
Acrocyanosis (bluish discoloration around the mouth)	Normal finding until skin has been exposed to the sun; does not mean cyanosis
Clubbing of fingers and toes	Cyanotic congenital heart disease Usually appears after 12 months of age Infective endocarditis Chronic liver disease Inflammatory bowel disease Chronic pulmonary disease Benign genetic variant
Dependent edema	High right heart pressure-tricuspid valve malfunction Right-sided heart failure
Hepatomegaly (infant and child)	Right heart failure Pulmonary edema related to left-to-right shunting (pulmonary congestion = hyperexpansion = pushing liver further below the costal margin)

Assessment	Significance
Splenomegaly	Congestive heart failure Infective endocarditis
Ascites	Congestive heart failure
Dextrocardia (heart on right side of chest)	Situs inversus totalis (all organs "switch" sides Heart shift alone = heart defects
Blue color on room air and on 100% O_2	Heart disease (lung disease = color changes from blue to pink when on 100% O_2)
60–62% pulse oximetry on room air and on 100% O_2	Heart disease (lung disease = pulse oximetry changes from 60% to 99% when on 100% O_2)
35–38 PaO_2 (mm Hg) on room air and on 100% O_2	Heart disease (lung disease = PaO_2 changes from 35 to 120 when on 100% O_2)

Left-to-Right Shunting Defects

Left-to-right shunting occurs when blood in the higher pressure left side of the heart flows through a defect in a septum to the lower pressure right side of the heart. Because the right side of the heart and pulmonary artery receive an excessive amount of blood, volume overload occurs, resulting in right ventricular hypertrophy, congestive heart failure (CHF), pulmonary hypertension, and frequent respiratory infections. Altered gas exchange occurs because of pulmonary artery congestion. This defect may not result in cyanosis because oxygenated blood is shunted back to the right side of the heart where it reenters the pulmonary circulation.

Atrial Septal Defects

The most common **atrial septal defect (ASD)** occurs more often in females than in males. ASD is located near the foramen ovale and results in blood flowing between the right and left atria, causing an enlarged right atrium and ventricle and an increased blood flow to the pulmonary artery. ASDs are classified according to where on the atrial septum they appear. Uncorrected, it can lead to pulmonary vascular disease by the time the child is 30 years old.

Most children with ASD are asymptomatic, whereas others may develop fatigue, palpitations, frequent respiratory infections, and cardiac hypertrophy. If the defect is small (less than 4 mm in diameter) it may close on its own; if not, when the child is 12 to 36 months old surgical or cardiac catheterization interventions to close the defect are performed. If the defect is not corrected, exercise intolerance and tachyarrhythmias may develop in adulthood.

Ventricular Septal Defects

Approximately 30% of congenital heart defects are simple **ventricular septal defects (VSDs)**. Small and moderate defects (less than 3 to 5 mm in diameter) account for 85–95% of all VSDs and are asymptomatic. Ninety percent of small and moderate sized VSDs close on their own by the time the child is 2 to 6 years of age. Large defects (6–10 mm in diameter) require surgical closure by 12 months of age to prevent pulmonary vascular disease. Infants with large VSDs are prone to develop CHF, frequent respiratory infections, dyspnea, fatigue, pulmonary hypertension, and failure to thrive by 3–6 months of age.

Patent Ductus Arteriosus

Patent ductus arteriosus (PDA) comprises approximately 10% of all congenital heart defects in full-term infants and is more common in girls than in boys and in preterm infants (20–60%). During fetal life blood is shunted from the pulmonary artery to the aorta (fetal gas exchange takes place at the placenta, not by breathing). Within 24 hours after birth high levels of oxygen in inspired air and decreased prostaglandin levels cause the ductus arteriosus to close. If it remains open, it is called a patent ductus arteriosus. PDA may accompany other heart defects, occur on its own, or be a life-sustaining measure in infants who have pulmonary atresia. If the PDA is not corrected, dyspnea on exertion, exercise intolerance, and CHF may develop by ages 30–40.

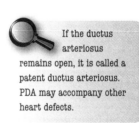
If the ductus arteriosus remains open, it is called a patent ductus arteriosus. PDA may accompany other heart defects.

Infants with a significant PDA have a rough continuous murmur, bounding pulses, increased pulmonary blood flow, and increased workload for the left side of the heart, resulting in CHF. A premature infant with PDA and respiratory distress syndrome presents with a soft murmur, increased peripheral pulses, increasing oxygen need, and/or CHF. Eighty to ninety percent of preterm infants weighing more than 1,200 g may achieve closure of their PDA after receiving indomethacin, but it does not close a PDA in a smaller preterm infant, a full-term infant, or child. Some research studies have demonstrated that ibuprofen may work as well as indomethacin in closing the PDA. Both drugs are prostaglandin synthesis inhibitors. PDA is usually closed surgically or during cardiac catheterization if the infant does not have pulmonary vascular obstruction and the PDA has not closed in response to medication.

DEFECTS OBSTRUCTING BLOOD FLOW

Narrowing of a blood vessel or valve partially decreases or may completely obstruct blood flow though a blood vessel or valve, resulting in increased pressure behind the obstruction. If the obstruction occurs on the left side of the heart, blood flow to the systemic circulation is impeded. If the obstruction occurs on the right side of the heart, blood flow to the pulmonary circulation is impeded. Either right- or left-sided obstruction causes an increased cardiac workload, decreased cardiac output, and CHF.

Defects Obstructing Blood Flow to the Right Side of the Heart

Pulmonary Stenosis

In **pulmonary stenosis** the pulmonic valve leaflets (cusps) are fused together and form a membrane with a small hole in the center. Because blood flow across the pulmonary valve is hindered, the right ventricle increases the amount of pumping pressure in an attempt to move blood into the pulmonary artery. Untreated right ventricular hypertrophy and right-sided congestive heart failure develop. If the child also has a ventricular septal defect the pressure is relieved and CHF does not develop. Children with severe pulmonic valve stenosis who also have a patent foramen ovale become cyanotic.

If the pulmonary stenosis is mild to moderate the child will be asymptomatic and have a systolic ejection murmur; however, severe stenosis produces cyanosis, CHF, and clubbing. Percutaneous balloon valvuloplasty is an effective treatment of choice; however, surgical repair is necessary if the balloon valvuloplasty is unsuccessful.

Defects Obstructing Blood Flow to the Left Side of the Heart

Coarctation (Narrowing) of the Aorta

Three times as many male newborns have **coarctation of the aorta** than do female newborns, and in females it is associated with Turner's syndrome. The coarctation usually occurs in the thoracic region of the aorta, rarely in the abdominal section. Eighty to 85% of infants with a bicuspid aortic valve (instead of the usual three cusps) also have coarctation of the aorta.

Infants with severe coarctation of the aorta have diminished or absent femoral pulses (because blood flow through the aorta is greatly diminished), metabolic acidosis, CHF, and shock. In about 40% of infants born with coarctation of the aorta, signs and symptoms develop between days 4 and 10 after birth when the ductus arteriosus closes. Immediate surgical repair is essential for infants with severe defects causing CHF. If the defect is corrected after age 5, the child is at risk for developing hypertension and myocardial dysfunction even if surgery is successful.

 If the defect is corrected after age 5, the child is at risk for developing hypertension and myocardial dysfunction even if surgery is successful.

Children with mild coarctation of the aorta are asymptomatic. The defect is discovered during a routine well child exam and presents as hypertension, diminished or absent leg pulses, leg cramping, and systolic murmur.

Aortic Stenosis

There are three types of aortic stenosis: valvular, subvalvular, and supravalvular. **Valvular aortic stenosis** (75%) occurs when the aortic valve contains one cusp diaphragm-like structure without defining commissures. **Subvalvular aortic stenosis** (23%) occurs when a fibrous ring develops just below the aortic valve. Many times the aortic valve and anterior cusp of the mitral valve are also deformed. **Supravalvular aor-**

tic stenosis (1–2%), which has a genetic component, occurs when the ascending aorta is constricted just above the coronary arteries.

Most children with mild to moderate aortic stenosis are asymptomatic except for exercise intolerance. In rare cases adolescents with aortic stenosis and hypertrophic cardiomyopathy may have sudden cardiac death. If surgical treatment is required, the initial procedure of choice is percutaneous balloon valvuloplasty. If this treatment is not successful, patients will require valve replacement.

Defects Resulting in a Decreased Pulmonary Blood Flow

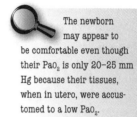

The newborn may appear to be comfortable even though their PaO_2 is only 20–25 mm Hg because their tissues, when in utero, were accustomed to a low PaO_2.

Incomplete cardiac development, abnormal placement of major blood vessels, or obstruction on the right side of the heart results in decreased pulmonary circulation. Without adequate pulmonary circulation gas exchange is severely limited, resulting in cyanosis, a low oxygen saturation level, increased workload for the heart, dyspnea, and activity intolerance. The newborn may appear to be comfortable even though their PaO_2 is only 20–25 mm Hg because their tissues, when in utero, were accustomed to a low PaO_2.

Tetralogy of Fallot
Tetralogy of Fallot (ToF) is composed of four structural abnormalities: a VSD, pulmonary stenosis, an overriding aorta, and right ventricular hypertrophy as a result of the pulmonary stenosis.

Defects Resulting in Increased Pulmonary Blood Flow

Defects that mix oxygen-rich blood and oxygen-poor blood, or which transpose major blood vessels, result in deoxygenated blood being pumped into the systemic circulation. Tissues do not receive adequate oxygen or nutrients and thus the infant appears cyanotic or gray and has severely decreased cardiac output, dyspnea, and possibly shock.

Transposition of the Great Arteries
Transposition of the great arteries (TGA), which occurs three times more often in males than in females, is the second most common cyan-

otic congenital heart defect in newborns. Infants without a PDA are very cyanotic because the aorta arises from the right ventricle, which receives deoxygenated blood from the systemic circulation. Infants with a VSD are less cyanotic because some oxygenated blood can mix with the deoxygenated blood, but these infants often develop CHF because of a high pulmonary blood flow. If the infant also has VSD and pulmonary stenosis, he or she will be severely cyanotic because only a small amount of blood ever reaches the lungs.

Newborns with transposition of the great arteries present as severely cyanotic at birth and are unresponsive to supplemental oxygen. These newborns are generally large (4 kg) and may not have a significant murmur or respiratory distress. Arterial switch operation (AOS), which has a 95% survival rate, is usually performed when the infant is less than 1 week old. During the arterial switch operation the arteries are switched, the coronary arteries reimplanted, atrial septum closed, and large VSD repaired, leaving the left ventricle as the systemic pumping ventricle. Developmental delays are thought to be prevented by relieving cyanosis promptly.

Newborns with transposition of the great arteries present as severely cyanotic at birth and are unresponsive to supplemental oxygen.

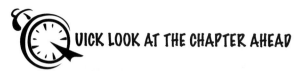

QUICK LOOK AT THE CHAPTER AHEAD

This chapter provides an overview of the etiology and effects of congestive heart failure.

26

Congestive Heart Failure

TERMS
- ☐ Cardiomyopathy
- ☐ Congestive heart failure (CHF)
- ☐ Dilated cardiomyopathy
- ☐ Hypertrophic cardiomyopathy
- ☐ Renin-angiotensin-aldosterone system
- ☐ Restrictive cardiomyopathy

Congestive heart failure (CHF) occurs when the heart fails as a pump and is therefore unable to meet the circulatory and metabolic requirements of the body. Right-sided CHF occurs when blood is not efficiently pumped to the pulmonary vasculature, resulting in a systemic backup of blood. Left-sided CHF occurs when blood cannot be pumped to the systemic circulation, resulting in pulmonary vasculature congestion.

A congenital heart defect is the most common cause of CHF and, if severe, causes symptoms of CHF at birth, whereas milder defects cause symptoms by the time the infant is 6 months old. Inadequate cardiac output triggers both hemodynamic and

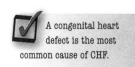

A congenital heart defect is the most common cause of CHF.

neurohumoral responses meant to compensate for the failing heart. Although congenital heart defects account for most cases of pediatric CHF, other causes include infection, dysrhythmias, drugs, severe anemia, and tumors.

In an attempt to reduce blood volume and cardiac workload, the heart chambers and blood vessels secrete natriuretic peptides, which promote diuresis. These peptides are classified as A-type natriuretic peptide (ANP), produced mainly by the atrial myocardium; B-type natriuretic peptide (BNP), produced by the ventricular myocardium; and C-type natriuretic peptide, produced by endothelial cells that line the blood vessels and also the kidneys. Peptide hormones are antagonists to the renin-aldosterone-angiotensin system and therefore limit aldosterone secretion and promote salt and water loss. They also lower blood pressure by promoting vasodilation by inhibiting the sympathetic nervous system and reducing circulating blood volume. Laboratory tests that measure these peptides are useful indicators of the success of treatment and/or level of cardiac decompensation.

Decreased cardiac output also triggers hemodynamic compensatory mechanisms. In response to low cardiac output the sympathetic nervous system is triggered, resulting in a rapid heart rate (to pump blood to the body quickly), stronger heart muscle contractions (to increase ejection fraction), increased stroke volume, and vasoconstriction (to return more blood to the heart). This compensatory mechanism makes the heart work harder by decreasing the amount of preload while increasing afterload and increasing cardiac muscle oxygen demands that cannot be met.

Stimulation of the **renin-angiotensin-aldosterone system** is the result of decreased blood flow to the kidneys and a decreased glomerular filtration rate. As a consequence salt and water are retained, increasing intravascular volume. In the beginning the system has a positive effect by increasing preload and cardiac output. Eventually, however, the heart muscle becomes fatigued from pressure overload, the lung tissue becomes edematous, and symptoms of CHF worsen. Long-term untreated CHF results in cardiac muscle remodeling and ventricular hypertrophy.

Management of CHF is aimed at correcting the congenital defect causing the heart failure and/or reducing the workload of the heart by administering positive inotropic medications, diuretics, oxygen therapy, and vasodilators. Table 26-1 lists the signs and symptoms of the types of congestive heart failure.

ACQUIRED HEART DISEASE

Rheumatic Heart Disease

Although treatment of strep throat with antibiotics has greatly reduced the number of rheumatic fever cases in the United States, Salt Lake City, Utah and Denver, Colorado, continue to have 30–50 pediatric cases of rheumatic fever yearly. The reason for this trend is unknown. In susceptible children an upper respiratory tract infection with group A β-hemolytic streptococci is the triggering event leading to rheumatic fever. Children and adolescents aged 5–15 years, females, and African-Americans are at highest risk for developing rheumatic fever within 1 to 5 weeks after an untreated strep throat. If more than one episode of strep throat is untreated, the child has an almost 50% chance of developing rheumatic fever.

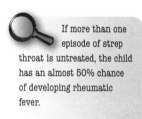

If more than one episode of strep throat is untreated, the child has an almost 50% chance of developing rheumatic fever.

The inflammatory process of rheumatic fever is set up by the sensitization of B lymphocytes by streptococcal antigens. Antistreptococcal antibodies then develop, leading to immune complexes that cross-react with antigens in cardiac tissue. A multiorgan inflammatory process involves connective tissue, the heart, joints, central nervous system, and subcutaneous tissue. Residual heart valve damage may follow a single episode of rheumatic fever and result in CHF.

Table 26-1 Signs and Symptoms of Congestive Heart Failure

Location	Sign and Symptoms
Right-sided CHF	Hepatomegaly (cardinal sign) Splenomegaly Periorbital/facial edema Neck vein distention (difficult to detect in infants; more reliable as child grows) Decreased urine output Delayed capillary refill
Left-sided CHF	Cyanosis Pallor Grunting respirations (increases end-expiratory pressure and helps prevent atelectasis) Retractions Head bobbing (infants) Nasal flaring (infants) Wet lung sounds Tachypnea Low oxygen saturation Use of accessory muscles (scapula and sternocleidomastoid) to breathe (detected mainly in older children)
Common signs and symptoms regardless of pump failure location	Fatigue Difficulty feeding (prolonged time needed to feed due to fatigue and dyspnea) Activity intolerance Slow weight gain Diaphoresis—head/neck (sympathetic nervous system stimulation) Irritability Resting tachycardia (above 150/min) Increased respiratory rate (above 50/min) Cool extremities Lethargy Third heart sound—gallop rhythm

The main signs and symptoms of rheumatic fever include carditis, multijoint pain, Sydenham chorea (St. Vitus' dance), rash on the trunk and extremities, and subcutaneous nodules over the joints, scalp, and spinal column. Streptococcal antibody titers are higher in children with rheumatic fever than they are in children with strep throat alone. Sydenham chorea is self-limiting but may not be manifested for months to years after the acute infection. Signs and symptoms include emotional instability and involuntary movements leading to ataxia, slurred speech, and muscle weakness.

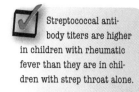
Streptococcal antibody titers are higher in children with rheumatic fever than they are in children with strep throat alone.

Mitral valve insufficiency is the most common valve disorder associated with rheumatic fever. Mitral valve stenosis, aortic valve insufficiency, and aortic stenosis may also occur.

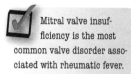
Mitral valve insufficiency is the most common valve disorder associated with rheumatic fever.

CARDIOMYOPATHY

Cardiomyopathy, a condition in which the heart muscle stretches and becomes weak, results in CHF. There are three main types of cardiomyopathy: dilated, hypertrophic, and restrictive.

Dilated Cardiomyopathy

Idiopathic **dilated cardiomyopathy** occurs most frequently, although long-term tachyarrhythmias, chronic heart inflammation, Duchenne muscular dystrophy, alcoholism, and inborn errors of metabolism (fatty acid oxidation) account for some cases of dilated cardiomyopathy. As dilated cardiomyopathy progresses the child develops classic signs of CHF, with an ejection fraction of around 40% (normal, 65–70%). Treatment begins by correcting the cause, such as medication to control arrhythmias, treatment of symptoms, and cardiac heart transplantation if other measures fail.

Hypertrophic Cardiomyopathy

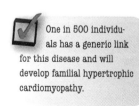
One in 500 individuals has a generic link for this disease and will develop familial hypertrophic cardiomyopathy.

Hypertrophic cardiomyopathy results in ventricular hypertrophy and ventricular septum hypertrophy, which causes an outflow obstruction. One in 500 individuals has a generic link for this disease and will develop familial hypertrophic cardiomyopathy. Signs and symptoms usually begin in older children and adolescents. Metabolic disorders such as glycogen storage disease (Pompe's disease) also cause hypertrophic cardiomyopathy. Because of an enzyme deficiency, glycogen cannot be metabolized correctly and is deposited in the myocardium. The infant with this disorder usually does not live past 12 months of age.

Although signs and symptoms of poor cardiac muscle perfusion, including exercise intolerance and angina, may occur, sudden cardiac death during a sports activity may be the first indication of the condition. Exercise stress testing can help diagnose the disorder. Treatment options include implantable cardiac defibrillators, beta-blockers, dual-chamber pacemakers, surgical myectomy (removal of part of the septum), and, for the adult, ethanol ablation of part of the septum that reduces outflow obstruction.

Restrictive Cardiomyopathy

Restrictive cardiomyopathy is rare in children in Western countries and is often idiopathic in nature. In parts of Africa, India, South and Central America, and Asia the condition is endemic. In restrictive cardiomyopathy the atria enlarge and the ventricles become stiff and rigid. The child develops severe CHF, and heart transplantation is required because other treatment options are limited.

SECTION X · REVIEW QUESTIONS

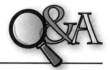

1. When teaching nursing students about cardiac anatomy and physiology the nurse makes several statements. Which of the following statements is correct?
   a. The heart secrets peptides, which help regulate blood volume.
   b. The systemic circulation originates from the right side of the heart.
   c. The systemic circulation carries oxygenated blood to all organs.
   d. Oxygenated blood returns to the left atria via the pulmonary artery.

2. Which of the following statements concerning natriuretic peptides is *true*?
   a. A-natriuretic peptide is produced by the ventricles.
   b. B-natriuretic peptide is produced by the atria.
   c. C-natriuretic peptide is produced by the endothelial cells lining the blood vessels.
   d. Natriuretic peptides are agonists for the renin-angiotensin-aldosterone system.

3. When explaining the structure of the heart the nurse should state which of the following?
   a. When the cardiac muscle fibers contract they create a squeezing motion.
   b. The muscle fibers between the atria and ventricles are arranged in a loop pattern.
   c. The endocardium lines the heart and creates the pericardial sac.
   d. The pericardial sac normally contains 1–3 mL of fluid.

4. Which of the following statements about the heart chambers is correct?
   a. The right side of the heart is a pressure pump.
   b. The atrial kick provides 40% of the blood going to the ventricles.
   c. Although smaller in size, the atria are thicker than the ventricles.
   d. During diastole blood trickles through the AV valves.

5. Which of the following statements about cardiac valves is correct?
    a. Cardiac valves move actively in response to pressure.
    b. The left atrioventricular valve is called the tricuspid valve.
    c. The function of the papillary muscle is to keep the closed atrioventricular valves in place.
    d. Semilunar valves prevent backflow of blood from the pulmonary vein to the right atria.

6. The ejection fraction is:
    a. Approximately 65%
    b. Defined as the amount of blood filling the atria during one contraction
    c. The amount of blood pumped to the general circulation by the left ventricle
    d. The percent of blood left in the ventricles after contraction

7. As an electrical impulse travels through myocardium cells
    a. Sodium binds to troponin
    b. Potassium moves into the cardiac cells
    c. Sodium moves out of cardiac cells
    d. Calcium is released from the cardiac cells

8. Preload is defined as the:
    a. Amount of blood in the ventricles at the end of systole
    b. End-diastolic volume
    c. Vascular resistance to the pumping action of the left ventricle
    d. Prediastolic volume

9. During a prenatal class the nurse explains to the expectant parents that their baby will take his or her first breath in response to (select all that apply):
    a. Hypoxia
    b. Reexpansion of the chest after a cesarean section
    c. A startle reflex in response to the delivery room's bright lights
    d. Changes in skin temperature upon delivery

10. During labor which of the following events takes place?
    a. Surfactant is produced.
    b. Rapid absorption of fluid present in the alveoli begins.
    c. The ductus arteriosus closes.
    d. Surfactant moves into the alveoli.

11. When an infant takes his or her first breath:
     a. Pulmonary artery blood flow decreases.
     b. Pulmonary artery resistance increases.
     c. The patent ductus arteriosus closes completely.
     d. Functional closure of the ductus arteriosus occurs.

12. The parents of newborn Sergio, who has a left-to-right shunting defect, ask the nurse to explain this defect. The nurse correctly explains that:
     a. Sergio will be cyanotic most of the time.
     b. There is a defect in the pulmonary artery valve.
     c. The right side of the heart will enlarge.
     d. The pressure in the pulmonary artery is low so blood cannot be oxygenated.

13. Newborn Amy has an atrial septal defect. The nurse explains to Amy's parents that:
     a. Blood flow to the pulmonary artery is decreased.
     b. Amy may have frequent respiratory infections.
     c. Surgery is required to correct the defect.
     d. Surgery to close the defect will be performed when Amy is 3–4 months old.

14. Newborn Carlos has a moderate sized ventricular septal defect. The nurse recognizes that this type of defect:
     a. Requires surgical closure in approximately 10% of cases
     b. Accounts for almost half of all congenital heart defects
     c. Is usually corrected by surgery by the time the infant is 4 weeks old
     d. Most likely results in symptoms such as CHF

15. Baby Shanese has a patent ductus arteriosus (PDA). The preceptor orienting a new registered nurse to the unit explains which of the following (select all that apply)?
     a. At birth, inspired oxygen and decreased prostaglandin levels usually cause the ductus arteriosus to close spontaneously.
     b. The nurse can expect to assess severe dyspnea in baby Shanese.
     c. PDA is much more common in boys than in girls.
     d. PDA causes severe hypoxia in infants who also have pulmonary atresia.

16. Research has demonstrated that indomethacin closes a PDA in
    a. Full-term infants
    b. Small children
    c. Preterm infants weighing more than 1,200 g
    d. Preterm infants weighing less than 1,200 g

17. Shortly after birth baby Scott was diagnosed with mild pulmonary stenosis. The nurse practitioner explains which of the following to his parents?
    a. Because of the defect he will develop left-sided congestive heart failure.
    b. His lips will appear bluish most of the time.
    c. His finger nails will have a clubbed appearance because of chronic hypoxia.
    d. The pulmonic valve cusps are fused.

18. Marco, an 8-year-old, is seen in the pediatrician's office for a well child visit. The office nurse suspects that Marco has a mild coarctation of the aorta when she assesses (select all that apply):
    a. Hypotension
    b. Bounding leg pulses
    c. Systolic murmur
    d. Leg cramping

19. Infant Marilyn's parents ask the nurse why the doctor has scheduled her for surgical correction of coarctation of the aorta. The nurse's reply is based on his knowledge that:
    a. If corrected after age 5, Marilyn's risk for developing hypertension and cardiac dysfunction increases.
    b. Marilyn is at risk for also developing a PDA.
    c. Infants tolerate anesthesia better than older children.
    d. Surgery is often unsuccessful if done after age 5.

20. The nurse notes that toddler Simon's chart indicates he has mild valvular aortic stenosis. She knows that this means Simon has:
    a. A stricture of the aorta just below the coronary arteries
    b. An aortic valve with one cusp-like structure
    c. A fibrous ring just below the aortic valve
    d. Many symptoms of CHF

21. Newborns who have a congenital anomaly resulting in decreased pulmonary blood flow present with:
    a. General discomfort
    b. Cyanosis
    c. Clubbing of the fingers
    d. Pao$_2$ between 80 and 85 mm Hg

22. Newborn Conseula was admitted to the newborn intensive care unit at birth because of transposition of the great arteries. The parents ask the nurse for information about this congenital disorder. The nurse correctly tells them which of the following?
    a. Transposition of the great arteries is a rare disorder that causes cyanosis.
    b. Conseula will probably have surgery when she is 12 months old.
    c. Developmental delays occur in almost all cases.
    d. Supplemental oxygen will not relieve Conseula's cyanosis.

23. Baby Keenan has right-sided CHF. The nurse will most likely assess:
    a. Bradycardia
    b. Heart murmur
    c. Enlarged liver
    d. Flat neck veins

24. While conducting a seminar on rheumatic fever, the nurse tells the audience that most cases of rheumatic fever per year in the United States occur in:
    a. New York City
    b. Dallas
    c. Boston
    d. Salt Lake City

25. The parents of LeVerne, a 10-year-old with strep throat, ask the nurse about rheumatic fever. The nurse correctly replies that children in which of the following groups are at highest risk for developing rheumatic fever?
    a. Males
    b. African-Americans
    c. Those aged 2–5
    d. Those with a first time infection

26. The nurse speaking at a community health fair explains that rheumatic heart disease is the result of (select all that apply):
    a. Immune complexes interacting with antigens in cardiac tissue
    b. Sensitization of helper T cells
    c. The development of streptococcal antigens
    d. Inflammatory process involving the heart, connective tissue, joints, central nervous system, and subcutaneous tissue

27. The school nurse tells parents attending a PTA meeting that the signs of rheumatic fever include:
    a. Rash on the palms of the hands and soles of the feet
    b. High streptococcal antibody titer
    c. Nodules on the face and hands
    d. Moist cough

28. The nurse caring for Samuel, an 11-year-old with dilated cardiomyopathy, asks his preceptor about the disorder. The preceptor correctly explains that dilated cardiomyopathy:
    a. Is most often caused by long-term tachyarrhythmias
    b. Results in shortened cardiac muscles
    c. Reduces the ejection fraction to approximately 40%
    d. Causes the ventricles to hypertrophy

29. Research has demonstrated that hypertrophic cardiomyopathy (select all that apply):
    a. Causes an outflow obstruction
    b. May cause sudden cardiac death during exercise
    c. Is sometimes successfully treated by implanting an automatic cardiac defibrillator
    d. Is very rare

ANSWERS AND RATIONALES

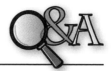

1. **The answer is a.** Rationale: Systemic circulation originates from the left side of the heart and oxygenates all organs except the lungs, and oxygenated blood returns from the lungs to the left atria via the pulmonary vein.

2. **The answer is c.** Rationale: A-natriuretic peptide is produced by the atrial myocardium, B-natriuretic peptide is produced by the ventricular myocardium, and natriuretic peptides are antagonists of the renin-angiotensin-aldosterone system.

3. **The answer is b.** Rationale: When the heart muscle fibers contract they create a wringing motion. The endocardium lines the internal myocardium and all blood vessels, creating one continuous circuit. The pericardial sac normally contains 15–50 mL of fluid.

4. **The answer is d.** Rationale: The atrial kick provides 20–30% of the blood going to the ventricles; the ventricles are thicker than the atria; and the right side of the heart is the volume pump, whereas the left side is the pressure pump.

5. **The answer is c.** Rationale: Valves move passively in response to pressure, the right AV valve is called the tricuspid valve, and the pulmonary semilunar valve prevents backflow of blood from the pulmonary artery to the right ventricle.

6. **The answer is a.** Rationale: Stroke volume is the amount of blood pumped from the ventricles during one contraction, and cardiac output is the amount of blood pumped to the general circulation by the ventricle each minute.

7. **The answer is d.** Rationale: Calcium moves out of cardiac cells and binds to troponin, sodium flows into cardiac cells, and potassium flows out of cardiac cells.

8. **The answer is b.** Rationale: Afterload is the vascular resistance to the pumping action of the left ventricle.

9. **The answers are a and d.** Rationale: The chest expands after a vaginal delivery.

10. **The answer is b.** Rationale: By 34 weeks' gestation surfactant production occurs, during labor fluid moves out of the alveoli, and the ductus arteriosus remains patent during labor.

11. **The answer is d.** Rationale: Pulmonary artery blood flow increases, pulmonary artery resistance decreases, and it takes from 1 to 3 weeks after birth for the ductus arteriosus to close completely.

12. **The answer is c.** Rationale: There is a septal defect, cyanosis may not be present, and an excessive amount of blood is pumped to the pulmonary artery.

13. **The answer is b.** Rationale: A small defect may close on its own; if not, surgery is performed when the infant is 12–36 months old. There is an increased blood flow to the pulmonary artery.

14. **The answer is a.** Rationale: Thirty percent of all congenital heart defects are ventricular septal defects, small and moderate sized defects do not cause symptoms and close on their own in 90% of the cases, and large defects cause symptoms such as CHF by the time the infant is 3–6 months old.

15. **The answers are a and b.** Rationale: PDA is more common in girls than in boys; it helps maintain life in infants who also have pulmonary atresia.

16. **The answer is c.**

17. **The answer is d.** Rationale: Children with severe pulmonary stenosis develop right-sided CHF and are cyanotic if they also have a patent foramen ovale. Children with a mild pulmonary stenosis are usually asymptomatic.

18. **The answers are c and d.** Rationale: Diminished leg pulses and hypertension are additional signs of mild coarctation of the aorta.

19. **The answer is a.** Rationale: Symptoms often develop when the ductus arteriosus closes, and CHF develops in severe cases if the condition is not surgically corrected.

20. **The answer is b.** Rationale: Supravalvular aortic stenosis causes a stricture of the aorta just above the coronary arteries, subvalvular aortic stenosis occurs when there is a fibrous ring just below the aortic valve, and mild valvular aortic stenosis is often asymptomatic.

21. **The answers are b and c.** Rationale: Infants may appear to be comfortable even with a PaO_2 between 20 and 25 mm Hg because they had a low PaO_2 while in utero.

22. **The answer is d.** Rationale: TGA is the second most common congenital cardiac defect causing cyanosis, surgery is usually performed within 1 week of birth, and prompt surgery helps prevent developmental delays because it increases oxygenation to the brain.

23. **The answer is c.** Rationale: The cardinal sign of right-sided CHF is hepatomegaly, compensatory mechanisms result in tachycardia, distended neck veins occur because of increased blood volume, and a gallop rhythm may be heard.

24. **The answer is d.** Rationale: Salt Lake City, Utah and Denver, Colorado, have the most cases of rheumatic fever per year (30–50 cases).

25. **The answer is b.** Rationale: Children and adolescents between the ages of 5 and 15, females, African-Americans, and children who have had more than one episode of untreated strep throat are at highest risk for developing rheumatic fever.

26. **The answers are a and d.** Rationale: Antistreptococcal antibodies develop in response to sensitization of B lymphocytes.

27. **The answer is b.** Rationale: Streptococcal antibody titers are higher in children with rheumatic fever than in those with only strep throat, a rash appears on the trunk and extremities, and subcutaneous nodules appear over the joints, scalp, and spinal column.

28. **The answer is c.** Rationale: Idiopathic dilated cardiomyopathy is the most common type; the heart muscle stretches, not shortens.

29. **The answers are a, b, and c.** Rationale: One in 500 people has a genetic link for hypertrophic cardiomyopathy and will develop this disorder.

XI

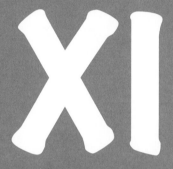

Diabetes Mellitus

Diabetes mellitus (DM), a chronic disease of altered fuel metabolism, is classified as **type 1 diabetes**/immune-mediated diabetes (formerly called juvenile diabetes or insulin-dependent diabetes mellitus), in which there is a lack of insulin production and ketosis, and **type 2 diabetes** (formerly called non–insulin-dependent diabetes mellitus), which results in a decreased sensitivity to insulin. Children may have a combination of type 1 and type 2 DM. Although type 1 DM is much more common in children than type 2, the incidence of type 2 DM is increasing rapidly in the pediatric population. Approximately 13,000 new cases of type 1 DM are diagnosed each year.

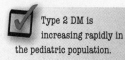

Type 2 DM is increasing rapidly in the pediatric population.

27

Diabetes Mellitus in the Pediatric Population

TERMS
- ☐ **Acanthosis nigricans**
- ☐ **C-peptide**
- ☐ **Glucogenesis**
- ☐ **Gluconeogenesis**
- ☐ **Glucosuria**
- ☐ **Glycogen**
- ☐ **Polydipsia**
- ☐ **Polyuria**
- ☐ **Proinsulin**
- ☐ **Type 1 diabetes**
- ☐ **Type 2 diabetes**

Glucose is used by all body tissue for energy, with the brain as a major consumer of glucose (25% of the total amount of glucose available). The brain and nervous system require a constant source of glucose for energy because they are unable to store glucose or to use fatty acids for fuel. Ingested food provides the body with more glucose than is needed. Approximately 66% of the glucose from each meal is stored in the liver as **glycogen** and some is converted to fat and stored. Between meals the liver releases glycogen, which is broken down into glucose (**glucogenesis**) to keep the serum glucose level constant (80–90 mg/dL). The liver can also manufacture glucose from amino acids, glycerol, and lactic acid (**gluconeogenesis**).

Insulin, produced in stages by pancreatic beta cells in the islets of Langerhans, allows glucose to enter cells for use as an energy source, promotes growth and development, decreases the production of glucose by the liver, increases protein synthesis, halts ketone production, and increases the production of very-low-density lipoproteins by the liver. The lipoproteins then transport triglycerides to fat tissue where they are stored.

During stage one of insulin production, preproinsulin is converted to **proinsulin**, a molecule composed of 81 amino acids. During stage two the beta cells remove a **C-peptide** structure from proinsulin to create insulin, which has a 51 amino acid structure. Because C-peptide is removed from each proinsulin molecule to create a unit of insulin, measuring the amount of C-peptide in the blood allows us to measure the amount of insulin produced daily by the beta cells. Approximately 40–50 units of insulin are released by the pancreas on a daily basis. In addition to the daily production, several hundred units are stored and can be released when the serum glucose level rises. Long-term untreated or under treated DM results in severe complications such as renal failure, cardiovascular disease, and blindness.

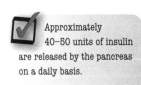

Approximately 40–50 units of insulin are released by the pancreas on a daily basis.

TYPE 1 DM

Type 1 DM is thought to be the result of a genetic predisposition to immunological damage, probably triggered by environmental factors such as viral infections and/or diet (Table 27-1). At present there is no

Table 27-1 Factors Associated With Type 1 DM

Factors (Theory)	Supporting Data for the Theory
Immunological damage	Cyclosporine (immunosuppressive agent) preserves islet tissue function for 1–2 years. White blood cells are frequently found in islet cells of newly diagnosed patients. White blood cells release free radicals, interleukin-1, tumor necrosis factor → damage to cells. Ninety percent of people who develop type 1 DM have antibodies to islet cells, insulin, and other antibodies present from months to years before signs and symptoms develop.
Environmental factors—diet	A diet very high in nitrates has been associated with type 1 DM.
Environmental factors—viral (trigger the autoimmune response)	Not all identical twins develop type 1 DM if the first twin has the disease; if it was purely genetic than 100% of all identical twins whose twin has type 1 DM would develop the disease. Forty percent of infants with congenital rubella develop either type 1 DM or glucose intolerance by age 20. Type 1*B* develops after a viral infection and the child does not have any indication of autoimmune disease (rare—affects children of African or Asian heritage more often than children in other ethnic groups).
Genetic factors Cell-surface molecules, called the human major histocompatibility complex (MHC), or human leukocyte antigens (HLA), are a group of genes found on chromosome 6. They produce cell-surface glycoproteins that enable the body to distinguish self-antigens from foreign antigens. HLA are identified by both letters and by numbers. Each child receives one HLA set from each parent. Antigens are substances that initiate the immune response. Antibodies are immunoglobins that are produced in response to antigens.	An identical twin has an approximately 50% chance of developing type 1 DM if the other identical twin has developed the disease. The incidence of type 1 DM in the general population is between 0.2% and 0.3%; however, 6% of siblings or children of people with type 1 DM also develop the disease. Susceptibility to type 1 DM is linked to HLA-DR3 and HLA-DR4 → children inherit an abnormal immune response to their own beta cells. Islet cell antibodies (ICAs) and insulin autoantibodies (IAAs) are found in some people years before DM develops. If neither antibody is detected, the risk of developing type 1 DM is 0%.

Table 27-1 Factors Associated With Type 1 DM (continued)

Factors (Theory)	Supporting Data for the Theory
Associated disease process	Children with cystic fibrosis are prone to develop type 1 DM because of the pancreatic damage that occurs with the disease.

way to prevent the development of type 1 DM. After approximately 90% of the insulin producing beta cells have been damaged, symptoms appear. This process of destruction takes several years, with most cases diagnosed when the child is either of school age or has reached adolescence.

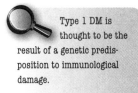

Type 1 DM is thought to be the result of a genetic predisposition to immunological damage.

Classic signs and symptoms of type 1 DM include excessive thirst (**polydipsia**), excessive urination (**polyuria**) as a result of osmotic diuresis (glucose pulls water into the bloodstream), and weight loss. Because the kidneys are unable to reabsorb all of the glucose when the serum level rises above 180 mg/dL, the excess glucose spills into the urine (**glucosuria**). As a result of osmotic diuresis the child becomes dehydrated and thus experiences excessive thirst in an effort to replace the lost water. DM and diabetes insipidus are the only two diseases that cause continued excessive urination even when the tongue and oral mucous membranes are dry. Weight loss occurs because cells cannot utilize glucose for energy and fat stores and protein are broken down for use as a fuel source.

DM may be discovered during routine screening when the child develops a minor illness and a routine urine sample reveals glucosuria (Table 27-2). DM is suspected in adolescent girls who develop a Candida vaginal infection. Blood tests are used to confirm DM. More than one sample is needed to confirm the disease because illness also raises blood glucose levels. (Stress causes the release of catecholamines, which prompt the liver to release glycogen.)

Treatment for type 1 DM includes insulin, diet, exercise, stress management, and blood glucose/ketone monitoring. Long-term untreated or under treated DM leads to macrovascular and microvascular complications. Macrovascular complications include coronary artery disease, and microvascular complications include retinopathy, nephropathy, and neuropathies.

Table 27-2 DM Serum Glucose Indicators

Indicator	Confirming Value
Random plasma glucose	Above 200 mg/dL
Fasting plasma glucose	Above 126 mg/dL
Two-hour postglucose load (1.75 g glucose/kg)	Above 200 mg/dL
Impaired fasting glucose (not yet diabetic)	110–125 mg/dL
Impaired 2-hr postglucose load (not yet diabetic)	140–200 mg/dL
HgA1c (measures serum glucose levels for the past 90 days—glucose attaches to red blood cells)	Desired value is below 7.5%
C-peptide (measures amount of insulin produced by the beta cells)	0.5 to 2.0 ng/mL (nanograms per milliliter) (values differ by laboratory)

 TYPE 2 DM

Type 2 DM is a chronic disease encompassing decreased insulin production, increased hepatic glucose production, and insulin receptor insensitivity. A genetic predisposition, obesity, insulin resistance (HgA1c between 10% and 12% [normal is below 6.5%]), and lack of exercise (environmental factors) are associated with the development of type 2 DM in children and adolescents (Table 27-3). Generally, children and adolescents with type 2 DM are diagnosed between the ages of 10 and 19. The Diabetes Prevention Study found that 30 minutes of exercise 5 days a week and a low-fat diet decreased the risk of developing type 2 DM by 58%. Children who are black, Hispanic, or American Indian have a higher prevalence of type 2 DM than children in other ethnic groups. Insensitivity to insulin has been associated with polycystic ovary disease. The child with type 2 DM may also have **acanthosis nigricans** in which the skin over the posterior neck, armpits, and elbows is thick and dark.

Treatment for type 2 DM includes lifestyle modifications (diet and exercise), stress

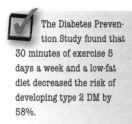

The Diabetes Prevention Study found that 30 minutes of exercise 5 days a week and a low-fat diet decreased the risk of developing type 2 DM by 58%.

reduction to reduce cortisol levels, and oral medication to increase insulin production by the beta cells and to increase receptor site sensitivity to insulin.

Table 27-3 Factors Associated With Type 2 DM

Factors (Theory)	Supporting Data for the Theory
Beta cell dysfunction, leading to impaired insulin production. Amyloid (insoluble fibrous protein) deposits decrease beta cell function. Hyperinsulinemia: beta cells become exhausted trying to secrete enough insulin to overcome insulin resistance.	First-degree relatives of those with type 2 DM had impaired glucose tolerance and beta cell dysfunction. First-degree relatives of those with type 2 DM who had normal glucose tolerance were found to have beta cell dysfunction. Islet amyloid polypeptide (amylin) has been isolated from amyloid deposits in the pancreas.
Insulin resistance/reduced insulin binding to receptor sites Insulin resistance triggers insulin production (adaptive response) to a point of beta cell exhaustion. Obesity (central) associated with insulin resistance. Insulin-resistant people have decreased blood flow to the capillaries and skeletal muscles → delivery of insulin to tissues is hampered.	Higher levels of insulin found in serum of individuals with type 2 DM. Obese children are 10 times more likely to develop type 2 DM than nonobese children. Fat cells produce cytokines (tumor necrosis factor), which impair insulin action. Recently, obese individuals have hyperinsulinemia, insulin resistance, and insulin hypersecretion compared with nonobese individuals. Insulin is a natural vasodilator. Forty-one percent of people with hypertension are also insulin resistant and have hyperinsulinemia.
Failure to suppress glucose production Normally, hypoglycemia stimulates the release of glucagons, which then stimulates the release of insulin, which then suppresses further glucose production. Normally, free fatty acids stimulate insulin secretion.	In type 2 DM glucose production by the liver is not contained. Insulin secretion is not stimulated by the release of free fatty acids in type 2 DM, so the liver over produces glucose, which cannot be utilized.
Stress response As a natural response to stress, cortisol raises blood glucose levels and enhances the effects of epinephrine.	Chronic stress results in higher than normal levels of cortisol and epinephrine. Epinephrine decreases the utilization of glucose. High serum cortisol levels leads to abdominal obesity → obesity is linked to type 2 DM.

Factors (Theory)	Supporting Data for the Theory
Genetics The tendency to develop type 2 DM is inherited.	First-degree relatives of people with type 2 DM have double the risk of developing the disease than do people without a family history of type 2 DM. A child whose parents both have DM has an 80% lifetime chance of developing type 2 DM. Fifty percent of the Pima Indian population (Arizona) have DM.

This chapter reviews complications of diabetes mellitus (DM), both acute and chronic. Acute complications of DM include hypoglycemia, ketonuria, ketonemia, diabetic ketoacidosis (DKA), and hyperglycemic hypersomolar nonketotic syndrome (HHNKS). Chronic complications of DM include macrovascular disease, microvascular disease, nephropathy, retinopathy, and neuropathy.

28

Complications:
Acute and Chronic

TERMS
- ☐ **Diabetic ketoacidosis**
- ☐ **Hemodilution**
- ☐ **Hypoglycemia**
- ☐ **Hyponatremia**
- ☐ **Ketonuria**
- ☐ **Ketonemia**
- ☐ **Kussmaul respirations**

ACUTE COMPLICATIONS

Hypoglycemia

When blood glucose falls below 60 mg/dL (below 70 mg/dL in preschool children) the child experiences **hypoglycemia** (insulin reaction). Causes of hypoglycemia include taking too much insulin, delaying or omitting meals, and high-energy activities such as playing hard or exercising vigorously without eating extra carbohydrates (exercise moves glucose into muscle cells). Hypoglycemia develops quickly, and the child presents with adrenergic signs such as hunger, weakness, shakiness, sweating, drowsiness, pallor, clammy skin, and headache and central nervous system signs such as irritability, tearfulness, euphoria, or temper tantrum-like behavior. A young child may tell the parent or caregiver that they feel "funny."

Hypoglycemia develops quickly, and the child presents with adrenergic signs such as hunger, weakness, shakiness, sweating, drowsiness, pallor, clammy skin, and headache and central nervous system signs such as irritability, tearfulness, euphoria, or temper tantrum–like behavior.

Giving the conscious child simple sugar, such as 4 ounces of juice, regular (not sugar-free) soda, or milk, reverses hypoglycemia. After 10 minutes the blood glucose should be rechecked. If it is still below 60 mg/dL, the juice, soda, or milk is repeated. If the serum glucose is above 60 mg/dL, solid food is given. If the child is unconscious, subcutaneous or intramuscular glucagon or intravenous glucose is administered. Left untreated, loss of consciousness, seizures, and brain damage occur.

Ketonuria, Ketonemia, and Diabetic Ketoacidosis (DKA)

If the child has an illness, even if it appears to be mild, or if they have a fasting glucose level above 240 mg/dL, the urine and/or serum ketone level(s) should be monitored. Blood ketone levels can be assessed by using the Precision Xtra® meter. If moderate or significant ketones in the urine are detected (**ketonuria**), if the serum ketone level is above 1.0 mmol/L (**ketonemia**), or if deep rapid respirations (**Kussmaul respirations**) are noted, the health care provider must be notified at once.

Diabetic ketoacidosis (DKA) (also known as metabolic acidosis), which has a 3–10% mortality rate, is indicated by a blood pH below 7.30, hyperglycemia (above 250 mg/dL), low serum bicarbonate (below 15 mEq/L), ketonemia, and ketonuria. It develops when there is a lack of insulin, resulting in the inability to use glucose for energy. DKA can result from a severe infection, stress, surgery, and an empty insulin pump or lack of subcutaneous insulin.

Serum glucose levels rise and counter-regulatory hormones are activated. Cortisol, glucagon, and catecholamines stimulate the liver to produce glucose, reduce the utilization of glucose by cells, and initiate lipolysis. Ketone byproducts of lipolysis build up in the bloodstream and are excreted by the kidneys, along with sodium bicarbonate.

Compensatory measures for combating metabolic acidosis include Kussmaul respirations. This type of respiratory pattern allows a large amount of carbon dioxide to be exhaled in an attempt to lower the amount of carbonic acid produced. When water in the blood combines with carbon dioxide carbonic acid is produced, adding to the already high acid load. By lowering the amount of carbon dioxide in the blood, less carbonic acid is produced. As acetone produced by ketosis is released from the bloodstream via respirations, the child's breath adopts the characteristic fruity odor of DKA. Severe hyperglycemia leads to polyuria, hypovolemia, and hypoperfusion and eventually causes lactic acidosis.

High serum levels of lipids, cholesterol, triglycerides, and free fatty acids are present because the body breaks down fat for an energy source when insulin is not available to move glucose into cells. Electrolyte imbalances also occur during DKA. Potassium shifts from inside the cell to outside the cell in response to metabolic acidosis, resulting in hyperkalemia. Low serum sodium (**hyponatremia**) occurs because water is pulled into the bloodstream in response to a high glucose load (high serum osmolarity). This increased water load in the bloodstream dilutes serum sodium levels (**hemodilution**). Serum sodium levels also drop because diuresis associated with severe hyperglycemia flushes sodium out of the body. In addition to a serum pH below 7.3, polyuria, dehydration, and thirst, a child with DKA also presents with nausea, vomiting, abdominal or chest pain, postural hypotension, tachycardia, and central nervous system depression. Chloride, phosphate, and magnesium levels will also be depleted.

Treatment for DKA includes intravenous insulin, fluid, salt and potassium replacement, correction of acidosis, and return to glucose, not fat, utilization for energy. As the hyperglycemia is corrected, potassium moves back into the cells, so intravenous potassium is given to prevent severe hypokalemia and dysrhythmias. Intracellular osmolality in the brain also increases in response to the severe hyperglycemia; therefore, to prevent cerebral edema and brain herniation from water rapidly infusing brain cells, fluid and glucose correction must be done gradually.

Hyperglycemic Hypersomolar Nonketotic Syndrome (HHNKS)

The mortality rate for hyperglycemic hypersomolar nonketotic syndrome (HHNKS) is 10–20%. This syndrome, which is caused by dehydration, is characterized by a high serum glucose level (800–2,400 mg/dL [hyperglycemic]), a high serum osmolality (340 mOsm/L [hyperosmolar]), and the absence of ketosis (nonketotic). Because children and adolescents with type 2 diabetes mellitus (DM) continue to have an endogenous supply of insulin, lipolysis is suppressed; however, dehydration and electrolyte imbalance are often severe in HHNKS.

Neurological signs such as hemiparesis, seizure, and aphasia are often mistaken for a brain attack (stroke). The child will complain of extreme thirst. Events that may lead to HHNKS include infection.

The treatment for HHNKS is similar to the treatment for DKA, and as in DKA fluid replacement cannot be rapid or cerebral edema results. It may take weeks before potassium stores are returned to normal.

 Neurological signs such as hemiparesis, seizure, and aphasia are often mistaken for a brain attack (stroke).

 # CHRONIC COMPLICATIONS

Macrovascular Disease

Under treated or untreated type 2 DM is considered an independent risk factor for coronary artery disease, cerebrovascular disease, and peripheral vascular disease. Because children and adolescents are developing type 2 DM at an alarming rate, they are at risk for developing these chronic complications of DM as adults.

The risk of macrovascular complications is not gender specific, with both men and women at risk for developing coronary artery disease, myocardial infarction (either silent or with typical presenting signs), angina, brain attack (cerebrovascular accident or stroke), peripheral vascular disease, and sudden death (Table 28-1). It has been estimated that up to 75% of people with type 2 DM will die because of macrovascular disease. The mortality rate after a myocardial infarction is higher in people with diabetes than in the general population.

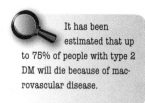

It has been estimated that up to 75% of people with type 2 DM will die because of macrovascular disease.

Microvascular Disease

Microvascular disease (nephropathy, retinopathy, and neuropathies) is thought to be caused by capillary vessel occlusion from protein deposits on vessel walls. Microcirculation is compromised by the narrow vessel walls.

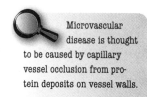

Microvascular disease is thought to be caused by capillary vessel occlusion from protein deposits on vessel walls.

Table 28-1 Macrovascular Disease Development Theory

Macrovascular Disease Development Theory	Supporting Data
People with DM have • A high lipid level with lipoproteins that are more likely to cause atherosclerosis • Increased platelet aggregation • Changes in blood vessel walls caused by hyperinsulinemia or exogenous insulin • Hypertension • Deposits of advanced glycosylation end products (proteins)	Lipoproteins are linked to atherosclerosis. Ruptured plaques lead to clot formation. Hypertension is the result of many factors, including vessel narrowing due to plaque buildup, fluid retention, and vasoconstriction. Advanced glycosylated end products may hinder the release of the natural vasodilator nitric oxide and thicken capillary basement wall membranes.
Cytomegalovirus (CMV)	CMV antibodies are higher in people with DM than in those without DM. CMV, which has been dormant in smooth muscle cells, reactivates because of the lowered immune response associated with DM. CMV then damages blood vessel walls and atherosclerosis results.
Syndrome X (insulin resistance, hyperinsulinemia)	Increased central obesity is associated with coronary artery disease. Hyperinsulinemia causes salt retention → salt retention causes water retention → salt and water retention cause hypertension → hypertension is associated with coronary artery disease.

Nephropathy

Nephropathy (renal disease) initially presents as microalbuminuria (30–300 mg albumin/24-hr specimen). Hypertension and hyperglycemia cause the glomerular membrane to thicken, which reduces filtration. Glomerulosclerosis allows protein to spill into the urine.

Nephropathy progresses slowly over a period of about 30 years in children who have type 1 DM and more quickly in those with type 2 DM (Table 28-2). Not all people with DM develop nephropathy, suggesting a genetic predisposition to developing this complication. Risk factors for developing nephropathy include family risk factors, poor glucose control (HbA1c above 8.1%), and systemic hypertension.

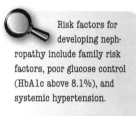
Risk factors for developing nephropathy include family risk factors, poor glucose control (HbA1c above 8.1%), and systemic hypertension.

Table 28-2 Stages of Nephropathy

Stage	Assessment
Stage 1 (diagnosis)	Enlarged kidneys Increased intraglomerular pressure Possibly the result of hypertension
Stage 2 (2 years of disease)	Initial decline in renal function but albumin excretion normal (below 20 µg/min or 30 mg/24 hr)
Stage 3 (7–15 years of disease)	Microalbuminuria (30–300 mg albumin/24 hr) Decrease in glomerular filtration rate if microalbuminuria significant Hypertension begins if not already present
Stage 4 (overt diabetic nephropathy)	Clinical proteinuria (assessed by urinalysis or dip stick) Microalbuminuria above 300 mg/24 hr Glomerular filtration rate declines Hypertension becomes more severe Aggressive treatment of HTN slows renal function decline but cannot reverse nephron destruction.
Stage 5	End-stage renal disease; dialysis required

Retinopathy

Retinopathy, which can develop in people as young as 20 years of age, is the result of blood vessel changes, red blood cell aggregation, scarring, retinal ischemia, and retinal detachment (Table 28-3); it develops more quickly in type 2 DM than in type 1 DM. Risk factors for developing retinopathy include poor glycemic control, hypertension, and hyperlipidemia.

Hyperglycemia causes the lens to change shape, leading to blurred vision. The lens changes shape because the high glucose content of aqueous humor pulls water out of the lens and causes myopia (nearsightedness). Vision can return to baseline in several weeks or months if glucose control is maintained.

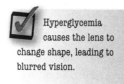 Hyperglycemia causes the lens to change shape, leading to blurred vision.

People with DM are also prone to develop cataracts and optic neuropathies. By the time type 2 DM is diagnosed, approximately 20% of those affected will have retinopathy. Children who have type 1 DM have an almost 100% chance of developing some degree of retinopathy after having the disease 20 or more years.

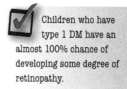 Children who have type 1 DM have an almost 100% chance of developing some degree of retinopathy.

Table 28-3 Stages of Retinopathy

Stages	Assessment Results
Nonproliferative	Retinal capillary microaneurysms Splinter hemorrhage Venous tortuosity Macular edema Hard exudates
Preproliferative	Areas of capillary nonperfusion Retinal hemorrhage Aneurysms Cotton wool spots
Proliferative	Neovascular vessel development Retinal detachment glaucoma

Neuropathy

People with DM may develop somatic and/or peripheral neuropathies. The two pathological processes responsible for neuropathy include blood vessel changes, leading to a decreased blood supply to the nerves, and demyelinization of nerve fibers, which slows down impulse conduction. Somatic neuropathy includes peripheral neuropathy, in which the person has a decreased perception of pain, vibration, sensation, position, and temperature. Some people with neuropathy complain of a severe burning pain in their extremities.

Autonomic neuropathy is characterized by malfunctions of the parasympathetic and sympathetic nervous systems, leading to decreased cardiac response, decreased gastric motility (gastroparesis), urinary retention, impotence, and impaired vasomotor reflexes, leading to vertigo.

SECTION XI · REVIEW QUESTIONS

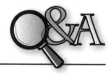

1. Which of the following organs is unable to store glucose for future use?
    a. Brain
    b. Liver
    c. Pancreas
    d. Stomach

2. Which of the following statements concerning glucose is *true*?
    a. All tissues except the muscles use glucose for energy.
    b. The liver is the major user of glucose.
    c. Glucose can be made from amino acids, glycerol, and lactic acid.
    d. Seventy percent of the glucose ingested at each meal is used, whereas 30% is stored as glycogen.

3. When conducting a community education program about diabetes mellitus, the nurse stresses that insulin (select all that apply):
    a. Is produced by the alpha cells of the islets of Langerhans
    b. Moves glucose into cells
    c. Increases the production of very-low-density lipoproteins
    d. Decreases protein synthesis

4. The nurse is analyzing lab results for Tommy, a 14-year-old who was admitted to rule out type 1 DM. Tommy's C-peptide laboratory value will tell the nurse:
    a. What Tommy's serum glucose has been for the past 90 days
    b. How well the liver is able to store glycogen
    c. How well Tommy's cells utilize insulin
    d. How much daily insulin is produced by Tommy's pancreas

5. The latest research concerning DM development theory indicates that:
    a. An identical twin has a 100% chance of developing DM if the other twin has the disease.
    b. A diet high in saturated fat leads to type 2 DM.
    c. Islet cell function can be maintained up to 24 months if cyclosporine is administered.
    d. Insulin antibodies are associated with the development of type 2 DM.

6. The school nurse leading a health education class stresses that:
   a. Type 1 DM can be prevented by limiting glucose in the diet.
   b. Type 2 DM is reaching epidemic proportions in young adults.
   c. Ninety percent of type 1 DM cases develop during the first 3 years of life.
   d. Signs of type 2 DM include excessive thirst.

7. Sara, a 16-year-old with type 1 DM, has a HgA1c of 10.6%. The clinic nurse tells Sara that her glucose control:
   a. Is at an optimal level
   b. Has improved since last month's reading of 9.2%
   c. Will prevent long-term complications as long as it remains around the present reading
   d. Requires further refinement

8. The pathophysiology of type 2 DM indicates that (select all that apply):
   a. Insulin production slows
   b. The liver produces excessive glucose
   c. Cells become less receptive to insulin
   d. C-peptide levels rise

9. During a public school board meeting the school nurse encourages the board members to fund gym classes because:
   a. Regular exercise reduces the risk of developing type 1 DM.
   b. The incidence of type 2 DM can be reduced by 30 minutes of exercise 5 days a week and following a low-fat diet.
   c. Children who exercise vigorously 3 days a week lower their risk of developing type 2 DM by 65%.
   d. Regular exercise increases HgA1c levels, indicating optimal glucose utilization by muscles.

10. The latest research concerning type 2 DM development theory indicates that:
    a. Obesity increases the risk of developing type 2 DM 10-fold.
    b. High serum cortisol levels indicate optimal beta cell function.
    c. The genetic link related to developing type 2 DM is weak.
    d. Alpha cells take over beta cell function in type 2 DM.

11. When explaining DM to the PTA, the school nurse stresses that:
    a. Type 1 DM only affects small children.
    b. Type 2 DM is not usual in adolescents and young adults.
    c. An adolescent can have both type 1 and type 2 DM.
    d. Type 2 DM is the result of an inflammatory reaction destroying the pancreas.

12. The school nurse suspects hypoglycemia when Jenice, an 8-year-old with type 1 DM, is brought to the nurse because she:
    a. Has a flushed face
    b. Has clammy skin
    c. Is hyperactive
    d. Is not hungry

13. When teaching caregivers about blood glucose monitoring, the nurse stresses that hypoglycemia occurs when the serum glucose is below _____mg/dL in a preschool child.
    a. 50
    b. 60
    c. 70
    d. 80

14. The purpose of Kussmaul respirations is to:
    a. Lower the serum pH below 7.3
    b. Increase the amount of oxygen inhaled
    c. Increase the serum pH above 7.5
    d. Reduce the serum acid load

15. The nurse is reviewing the causes of DKA with the parents of a child with type 1 DM. The nurse includes which of the following as causes of DKA (select all that apply)?
    a. Eating snacks high in glucose
    b. Kinked insulin pump tubing
    c. Illness
    d. Playing sports which require running

16. Metabolic acidosis causes:
    a. Potassium to move into the extracellular space
    b. Sodium to be retained by the kidneys
    c. Serum bicarbonate levels to rise
    d. Serum magnesium levels to rise

17. The nurse conducting a class on DM for teachers stresses that a child with DKA exhibits (select all that apply):
    a. Nausea and vomiting
    b. High blood pressure
    c. Slow pulse rate
    d. Thirst

18. A child with DKA has a fruity odor to their breath because:
    a. The blood glucose level is high.
    b. Dehydration occurs.
    c. Carbon dioxide is exhaled in large amounts.
    d. Acetone is exhaled.

19. An adolescent with hyperglycemic hyperosmolar nonketonic syndrome will have which of the following laboratory values?
    a. Serum glucose of 250–400
    b. Low serum osmolality
    c. Serum glucose above 800
    d. Serum pH below 7.3

20. Kenisha, a 20-year-old with type 2 DM, is in danger of developing hyperglycemic hyperosmolar nonketonic syndrome if:
    a. Her insulin pump is empty.
    b. She exercises vigorously on a hot day and does not drink fluids.
    c. She has a hot fudge sundae at a picnic.
    d. Her nighttime snack is high in sugar.

21. Which of the following statements about macrovascular disease is correct?
    a. More men with type 2 DM than women with type 2 DM develop coronary artery disease.
    b. Adolescents with type 2 DM have a low risk of developing macrovascular disease.
    c. People with type 2 DM and macrovascular disease are more likely to die of a myocardial infarction than people in the general population.
    d. Approximately 55% of people with type 2 DM will die of macrovascular disease.

22. Macrovascular disease is thought to develop in people with type 2 DM because (select all that apply):
    a. Their serum lipid levels are high.
    b. They are likely to have hypertension.
    c. Their platelets stick together easily.
    d. They are likely to have atherosclerosis.

23. Microvascular disease develops in people with DM because:
   a. Protein deposits on capillary walls cause occlusion.
   b. They are prone to hypotension.
   c. They are prone to develop salt and water retention.
   d. Large vessels are narrowed by fat deposits.

24. To reduce their chance of developing nephropathy, an adolescent with type 1 DM should maintain their:
   a. HgA1c between 8.2% and 8.9%
   b. Blood pressure at a normotensive state
   c. Total cholesterol below 210
   d. Albuminuria below 30 mg/24 hour

25. Which of the following statements concerning retinopathy is correct (select all that apply)?
   a. Retinopathy develops more quickly in type 1 DM than in type 2 DM.
   b. Retinopathy is strongly correlated with a HgA1c below 6.5%.
   c. Retinopathy does not develop before age 40.
   d. Retinopathy includes cataracts and retinal detachment.

26. Which of the following statements concerning neuropathy is correct?
   a. Somatic neuropathy results in gastroparesis.
   b. Pain that occurs as a result of autonomic neuropathy is associated with increased pain impulse conduction.
   c. Somatic neuropathy can cause sensations such as vibration.
   d. Autonomic neuropathy may result in tachycardia.

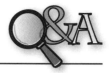

ANSWERS AND RATIONALES

1.   **The answer is a.** Rationale: The brain and nervous system cannot store glucose.

2.   **The answer is c.** Rationale: The brain is the major consumer of glucose, muscle tissue utilizes glucose for energy, and two thirds of the glucose from each meal is stored for later use. During gluconeogenesis the liver converts amino acids, glycerol, and lactic acid to glucose.

3.   **The answers are b and c.** Rationale: The beta cells produce insulin, and insulin increases protein synthesis.

4.   **The answer is d.** Rationale: HgA1c indicates serum glucose levels for the past 90 days, whereas C-peptide indicates daily insulin production.

5.   **The answer is c.** Rationale: An identical twin has a 50% chance of developing DM if the other twin has the disease, type 2 DM is associated with hypercholesterolemia but is not caused by a high-fat diet, and insulin antibodies are an indication of type 1 DM, an autoimmune disease.

6.   **The answer is b.** Rationale: Limiting dietary glucose does not prevent type 1 DM; the majority of type 1 DM cases involve school-aged children and adolescence, and thirst is a cardinal sign of type 1 DM.

7.   **The answer is d.** Rationale: The optimal level of HgA1c is below 7%, and a rising level indicates poor glucose control.

8.   **The answers are a, b, and c.** Rationale: C-peptide levels rise for a short time in people with type 2 DM but then fall as beta cells become exhausted and insulin production slows.

9.   **The answer is b.** Rationale: Exercise does not prevent type 1 DM, an autoimmune disease, but it will help prevent the development of type 2 DM; 30 minutes of exercise 5 times a week has been shown to reduce the risk of developing type 2 DM by almost 60%.

10. **The answer is a.** Rationale: High serum cortisol indicates abdominal obesity, a risk factor for developing type 2 DM; the genetic link for developing type 2 DM is strong (80% of children whose parents have type 2 DM will develop the disease).

11. **The answer is c.** Rationale: Children can have both type 1 DM, an autoimmune disease, and type 2 DM, insulin resistance. These children often take an oral hypoglycemic to decrease insulin resistance and insulin to replace what their beta cells can no longer produce.

12. **The answer is b.** Rationale: The child with hypoglycemia presents as pale, drowsy, and hungry.

13. **The answer is c.** Rationale: A blood glucose below 60 in a child or below 70 in a preschool-aged child indicates hypoglycemia.

14. **The answer is d.** Rationale: Deep rapid Kussmaul respirations rid the body of carbon dioxide so that less carbonic acid is produced, thereby reducing the body's acid load; the goal is to return the pH to WNL of 7.35–7.45.

15. **The answers are b and c.** Rationale: DKA is caused by a lack of insulin such as would occur with kinked insulin pump tubing and/ or by illness, which raises the blood glucose level.

16. **The answer is a.** Rationale: Metabolic acidosis moves potassium out of cells into the extracellular space.

17. **The answers are a and d**. Rationale: The child with DKA will have hypotension and tachycardia.

18. **The answer is d.** Rationale: As fat is utilized for energy acetone is produced, which has a fruity odor; a high blood glucose level alone will not produce acetone; carbon dioxide is odorless.

19. **The answer is c.** Rationale: HHNKS does not result in ketoacidosis; the serum osmolality will be high because of the glucose load.

20. **The answer is b.** Rationale: Dehydration leads to HHNKS, in type 2 DM insulin continues to be produced by the beta cells, and an insulin pump is not used.

21. **The answer is c.** Rationale: Men and women are equally at risk for macrovascular disease, adolescents with type 2 DM are at high risk for developing macrovascular disease, and up to 75% of people with type 2 DM die of macrovascular disease.

22. **The answers are a, b, c, and d**.

23. **The answer is a.** Rationale: As capillary size diminishes due to protein deposits, circulation is impaired.

24. **The answer is b.** Rationale: Hypertension and uncontrolled DM cause nephropathy, a HgA1c indicates poor glucose control, and albumin in the urine indicates renal damage.

25. **The answers are a and d.** Rationale: Retinopathy can develop as early as 20 years of age, and a HgA1c of 6.5% indicates excellent glucose control and lowers the risk of developing retinopathy.

26. **The answer is c.** Rationale: Autonomic neuropathy leads to gastroparesis and a decreased cardiac response, and pain conduction slows with neuropathy.

XII

Eye and Ear Disorders

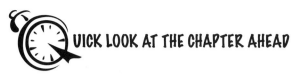

QUICK LOOK AT THE CHAPTER AHEAD

This chapter discusses common eye injuries and disorders associated with infancy and childhood.

29

Vision Development and Disorders of the Newborn Infant

TERMS

- ☐ Acquired glaucoma
- ☐ Angle-closure glaucoma
- ☐ Aqueous humor
- ☐ Astigmatism
- ☐ Barkan membrane
- ☐ Buphthalmos
- ☐ Congenital glaucoma
- ☐ Deprivation amblyopia
- ☐ Glaucoma
- ☐ Hyperopia
- ☐ Juvenile glaucoma
- ☐ Myopia
- ☐ Open-angle glaucoma
- ☐ Refractive amblyopia
- ☐ Secondary glaucoma
- ☐ Strabismic amblyopia
- ☐ Strabismus

243

Myelination of the optic nerve is not complete until the infant's eyes have been exposed to light for approximately 10 weeks; therefore although the newborn can see at birth, his or her visual acuity is usually between 20/100 and 20/400, making him or her hyperoptic (farsighted). Newborns cannot distinguish color and detail clearly. The infant sees best when objects are about 8 inches from his or her eyes. By age 2 or 3 the child's visual acuity is 20/50, and by age 6 or 7 it is 20/20. It takes about 6 weeks for the lacrimal glands to mature, so although the newborn cries no tears are produced until he or she is approximately 1½ months old. The newborn's sclera is thin, translucent, and bluish tinged, with a blue or gray iris. By 6 months of age the infant's eye color matures and becomes permanent.

During the birth process a corneal tear or subconjunctival hemorrhage may occur. Newborn eye assessment includes observing for persistent and irregular uncoordinated eye movements and leukokoria (white pupil). If warranted, an ophthalmologist assesses the infant for iris abnormalities, including Brushfield spots associated with trisomy 21, colobomas (gap in the optic nerve or other eye structure), red reflex abnormalities, and chorioretinitis (congenital viral infection) (Table 29-1).

 ## ECCHYMOSIS

A child may sustain orbital and soft tissue ecchymosis of the eyelid (black eye) related to a sport or playground injury, to a physical altercation with another child, or to child abuse. Because it is possible that an orbital fracture has occurred, eye injuries must be assessed, including eye movement and intraocular pressure (IOP). Cold compresses or ice packs applied for 5–10 minutes at a time may help reduce hemorrhage and edema.

Safety goggles should be worn by the child when playing sports (e.g., hockey, baseball, tennis, and racquetball) or when conducting experiments in chemistry or industrial arts classes to prevent eye injuries. Avoidance of extreme sports, such as bungee jumping, and prohibiting children from playing with fireworks or participating in paint ball games may also help prevent eye injuries.

 ## BURNS

Eyelid burns may occur because of contact with a curling iron or a lighted cigarette. The conjunctiva and cornea may also be burned by thermal, chemical, or radiant energy. Ultraviolet keratitis may occur when skiing on a bright day without wearing goggles. Exposure to exploding batteries, drain cleaner, and bleach can cause chemical burns, which require immediate eye irrigation and emergency care. Alkaline agents

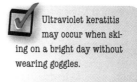

Ultraviolet keratitis may occur when skiing on a bright day without wearing goggles.

Table 29-1 Common Signs and Symptoms of Eye Disease

Signs	Meaning
Redness (injection)	Superficial or penetrating foreign bodies Infection Allergy Conjunctivitis associated with Stevens-Johnson syndrome or Kawasaki's disease Irritating agents, trauma Vascular abnormalities Tumor (rare)
Tearing	Nasolacrimal obstruction (infants) Congenital glaucoma Inflammation, allergy Viral disease Conjunctival and corneal irritation
Discharge	Bacterial conjunctivitis (purulent) Nasolacrimal obstruction (mucopurulent, infants/toddlers) Viral infection, iritis, superficial foreign bodies, nasolacrimal obstruction (watery) Allergic conjunctivitis, nasolacrimal obstruction (mucoid)
Pain and foreign body sensation	Foreign bodies Corneal abrasion Lacerations Acute infection, iritis Angle-closure glaucoma Headache (large refractive errors, poor accommodation, sinus disease) Trichiasis (in-turned eyelash) Contact lens problems
Photophobia	Corneal abrasions, foreign bodies Iritis Squinting of one eye in bright light sign of intermittent strabismus Present in infants/children with glaucoma, albinism, retinal dystrophies and aniridia (underdeveloped eye) Common after ocular surgery Common after pupil dilation Present with migraine headache, meningitis, optic neuritis

Table 29-1 Common Signs and Symptoms of Eye Disease (continued)

Signs	Meaning
Leukocoria (white pupil)	Retinoblastoma Retinopathy of prematurity Papillary membrane Cataract Vitreous opacity Retinal detachment, retinal dysplasia *Toxocara* infection (roundworm)
Brushfield spots (speckled iris)	Small, white, slightly elevated spots on the surface of the iris Ring pattern Normal or associated with trisomy 21 (Down's syndrome)

cause a deeper burn than do acidic agents because alkaline substances penetrate deeper into tissue.

NONACCIDENTAL TRAUMA AND SHAKEN BABY SYNDROME

Retinal hemorrhage and subdural hematoma are features of nonaccidental trauma and shaken baby syndrome and should always be investigated thoroughly. How severe the retinal hemorrhage presents is generally a sign of how severely the brain is damaged. Other reasons a retinal hemorrhage may occur include blood disorders.

Retinal hemorrhage and subdural hematoma are features of nonaccidental trauma and shaken baby syndrome.

REFRACTIVE ERRORS

Three common errors of refraction are **myopia** (nearsightedness), **hyperopia** (farsightedness), and **astigmatism** (irregularly shaped cornea or lens). These conditions occur most frequently in children born prematurely, those with Down's syndrome, those with parents who have refractive errors, and those with conditions such as Marfan's syndrome, an inherited connective tissue disorder. In approximately half of the children with Marfan's syndrome the lens of the eye is off center. They many also have myopia, cataracts, or retinal detachment. Glasses and contact lenses can correct all three errors. Laser correction is not recommended for most children but is an option for adolescents.

Myopia

A child who has myopia (nearsightedness) sees close objects clearly, but more distant objects are blurred because light rays focus in front of the retina. The child with myopia may complain of headaches and may squint to improve distance vision clarity. Myopia usually begins around age 8 and progresses into young adulthood.

Hyperopia

A child who has hyperopia (farsightedness) can see distant objects clearly but may see closer objects with blurred vision because light rays focus behind the retina. Hyperopia is common until a child is about 10 years of age. If severe and left uncorrected, the child may develop crossed eyes (esotropia) and amblyopia. Hyperopia is common in infants, but self corrects by the time the baby is a toddler.

Astigmatism

Normally, the cornea (crystalline lens) is perfectly spherical. If it is not, then objects will appear out of focus or blurred. If the astigmatism is severe and left untreated, amblyopia may result.

AMBLYOPIA

Visual development (clear retinal image) is a learned function that occurs during the first 10 years of life and depends on well-aligned eyes and a normal visual field. If a child has an eye disease or refractive error that is not corrected, then amblyopia or decreased vision results. Amblyopia may

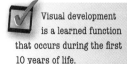
Visual development is a learned function that occurs during the first 10 years of life.

occur in one or both eyes and is present in approximately 3% to 7% of children.

The types of amblyopia include strabismic, refractive, and deprivation. **Strabismic amblyopia**, commonly called "lazy eye," occurs when one eye becomes stronger, subduing the image of the weaker eye. **Refractive amblyopia** may occur in one or both eyes if the refractive error is not corrected. **Deprivation amblyopia** occurs when a dense cataract or complete ptosis occurs, preventing the retina of the affected eye from receiving an image.

Treatment varies according to the cause and includes correction of refractive errors or surgery to remove cataracts. Once the cause is corrected or removed, the "good" eye is patched to force the weaker eye to process visual input and improve vision.

 ## STRABISMUS

By the time an infant is 5 to 6 months old their eye muscles should be of equal strength, producing constantly well-aligned eyes when looking at an object. **Strabismus**, or misalignment of the eyes, occurs in 2–3% of children and is classified as esotropia (inward deviation, or "crossed eyes") or exotropia (outward deviation). Esotropia is classified as congenital or acquired. Congenital esotropia occurs during the first year of life, is obvious when looking at the infant, and is corrected by surgery. Congenital esotropia can also be related to syndromes or central nervous system conditions such as intracranial hemorrhage.

Acquired esotropia is commonly caused by an accommodation error and begins when the child is between 2 and 5 years of age. In this type of esotropia the child may have myopia or hyperopia. Treatment includes glasses (perhaps bifocals), amblyopia treatment, and/or surgery. A child past age 5 who develops esotropia should be screened for central nervous system diseases such as hydrocephalus, idiopathic intracranial hypertension, and tumors.

A child past age 5 who develops esotropia should be screened for central nervous system diseases such as hydrocephalus, idiopathic intracranial hypertension, and tumors.

Infants rarely exhibit exotropia, and any child who exhibits constant exotropia should have a complete neurological workup to detect an underlying central nervous system disorder. Children older than 2 years of age may develop intermittent exotropia, which is usually treated with surgery, patching, eye exercises, and sometimes glasses.

GLAUCOMA

Increased IOP causes **glaucoma** by damaging the optic nerve; left untreated, glaucoma leads to loss of peripheral vision and blindness. Glaucoma is generally classified as open angle (also chronic or simple) or angle closure (also acute, closed angle, or narrow angle). Causes of glaucoma include infections, trauma, tumors, and hemorrhage; however, the most common cause is narrowing or blockage of the aqueous outflow channel.

Aqueous humor, a thin watery fluid continually produced by the ciliary body, fills the space between the cornea and the iris (anterior chamber). Its functions include feeding the cornea and lens and giving the front of the eye shape. Usually, aqueous humor flows freely from the posterior chamber of the eye through the pupil and into the anterior chamber. It leaves the anterior chamber via a trabecular mesh (canals) and enters the Canal of Schlemm, which connects to the bloodstream. When the production and absorption of aqueous humor is balanced, the IOP is between 8 and 21 mm Hg.

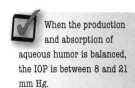

When the production and absorption of aqueous humor is balanced, the IOP is between 8 and 21 mm Hg.

In **open-angle glaucoma** the anterior chamber angle is open but there is an obstruction in the trabecular mesh leading to the Canal of Schlemm. In **angle-closure glaucoma** the anterior chamber is narrowed or closed, preventing the outflow of aqueous humor. Causes of angle-closure glaucoma include thickening of the lens or a forward movement of the lens, resulting in the lens pressing against the iris.

Congenital Glaucoma

Congenital glaucoma, an inherited disorder, occurs in 1 in 5,000 to 10,000 births. Children with siblings or parents with congenital glaucoma should be screened for the disorder. Photophobia, blepharos-pasm, and tearing are usual presenting symptoms and may be severe. The infant or toddler up to age 3 may also present with enlargement of the globe of the eye, called **buphthalmos**, and corneal clouding. IOP is increased because of blockage in the aqueous humor outflow channel caused by a membrane covering the trabecular channels (**Barkan membrane**) or by a thick iris. After age 3 glaucoma generally presents as optic nerve changes only. The most effective treatment for congenital glaucoma is surgery.

Secondary Glaucoma

Glaucoma that occurs after 3 years of age is termed **secondary glaucoma,** and it may be either open angle or angle closure. Secondary open-angle glaucoma occurs when eye disease causes the IOP to rise but the anterior chamber angle remains open.

Juvenile glaucoma is a type of open-angle glaucoma that develops after age 3 but before age 20. It may be an inherited disorder and is more common in children who have myopia (nearsightedness). The treatment for juvenile glaucoma is either medication or surgery. Because open-angle glaucoma develops over many years, it generally does not cause symptoms until peripheral vision is lost. Other signs and symptoms include seeing halos around lights, blurring of vision, myopia, and difficulty seeing in the dark.

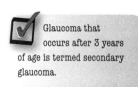
Glaucoma that occurs after 3 years of age is termed secondary glaucoma.

Acquired glaucoma is another type of secondary glaucoma and may be caused by trauma or infection or by cataract removal. If there is an acute rise in IOP, the child will complain of severe eye pain, blurred vision, seeing halos around lights, a cloudy cornea, nausea, and vomiting.

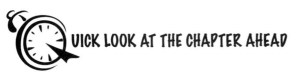

This chapter provides an overview of commonly occurring eye disorders including infections and conditions which may lead to blindness.

30

Eye Disorders

TERMS
- [ ] Blepharitis
- [ ] Cataracts
- [ ] Conjunctiva

DISEASES OF THE EYELIDS

Blepharitis

Blepharitis, inflammation of the lid margin, may be caused by a bacterial infection, commonly *Staphylococcus.* Crusts appear at the base of the eyelashes, along with erythema (redness) and in severe cases corneal ulcers. Bacterial blepharitis is treated with topical antibiotics and lid washes with a nonburning baby shampoo.

Another cause of blepharitis is a louse infestation (*Phthirus pubis*). Use of a magnifying glass allows visualization of nits and adult lice on the eyelashes. Removal of the parasites and topical application of phospholine iodide or 1% mercuric oxide is the recommended treatment.

A localized infection of the sebaceous glands of the eyelid (hordeolum) produces red, painful, localized swelling, whereas a localized infection of the oil-secreting glands of the eyelid (chalazion) produces a painless localized swelling on the eyelid.

DISEASES OF THE CONJUNCTIVA

Ophthalmia Neonatorum

Conjunctivitis in the newborn (ophthalmia neonatorum) may occur during the first 4 weeks of age and presents as redness, swelling, and discharge of the eyelids and conjunctiva. Common causes of ophthalmia neonatorum include silver nitrate drops used at birth, viral infection (herpes simplex), or bacterial infection (gonococcal, staphylococcal, or chlamydial). If caused by *Neisseria gonorrhoeae* vision loss may occur. It is important to note that silver nitrate drops do not protect the infant from acquiring a chlamydia infection during a vaginal birth. Treatment is achieved by specific antibiotics that target the responsible organism.

 It is important to note that silver nitrate drops do not protect the infant from acquiring a chlamydia infection during a vaginal birth.

DISEASES OF THE EYELIDS

Blepharitis

Blepharitis, inflammation of the lid margin, may be caused by a bacterial infection, commonly *Staphylococcus*. Crusts appear at the base of the eyelashes, along with erythema (redness) and in severe cases corneal ulcers. Bacterial blepharitis is treated with topical antibiotics and lid washes with a nonburning baby shampoo.

Another cause of blepharitis is a louse infestation (*Phthirus pubis*). Use of a magnifying glass allows visualization of nits and adult lice on the eyelashes. Removal of the parasites and topical application of phospholine iodide or 1% mercuric oxide is the recommended treatment.

A localized infection of the sebaceous glands of the eyelid (hordeolum) produces red, painful, localized swelling, whereas a localized infection of the oil-secreting glands of the eyelid (chalazion) produces a painless localized swelling on the eyelid.

DISEASES OF THE CONJUNCTIVA

Ophthalmia Neonatorum

Conjunctivitis in the newborn (ophthalmia neonatorum) may occur during the first 4 weeks of age and presents as redness, swelling, and discharge of the eyelids and conjunctiva. Common causes of ophthalmia neonatorum include silver nitrate drops used at birth, viral infection (herpes simplex), or bacterial infection (gonococcal, staphylococcal, or chlamydial). If caused by *Neisseria gonorrhoeae* vision loss may occur. It is important to note that silver nitrate drops do not protect the infant from acquiring a chlamydia infection during a vaginal birth. Treatment is achieved by specific antibiotics that target the responsible organism.

 It is important to note that silver nitrate drops do not protect the infant from acquiring a chlamydia infection during a vaginal birth.

Infants rarely exhibit exotropia, and any child who exhibits constant exotropia should have a complete neurological workup to detect an underlying central nervous system disorder. Children older than 2 years of age may develop intermittent exotropia, which is usually treated with surgery, patching, eye exercises, and sometimes glasses.

GLAUCOMA

Increased IOP causes **glaucoma** by damaging the optic nerve; left untreated, glaucoma leads to loss of peripheral vision and blindness. Glaucoma is generally classified as open angle (also chronic or simple) or angle closure (also acute, closed angle, or narrow angle). Causes of glaucoma include infections, trauma, tumors, and hemorrhage; however, the most common cause is narrowing or blockage of the aqueous outflow channel.

Aqueous humor, a thin watery fluid continually produced by the ciliary body, fills the space between the cornea and the iris (anterior chamber). Its functions include feeding the cornea and lens and giving the front of the eye shape. Usually, aqueous humor flows freely from the posterior chamber of the eye through the pupil and into the anterior chamber. It leaves the anterior chamber via a trabecular mesh (canals) and enters the Canal of Schlemm, which connects to the bloodstream. When the production and absorption of aqueous humor is balanced, the IOP is between 8 and 21 mm Hg.

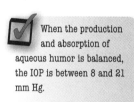 When the production and absorption of aqueous humor is balanced, the IOP is between 8 and 21 mm Hg.

In **open-angle glaucoma** the anterior chamber angle is open but there is an obstruction in the trabecular mesh leading to the Canal of Schlemm. In **angle-closure glaucoma** the anterior chamber is narrowed or closed, preventing the outflow of aqueous humor. Causes of angle-closure glaucoma include thickening of the lens or a forward movement of the lens, resulting in the lens pressing against the iris.

Congenital Glaucoma

Congenital glaucoma, an inherited disorder, occurs in 1 in 5,000 to 10,000 births. Children with siblings or parents with congenital glaucoma should be screened for the disorder. Photophobia, blepharospasm, and tearing are usual presenting symptoms and may be severe. The infant or toddler up to age 3 may also present with enlargement of the globe of the eye, called **buphthalmos**, and corneal clouding. IOP is increased because of blockage in the aqueous humor outflow channel caused by a membrane covering the trabecular channels (**Barkan membrane**) or by a thick iris. After age 3 glaucoma generally presents as optic nerve changes only. The most effective treatment for congenital glaucoma is surgery.

Secondary Glaucoma

Glaucoma that occurs after 3 years of age is termed **secondary glaucoma,** and it may be either open angle or angle closure. Secondary open-angle glaucoma occurs when eye disease causes the IOP to rise but the anterior chamber angle remains open.

   Juvenile glaucoma is a type of open-angle glaucoma that develops after age 3 but before age 20. It may be an inherited disorder and is more common in children who have myopia (nearsightedness). The treatment for juvenile glaucoma is either medication or surgery. Because open-angle glaucoma develops over many years, it generally does not cause symptoms until peripheral vision is lost. Other signs and symptoms include seeing halos around lights, blurring of vision, myopia, and difficulty seeing in the dark.

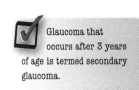 Glaucoma that occurs after 3 years of age is termed secondary glaucoma.

   Acquired glaucoma is another type of secondary glaucoma and may be caused by trauma or infection or by cataract removal. If there is an acute rise in IOP, the child will complain of severe eye pain, blurred vision, seeing halos around lights, a cloudy cornea, nausea, and vomiting.

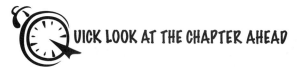

QUICK LOOK AT THE CHAPTER AHEAD

This chapter provides an overview of commonly occurring eye disorders including infections and conditions which may lead to blindness.

30

Eye Disorders

TERMS
- ☐ **Blepharitis**
- ☐ **Cataracts**
- ☐ **Conjunctiva**

Bacterial Conjunctivitis

The **conjunctiva**, which lines the posterior surface of the eyelids and anterior surface of the cornea, is a thin transparent mucous membrane. When this area becomes inflamed in response to exposure to viruses, bacteria, chemicals, or allergens it is called conjunctivitis. Bacterial conjunctivitis, which produces a purulent discharge, may affect one or both eyes, may be caused by a local or systemic infection, and is highly contagious. Bacteria commonly responsible for the infection include *Staphylococcus aureus*, *Bartonella henselae* (responsible for cat-scratch fever) and *Haemophilus*.

Children and adolescents who do not care for their contact lenses properly are at risk for developing bacterial conjunctivitis. Infections are treated by the application of topical antibiotics or systemic antibiotics if the causative pathogen is *Chlamydia trachomatis, N. gonorrhoeae,* or *Neisseria meningitides.*

Children and adolescents who do not care for their contact lenses properly are at risk for developing bacterial conjunctivitis.

Viral Conjunctivitis

Adenovirus infections are highly contagious, a common cause of many upper respiratory infections (URIs) during childhood, and may cause conjunctivitis. Older children may acquire the infection during the summer by swimming in lakes and pools, by sharing towels and toys, and by direct contact with an infected individual. In younger children the viruses may cause pharyngitis and conjunctivitis. Outbreaks commonly occur in daycare centers and schools. The child with this viral infection is considered contagious for approximately 2 weeks from the onset of symptoms (red eyes and tearing) and should not attend school or daycare during that time frame. A child in the prodromal stage (onset) of measles may develop conjunctivitis, as may a child with a herpes simplex infection.

When did your child's symptoms develop?

Allergic Conjunctivitis

Exposure to seasonal allergens, such as those that cause hay fever, is a common cause of allergic conjunctivitis.

Exposure to seasonal allergens, such as those that cause hay fever, is a common cause of allergic conjunctivitis. The child presents with an itchy red conjunctiva and mucoid discharge. Eye drops containing mast cell stabilizers, topical vasoconstrictors, and/or antihistamines are the treatment of choice.

DISORDERS OF THE CORNEA

Keratitis

Keratitis, inflammation of the cornea, can be caused by viruses such as herpes simplex, herpes zoster, or adenoviruses. Recurrent herpes simplex infections can lead to blindness. Topical antivirals and possibly systemic corticosteroids may be used to treat a herpes simplex infection, although the infection may become worse when steroids are used. Herpes zoster infections of the eye are generally treated with an oral antiviral agent. Treatment for adenoviruses is not warranted because they are self-limiting; however, they are also highly contagious.

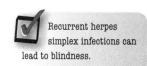

Recurrent herpes simplex infections can lead to blindness.

Contact lens wearers may develop *Acanthamoeba* keratitis (caused by an ameboid protozoan), leading to blindness. Using a contaminated contact lens solution; wearing contacts when swimming in pools, lakes, or seawater; storing contact lenses in homemade solutions; and poor contact lens hygiene are all causes of this condition. Signs and symptoms include severe eye pain and redness but little discharge. Microscopic examination of the cells taken from the cornea confirms the diagnosis. Year-long treatment with antibiotics and antifungals is necessary. If corneal scarring occurs, corneal transplantation may be required.

Contact lens wearers may develop *Acanthamoeba* keratitis (caused by an ameboid protozoan), leading to blindness. Using a contaminated contact lens solution; wearing contacts when swimming in pools, lakes, or seawater; storing contact lenses in homemade solutions; and poor contact lens hygiene are all causes of this condition.

DISORDERS OF THE LENS

Cataracts

Cataracts, or cloudiness of the eye lens, may affect one or both eyes, may be congenital, or may be related to chromosomal abnormalities or systemic disease such as infection. Children younger than 9 years of age may develop deprivation amblyopia if the cataract is not diagnosed and treated early. Contact lenses, glasses, and in some cases cataract extraction and intraocular lens implantation are treatment choices to improve vision.

DISORDERS OF THE RETINA

Retinopathy of Prematurity

Infants born before 28 weeks' gestation and weighing less than 1,250 g are at risk for developing retinopathy of prematurity (ROP) and possible strabismus, amblyopia, myopia, glaucoma, and partial or total blindness. ROP is a result of abnormal peripheral retinal vascularization, including arteriole constriction and propagation of abnormal blood vessels, which leads to retinal detachment. In the full-term newborn, normal retinal vascularization occurs by 32 weeks' gestation. ROP, which affects approximately 12.5% of infants born between 23 and 26 weeks' gestation, develops more often in white newborns than in African-American newborns. Risk factors associated with ROP in addition to low birth weight and prematurity include artificial ventilation, bronchopulmonary dysplasia, sepsis, apnea, multiple blood transfusions, acidosis, shock, heart disease, infection, and bradycardia.

Whether or not a premature infant develops blindness because of ROP appears to be more highly correlated with birth weight and gestational age than with supplemental oxygen administration. Infants weighing less than 1,500 g and born less than 33 weeks' gestation have the highest risk of developing retinal detachment and blindness. The role that exposure to nursery ambient light plays in the development of ROP is inconclusive. The most recent research is focusing on the role vascular endothelial growth factor plays in ROP.

Retinoblastoma

The most common intraocular malignancy of childhood is retinoblastoma, which may be autosomal dominant (inherited) or spontaneous and may present as one or more tumors in one or both eyes. Children with the autosomal dominant type are also at risk for developing pineal tumors, osteosarcoma, and other soft tissue sarcomas.

Retinoblastoma may present as leukocoria (white lens), strabismus, red eye, glaucoma, or pseudohypopyon (pus-like material in the anterior chamber). The newest treatment, chemoreduction of the tumor, is aimed at preserving sight, although for large tumors enucleation (removal of the eye) is required. Genetic testing is recommended for all family members to help determine future reproductive risks.

Retinal Detachment

Retinal detachment in children is not common but can occur related to trauma, ROP, Marfan's syndrome, and Stickler's syndrome. If the child is old enough to verbalize symptoms, he or she may complain of seeing floaters and flashing lights and loss of visual fields. Younger children may be diagnosed after being referred to an ophthalmologist because they failed a vision test or have developed strabismus or leukocoria (white lens). Regardless of the cause, the treatment of retinal detachment is surgery.

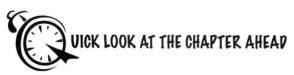

QUICK LOOK AT THE CHAPTER AHEAD

This chapter discusses the etiology of internal and external ear infections which commonly occur in childhood.

31

Ear Disorders

TERMS
☐ Eustachian tube
☐ Middle ear
☐ Otitis externa
☐ Otitis media

257

MIDDLE EAR STRUCTURE

The **middle ear** is a pea-sized, sealed, air-filled cavity that gives the paper-thin eardrum the ability to vibrate easily (compliance) and to transmit sound waves from the three tiny bones in the middle ear to the inner ear and then to the brain for processing. The **eustachian tube,** composed of membrane and cartilage, is a narrow tube that allows air to enter behind the sealed eardrum from the back of the nose and replace the air that is normally absorbed by the body from the middle ear. It also equalizes pressure on both sides of the eardrum and drains fluid from the middle ear. Equal pressure on both sides of the eardrum is necessary for compliance to occur. If the tube is blocked by edema or thick secretions, a vacuum develops that pulls fluid and nasopharyngeal secretions/pathogens into the middle ear. Yawning, sneezing, or swallowing results in intermittent opening of the eustachian tube, allowing fluid from the middle ear to drain and pressure to be equalized.

In children the eustachian tube is short (average length 18 mm) and lies horizontally at an approximate 10-degree angle, thereby allowing reflux of nasopharyngeal secretions into the middle ear. By adolescence the average length of the eustachian tube has increased to 31–38 mm and the angle has increased to about 45 degrees, thereby making otitis media much less common as the child matures. Adults also have a more rigid eustachian tube than do children. A floppy tube increases the likelihood of developing acute otitis media (AOM).

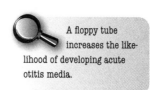

A floppy tube increases the likelihood of developing acute otitis media.

EAR INFECTIONS

Ear infections may involve the outer ear (otitis externa), middle ear (otitis media), mastoid bone (mastoiditis), and/or the inner ear (labyrinthitis).

Otitis Externa

Inflammation of the skin lining the ear canal and surrounding soft tissue is called **otitis externa**. Cerumen (ear wax) provides a protective function, and if it is lost maceration of the underlying skin is possible, leading to otitis externa. Trauma to the ear canal can also occur because of drainage from a perforated tympanic membrane or from tympanic drainage tubes, the insertion of cotton-tipped applicators to clean the ear canal, poorly fitting ear plugs used when swimming, dermatitis from hair spray, ear drops, and infection from *Staphylococcus aureus* or *Pseudomonas aeruginosa*.

The child with otitis externa complains of pain and itching in the ear, especially when they chew, but hearing is normal. Attempts to inspect the ear canal are met with resistance, and drainage is usually scant. The ear canal, if visualized, appears edematous.

If the tympanic membrane can be seen and is intact, the moist cerumen and desquamated epithelium is removed by ear irrigation, and then topical antibiotic drops are instilled two or three times a day. The role of corticosteroid ear drops is unclear. If the child has systemic symptoms such as a fever, oral antibiotics, in addition to antibiotic ear drops, may be needed. Parents should be advised not to let the child swim or use cotton ear plugs during the acute phase. Prophylactic measures in a child who is prone to develop otitis externa and who has an intact tympanic membrane include instilling two to three gtts of a 1:1 solution of white vinegar and 70% ethyl alcohol into the ears before and after swimming.

> Trauma to the ear canal can also occur because of drainage from a perforated tympanic membrane or from tympanic drainage tubes, the insertion of cotton-tipped applicators to clean the ear canal, poorly fitting ear plugs used when swimming, dermatitis from hair spray, ear drops, and infection from *Staphylococcus aureus* or *Pseudomonas aeruginosa*.

Otitis Media

Otitis media is an inflammation of the middle ear. AOM is the term used to describe an infection of the middle ear and is the most common bacterial illness in children. *Streptococcus pneumoniae, Haemophilus influenzae,* and *Moraxella catarrhalis* are the bacteria responsible for most cases of bacterial otitis media. Signs and symptoms of AOM include a sudden onset of ear pain, erythema of the tympanic membrane, and middle ear effusion (bulging of the tympanic membrane, decreased mobility of the membrane, and otorrhea). Otitis media with effusion is defined as fluid in the middle ear that is not accompanied by infection and the inflammatory process.

Several factors, including bacterial nasopharyngeal colonization, frequent upper respiratory infections (URIs), exposure to cigarette smoke, allergies, immunocompromised status, possible genetic susceptibility, male gender, use of a pacifier for several hours per day, and a short eustachian tube, make AOM common in children.

Infants and children in daycare acquire different serotypes of nasopharyngeal pathogens and thus develop AOM more frequently than infants and children not in daycare. Approximately 70% of infants younger than 12 months of age will have at least one episode of AOM, especially between 6 and 12 months of age. Use of a pacifier raises the soft palate, allowing nasopharyngeal pathogens to enter the eustachian tube.

Viral respiratory infections play a role in AOM by increasing the colonization of the nasopharynx with viruses causing edema of the adenoids and hindering eustachian tube function. Children who are bottle fed, exposed to cigarette smoke, placed in daycare, or have siblings are at risk for developing frequent viral respiratory infections and AOM.

> Viral respiratory infections play a role in AOM by increasing the colonization of the nasopharynx with viruses causing edema of the adenoids and hindering eustachian tube function.

Effects of exposure to cigarette smoke include stronger pathogen attachment to the middle ear and production of an inflammatory response that hinders eustachian tube function. Smoking also hinders normal ciliary action in the eustachian tube so that it does not drain the middle ear effectively. The impact of exposing children ages 12 to 18 months to cigarette smoke is significant. Exposure to each pack of cigarettes smoked by someone in the home and/or car increases the duration of otitis media by 11%.

Breast-feeding lowers the risk of developing AOM by reducing the number of URIs an infant develops. IgA antibodies are passed to the child via breast milk, thus reducing colonization with pathogens associated with AOM. Breast-fed infants are also less likely to aspirate contaminated secretions because of the position assumed during breast-feeding compared with infants who are bottle fed in a supine position.

Symptoms of AOM include ear pain, fever irritability, anorexia, and vomiting. The nonverbal child frequently pulls on the infected ear and is fussy. The tympanic membrane bulges and is a yellow, white, or bright red color and exudates may be present. Some children develop persistent otorrhea lasting more than 6 weeks. It is important to note that AOM is overdiagnosed due to assessment failures. To diagnosis AOM correctly, the child's tympanic membrane must be visible and a pneumatic otoscopy performed. A red tympanic membrane is not sufficient to diagnose

AOM because a red membrane may be the result of a viral URI, crying, or trauma caused when trying to remove cerumen to visualize the tympanic membrane.

Antibiotic therapy for the treatment of AOM is controversial. Since 1990 increasingly resistant organisms have been isolated and efficacy of routine oral antibiotic therapy called into question for children over 2 years of age. The current recommendation is for children 2 years of age and younger (or those in daycare) to receive oral antibiotic therapy for AOM for 10 days due to the risk of complications if left untreated. Improvement in AOM occurs without treatment due to the body's own defense mechanisms and therefore some health care providers have adopted a watch and wait approach for children over 2 years of age rather than automatically prescribing oral antibiotics.

> Antibiotic therapy for the treatment of AOM is controversial. Since 1990 increasingly resistant organisms have been isolated and efficacy of routine oral antibiotic therapy called into question for children over 2 years of age.

If symptoms fail to resolve in 48–72 hours or if pain persists, the child aged 2 or older who is not in daycare should be reassessed and oral antibiotics prescribed for 5 days. Effective pain relief may negate the need for antibiotic therapy. Auralgan ear drops (benzocaine and antipyrine) have been shown to relieve pain in children older than age 2.

Children with persistent AOM, those younger than 48 months with painful bulging of the tympanic membrane, or those experiencing hearing loss may require tympanocentesis or myringotomy with tube placement. These procedures allow the fluid behind the tympanic membrane to drain and AOM to resolve. The heptavalent vaccine (Prevnar) has been shown to reduce AOM caused by certain bacterial strains by up to 57% and is recommended for children ages 2 to 5 with a history of recurrent AOM.

SECTION XII • REVIEW QUESTIONS

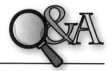

1. Vivian, who delivered 12 hours ago, asks the nurse working in the newborn nursery about her baby's eyes and vision. Which statement by the nurse is correct?
   a. All newborns are nearsighted at birth.
   b. Your baby can see objects if they are about 2 feet away.
   c. Your baby will have blue eyes as he does now.
   d. Even though your baby will cry, he will not produce tears until he is about 6 weeks old.

2. The school nurse is conducting a health education class. She stresses that to avoid eye injury the child/adolescent should (select all that apply):
   a. Wear goggles when skiing
   b. Avoid extreme sports
   c. Avoid playing contact sports such as baseball
   d. Avoid playing sports such as tennis

3. The school nurse is explaining vision screening to the teachers. Which statement by the nurse is correct?
   a. Children who have myopia are farsighted.
   b. Hyperopia cannot be corrected easily.
   c. The term astigmatism means the child has an irregularly shaped cornea.
   d. Laser vision correction is recommended for children age 9 and above.

4. Yesenia, a 6-year-old, has been diagnosed with strabismic amblyopia. When explaining this condition to Yesenia's parents the nurse should stress that:
   a. Amblyopia is always present in both eyes.
   b. The image from the weaker eye is being subdued by vision from the stronger eye.
   c. Surgery is required to correct the condition.
   d. The weaker eye is patched to strengthen it.

5. During a well baby visit, Jasmine asks the nurse if her 3-month-old baby's eyes will always be crossed. The nurse correctly explains that strabismus is:
   a. Usually self-corrected by the time the infant is 8 weeks old
   b. Is most common between the ages of 5 and 7 years
   c. Called esotropia if the deviation is inward
   d. Is caused by equally strong eye muscles in both eyes

6. The ophthalmologist diagnosed Maria, a 9-year-old, with myopia. When explaining this condition to Maria's parents the school nurse should explain that:
   a. Maria is able to see close objects clearly, but distant objects appear blurred.
   b. Myopia occurs because light rays focus in back of the retina.
   c. Maria can see distant objects clearly but words in a book appear blurry.
   d. Maria's vision will correct to 20/20 during adolescence.

7. Which of the following statements concerning glaucoma is correct?
   a. If left untreated, glaucoma leads to the loss of central vision.
   b. Normal intraocular pressure is between 12 and 25 mm Hg.
   c. Scant aqueous humor production by the ciliary body causes glaucoma.
   d. Congenital glaucoma is an inherited disorder.

8. When explaining ophthalmia neonatorum during orientation to the newborn nursery, the nurse correctly states that:
   a. Causes include silver nitrate drops or a viral infection.
   b. The condition self-corrects by age 14 days.
   c. If caused by chlamydia, blindness may result.
   d. Inflammation of the eye is a presenting sign.

9. Marcos, a 16-year-old, was diagnosed with bacterial conjunctivitis. When questioning Marcos the school nurse should ask him if he:
   a. Recently swam in a public swimming pool
   b. Has noted any drainage from his eyes
   c. Wears glasses
   d. Has recently had an upper respiratory infection

10. The nurse conducting a community health education class is asked how someone might develop *Acanthamoeba* keratitis. The nurse correctly responds that this condition may be caused by (select all that apply):
    a. Infection with herpes virus
    b. A contaminated contact lens solution
    c. Wearing contact lenses when swimming in a lake
    d. Using a homemade cleaning solution to clean contact lenses

11. Alanna delivered a premature infant 3 days ago. When visiting the newborn intensive care nursery she asks the nurse about retinopathy of prematurity. The nurse correctly explains that this condition:
    a. Is a risk for infants born before 35 weeks' gestation
    b. Is more common in African-American newborns than in white newborns
    c. Results from abnormal blood vessel development in the eye
    d. Affects almost all newborns who need supplemental oxygen after birth

12. Which of the following statements concerning the eustachian tube is correct?
    a. The eustachian tube lies at a 45-degree angle in children.
    b. The eustachian tube is floppy in children.
    c. The eustachian tube drains air from the middle ear.
    d. Swallowing closes the eustachian tube.

13. The camp nurse explains to Jose that otitis externa:
    a. Is an inflammation of the eardrum
    b. Will result in moderate temporary hearing loss
    c. Is caused by wax buildup in the ear
    d. May be caused by using poorly fitting ear plugs when swimming

14. During a well baby visit Elise, a first-time mother, asks the nurse how she will know if her baby develops otitis media. The nurse tells Elise that her baby might:
    a. Pull on the infected ear
    b. Sleep more than usual
    c. Want to eat more frequently than usual
    d. Have loose stools

15. When presenting a class to new parents concerning acute otitis media, the nurse stresses that risk factors for the development of acute otitis media include (select all that apply):
    a. Exposure to cigarette smoke
    b. The child's gender
    c. The child's age
    d. Participation in daycare

16. During a well baby visit the parents of Vanessa, a 5-month-old infant, ask the nurse if giving Vanessa a pacifier is recommended. The nurse replies that a pacifier:
    a. Promotes a strong swallowing reflex
    b. Increases the risk of developing acute otitis media
    c. Decreases the amount of formula Vanessa takes at each feeding
    d. Is safe to use up to 6 hours a day

17. During a La Leche meeting the nurse explains to the mothers that infants who are breast-fed have a reduced risk of developing acute otitis media compared with bottle-fed infants because breast-feeding (select all that apply):
    a. Reduces the frequency of upper respiratory infections
    b. Lowers the soft palate
    c. Passes IgA antibodies from mother to the infant
    d. Reduces the risk of aspiration

18. LaShone, the mother of a month-old infant, smokes a pack of cigarettes per day. The nurse encourages LaShone not to expose her infant to cigarette smoke because exposure to cigarette smoke:
    a. Increases the duration of acute otitis media by 30%
    b. Makes the eustachian tube floppy
    c. Inhibits eustachian tube ciliary action
    d. Reduces the infant's appetite

19. The nurse working in the pediatric clinic explains to the parents of Lee, a 4-month-old infant, that a red tympanic membrane may indicate (select all that apply):
    a. An ear infection
    b. A response to crying
    c. Ear drum trauma
    d. Hearing loss

20. Research has demonstrated that antibiotic treatment for acute otitis media:
   a. Should be instituted for all children under the age of 5
   b. Is indicated if ear pain lasts longer than 72 hours
   c. Should be given prophylactically to children younger than 24 months who are in daycare
   d. Has resulted in a decrease in resistant pathogens because of the high compliance rate

ANSWERS AND RATIONALES

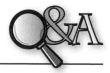

1. **The answer is d.** Rationale: At birth newborns are farsighted. They see best if objects are about 8 inches from their face. Newborns have a blue or gray eye color at birth—permanent eye color develops by 6 months of age.

2. **The answers are a and b.** Rationale: Exposure to sun glare and ultraviolet light may cause keratitis, extreme sports such as bungee jumping should be avoided, and sports such as tennis and baseball can be safely enjoyed if safety equipment is used and the rules of the game are followed.

3. **The answer is c.** Rationale: Myopia means nearsighted, hyperopia (farsightedness) is easily corrected with glasses/contact lenses, and laser vision is not recommended for children as young as 9.

4. **The answer is b.** Rationale: Strabismic amblyopia (lazy eye) results when vision from the stronger eye subdues vision from the weaker eye; the stronger eye will be patched to force the weaker eye to relay images to the retina.

5. **The answer is c.** Rationale: Eye muscles of unequal strength cause strabismus, by age 5–6 months the infants eyes should be well aligned when looking at an object, and after age 5 strabismus may indicate neurological disease.

6. **The answer is a.** Rationale: Hyperopia causes close objects to be blurred, myopia usually begins around age 8, and hyperopia causes light rays to focus behind the retina.

7. **The answer is d.** Rationale: Glaucoma leads to a loss of peripheral vision and blindness, the production of too much aqueous humor is one cause of glaucoma, and normal IOP is between 8 and 21 mm Hg.

8. **The answer is a.** Rationale: This condition may present anytime during the first month of life, infection with *Neisseria gonorrhoeae* may lead to blindness, and the conjunctiva and eyelids are inflamed.

9. **The answer is b.** Rationale: Purulent discharge is a common symptom of bacterial conjunctivitis and may develop if the

adolescent does not care for contact lenses properly; viral conjunctivitis may develop after swimming in a public pool or after an upper respiratory infection.

10. **The answers are b, c, and d.** Rationale: Keratitis may be caused by a herpes infection; however, *Acanthamoeba* keratitis is caused by a protozoan infection. Poor contact hygiene and wearing contacts when swimming are common causes of the infection.

11. **The answer is c.** Rationale: ROP affects white infants more often than African-American infants, is a risk for infants born before 33 weeks' gestation, and is more highly correlated with birth weight and gestational age than supplemental oxygen use.

12. **The answer is b.** Rationale: The eustachian tube lies at a 10-degree angle in children, opens during swallowing, and drains fluid from the middle ear.

13. **The answer is d.** Rationale: Otitis externa is an inflammation of the lining of the ear canal and surrounding soft tissue, ear wax protects these structures, and pain and itching occur but not hearing loss.

14. **The answer is a.** Rationale: Symptoms of otitis media include anorexia and fussiness.

15. **The answers are a, b, c, and d.**

16. **The answer is b.** Rationale: Use of a pacifier increases the risk of developing acute otitis media because the soft palate is raised, allowing bacteria to enter the middle ear via the eustachian tube.

17. **The answers are a, c, and d.**

18. **The answer is c.** Rationale: Exposure to each pack of cigarette smoke increases the duration of AOM by 11%, eustachian tube ciliary action is reduced, and pathogen attachment to the middle ear is strengthened.

19. **The answers are a, b, and c.** Rationale: Hearing loss is not indicated by a red tympanic membrane.

20. **The answer is b.** Rationale: Resistance to antibiotics is increasing, treatment is recommended for children younger than 24 months because of the risk of complications if left untreated, and antibiotics are not used prophylactically.

XIII

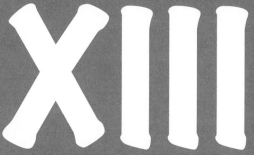

Gastrointestinal Disorders

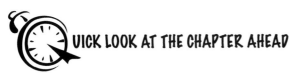

QUICK LOOK AT THE CHAPTER AHEAD

The four common disorders in the gastrointestinal (GI) system are motility, inflammatory, structural, and obstructive. Complications related to these include malabsorption, fluid and electrolyte disturbances, malnutrition, and poor growth. Examples of each of the four disorders are discussed.

32

Gastrointestinal Disorders

TERMS
- ☐ Enterocolitis
- ☐ Fistula
- ☐ Gastroenteritis
- ☐ Hirschsprung's disease
- ☐ Intussusception
- ☐ Logan's bow
- ☐ Pyloric stenosis
- ☐ Pyloromyotomy

PYLORIC STENOSIS

Pyloric stenosis is the most common upper GI disorder requiring surgery during the neonatal period (Figure 32-1). It is often seen in male infants between the ages of 1 and 6 months. It is common in first-born white males, less common among African-Americans, and rare in Asians. Increased gastrin secretion in the last trimester by the mother has been found to increase the chance of having pyloric stenosis.

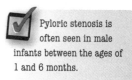
Pyloric stenosis is often seen in male infants between the ages of 1 and 6 months.

Pathophysiology

Pyloric stenosis, an example of an obstructive disorder, occurs when the muscle at the pylorus narrows and thickens due to an increase in cell size and cell number. Hypertrophy and hyperplasia cause the circular mus-

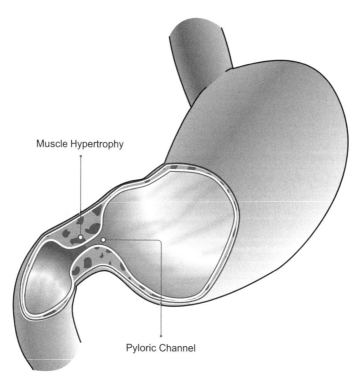

Muscle Hypertrophy

Pyloric Channel

Figure 32-1 Pyloric stenosis.

cle of the pylorus to thicken. Swelling and inflammation reduce the opening and could result in complete obstruction.

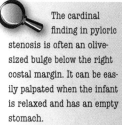

The cardinal finding in pyloric stenosis is often an olive-sized bulge below the right costal margin. It can be easily palpated when the infant is relaxed and has an empty stomach.

The cardinal finding in pyloric stenosis is often an olive-sized bulge below the right costal margin. It can be easily palpated when the infant is relaxed and has an empty stomach. Other significant symptoms include projective vomiting during or shortly after feedings, constipation, poor weight gain, and often dehydration and lethargy as the symptoms progress. If undetected, severe fluid and electrolyte imbalances can occur, such as metabolic alkalosis, often leading to chronic malnutrition and fatalities.

Treatment

Pyloric stenosis is treated by intravenous therapy to correct the electrolyte imbalances, nothing by mouth before surgery, and surgical treatment, called a **pyloromyotomy,** in which the muscles are split and separated. Feedings are usually begun 4–6 hours after surgery, and the procedure has a high success rate.

HIRSCHSPRUNG'S DISEASE

Hirschsprung's disease is a motility disorder that commonly coexists with other congenital anomalies, particularly Down's syndrome (Figure 32-2). It is four times more common in males and accounts for about one fourth of all cases of neonatal obstruction.

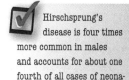

Hirschsprung's disease is four times more common in males and accounts for about one fourth of all cases of neonatal obstruction.

Pathophysiology

Hirschsprung's disease, also called congenital aganglionic megacolon, results from an absence of ganglion cells in one or more segments of the colon. The aganglionic segment is narrowed, with a dilated portion of the proximal normal colon. Lack of enervation causes peristalsis, and stool accumulates in the distal portion of the colon, resulting in obstruction. As

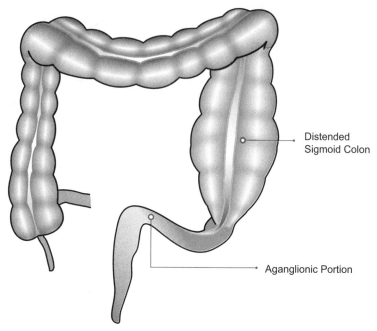

Distended
Sigmoid Colon

Aganglionic Portion

Figure 32-2 Hirschsprung's disease.

a result, findings include liquid or ribbon-like stool, distended abdomen, signs of dehydration, and often **enterocolitis**, inflammation of the small intestine and colon. In the newborn period, the newborn may fail to pass meconium within 24 to 48 hours after birth. A rectal biopsy confirms diagnosis by showing the absence of ganglionic cells.

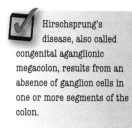

Hirschsprung's disease, also called congenital aganglionic megacolon, results from an absence of ganglion cells in one or more segments of the colon.

Treatment

Surgical resection of the aganglionic segment is the treatment of choice and is usually delayed until the child is around 6 months old. Initially, a colostomy may be created proximal to the aganglionic section to relieve obstruction. This allows the child to gain weight, gives the bowel a rest, and provides a means for the child to defecate. A second procedure would reverse the colostomy and resect or remove the involved area. This procedure is performed when the child is between 6 and 15 months of age or weighs between 18 and 20 pounds.

INTUSSUSCEPTION

Intussusception is the most frequent cause of intestinal obstruction in the first 2 years of life, peaking between the third and ninth month of life (Figure 32-3). It is twice as common in males as females, and in most cases the cause is unknown.

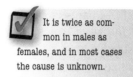
It is twice as common in males as females, and in most cases the cause is unknown.

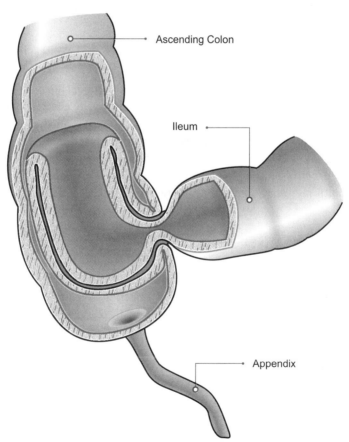

Figure 32-3 Intussusception.

Pathophysiology

Intussusception occurs in the lower gastrointestinal tract as one segment of the bowel telescopes into the lumen of the adjacent section of intestine. The walls of the bowel press against each other, become inflamed and edematous, and may cause bleeding. A cardinal sign in about one half of infants is current jelly–like stools caused by blood and mucus in the stool. As it progresses, abdominal distention and vomiting occur, eventually leading to necrosis and perforation if left untreated. The infant may appear lethargic and listless with risk of weak thready pulse, shallow respirations, and a marked elevation in temperature.

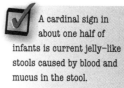 A cardinal sign in about one half of infants is current jelly–like stools caused by blood and mucus in the stool.

Treatment

Nonsurgical emergency intervention is the treatment of choice for intussusception. Studies have shown that the water-soluble contrast and air enema reduce the risk of bowel perforation and are safer than barium enemas. Successful reduction rates have been reported in 90% of cases using air and in 65–85% of cases for barium or water-soluble contrast. Any evidence of acute signs and symptoms such as perforation, shock, or peritonitis require prompt surgical intervention to be instituted.

 # GASTROENTERITIS

Acute **gastroenteritis** is an inflammation of the mucous membranes of the stomach and intestines caused by infectious agents that come on quickly, often with few other symptoms. It is the leading cause of illness in children younger than 5 years of age.

Pathophysiology

A variety of viruses, bacteria, and parasites causes gastroenteritis (Table 32-1). It is thought that the causative agent destroys or damages the epithelial cells lining the intestines, causing diarrhea, vomiting, dehydration, and electrolyte imbalances. The result is a decreased surface area and less capacity to absorb fluid and electrolytes.

Table 32-1 Infectious Causes of Acute Gastroenteritis

Viruses	Bacteria	Parasites
Rotavirus	*Escherichia coli*	*Giardia lamblia*
Adenovirus	*Shigella*	*Cryptosporidium*
Norwalk	*Salmonella*	*Entamoeba histolytica*
	Campylobacter jejuni	
	Clostridium difficile	
	Yersinia enterocolitica	

Treatment

Treatment is aimed at restoring the fluid and electrolyte balance and preventing complications. The decision about the type of management depends on the underlying agent, the age of the child, and the degree of dehydration the child presents with. Oral rehydration solutions such as Pedialyte, Infalyte, and Rehydralyte are preferred over water, carbonated beverages, and fruit juices because these do not contain the needed electrolytes. The timing and amount of fluid replacement varies depending on the age of the child and the degree of dehydration. Advancement to formula, breast milk, and a regular diet should proceed slowly and as tolerated.

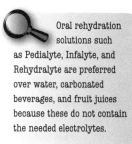

Oral rehydration solutions such as Pedialyte, Infalyte, and Rehydralyte are preferred over water, carbonated beverages, and fruit juices because these do not contain the needed electrolytes.

INFLAMMATORY BOWEL DISEASE

Inflammatory bowel disease encompasses two disorders: Crohn's disease and ulcerative colitis. The incidence and frequency of the two disorders varies greatly from geographical location and ethnic background. However, some researchers hypothesize that complex genetic and unidentified environmental factors play a role in the etiology. The greatest risk factor is having an immediate relative with inflammatory bowel disease; coming from Jewish or middle European origin and living in an urban

The greatest risk factor is having an immediate relative with inflammatory bowel disease; coming from Jewish or middle European origin and living in an urban environment increase the risk. Men and women are affected equally.

environment increase the risk. Men and women are affected equally. Statistics have shown an increase in the diagnosis and incidence of young adults and adolescents diagnosed with inflammatory bowel disease, but no definitive reasons have been determined.

Pathophysiology

Crohn's disease and ulcerative colitis are often discussed together, but they do have specific signs and symptoms and etiology (Table 32-2). Crohn's disease most commonly affects the terminal ileum (30–70%), involves the ileum and colon in 60% of the cases, and is limited to only the colon in a small percentage of cases. Most children present with abdominal pain, diarrhea, weight loss, and anorexia, often with marked growth retardation. The abdominal pain may be crampy, diarrhea may contain occult blood, and urgency to defecate may also be present.

A characteristic feature of Crohn's disease is the demarcated granulomatous lesions that are surrounded by normal mucosal tissue. All layers of the bowel are affected, and after a while the bowel often becomes thickened and inflexible. Another characteristic feature is that the lesions often "skip" segments of bowel, being interspersed with normal segments of bowel. Because Crohn's disease usually involves the submucosal layer more than the mucosal layer, there is often less bloody diarrhea.

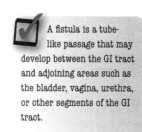

A fistula is a tube-like passage that may develop between the GI tract and adjoining areas such as the bladder, vagina, urethra, or other segments of the GI tract.

A common complication of Crohn's disease is the formation of fistulas. A **fistula** is a tube-like passage that may develop between the GI tract and adjoining areas such as the bladder, vagina, urethra, or other segments of the GI tract.

Ulcerative colitis is usually confined to the rectum and colon. The disease usually begins in the rectum, progressing proximally and continuously, affecting primarily the mucosal layer. One characteristic of the disease is the presence of lesions that lead to the formation of minute hemorrhages. These lesions may become necrotic and ulcerate. Signs and symptoms include gross rectal bleeding, severe diarrhea, mild to moderate anorexia and weight loss, and mild growth retardation.

Table 32-1 Comparison of the Two Types of Inflammatory Bowel Disease

	Crohn's Disease	**Ulcerative Colitis**
Pathology	Primarily submucosal Skips lesions May affect entire GI tract	Primarily mucosal Continuous lesions Affects colon and rectum
Characteristics	Mild to moderate diarrhea Crampy abdominal pain Severe weight loss, growth retardation Fistulas, strictures, and perianal abscesses common Development of cancer rare	Severe diarrhea Mild abdominal pain Mild weight loss, growth retardation Fistulas, strictures, and perianal abscesses common Development of cancer common

Treatment

The goals of treatment for inflammatory bowel disease are to reduce inflammation, promote healing, and maintain adequate nutrition. Diet is addressed by promoting high-calorie high-protein foods and by avoiding high-fat, spicy, lactose-containing, and gas-forming foods. Liquid supplements may provide additional calories and vitamins and minerals. At times, nutritional supplementation in the form of total parenteral nutrition may be instituted.

Medications include corticosteroids, antibiotics, aminosalicylates, and immunosuppressants. As a last resort when the disease does not respond to medical management, surgical intervention may also be indicated.

 ## CLEFT LIP AND CLEFT PALATE

Cleft lip and cleft palate are examples of structural defects that may occur together or separately. They are the most common congenital craniofacial deformity and may be associated with an underlying syndrome. Incomplete fusion of the lip occurs in approximately 1 in 700 births, whereas incomplete fusion of the palate occurs in 1 in 2,000 births.

> Incomplete fusion of the lip occurs in approximately 1 in 700 births, whereas incomplete fusion of the palate occurs in 1 in 2,000 births.

Several etiologic and genetic factors have been associated with the incidence of cleft lip and cleft palate. They are maternal use of tobacco, certain medications, and folic acid deficiency.

Pathophysiology

During the sixth week of gestation, a cleft lip occurs if the median nasal and premaxillary prominences fail to fuse with the lateral maxillary prominences. A cleft lip is described as unilateral or bilateral and incomplete or complete. This classification depends on whether or not the cleft extends into the nasal cavity. Cleft lip is usually below the center of one nostril. The greater the cleft lip, the greater the chance the teeth near the cleft lip are missing or malformed.

A cleft palate occurs if the palatine shelves failed to fuse between the 6th to 12th week of gestation. This happens if the tongue fails to descend soon enough or if there is a delay in the fusion. A cleft palate involves either the primary palate or the secondary palate (hard and soft palate).

Treatment

Management of a cleft lip includes a surgical Z-plasty within the first few weeks of life if there are no respiratory, oral, or systemic infections present. The goal is to close the cleft with minimal scaring and impact on growth and development. After surgery, the infant may have a **Logan's bow,** which is a small metal strip that protects the suture line, along with arm restraints to prevent the child from touching and pulling at the incision.

Management for the cleft palate is more involved. It includes a team of multidisciplinary professionals that include speech and language pathologists, orthodontists and dentists, plastic surgery, audiology, nursing, and medicine. Surgery techniques have changed over time, and there is a variation in timing in which surgery may be done. Some surgeons may wait until the child is 1 year of age, whereas others may opt to perform the surgery earlier to minimize faulty speech habits, hearing problems, and dental problems. After surgery, there is an increased risk of recurrent infection in the paranasal sinuses and middle ear.

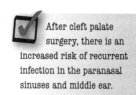

After cleft palate surgery, there is an increased risk of recurrent infection in the paranasal sinuses and middle ear.

SECTION XIII • REVIEW QUESTIONS

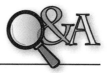

1. A mother asks the nurse to clarify for her what Hirschsprung's disease is. Which of the following is correct?
   a. Atrophy at the junction of the small and large intestine
   b. Absence of nerve innervation in the distal colon
   c. Atresia in the small intestine
   d. Lack of sphincter control

2. What is a cardinal sign seen with intussusception?
   a. Vomiting
   b. Severe abdominal pain
   c. Edema
   d. Weight loss

3. An infant is diagnosed with gastroenteritis. The clinic nurse tells the father to feed his baby:
   a. Diluted fruit juice
   b. Water
   c. Half-strength formula
   d. Pedialyte

4. Which of the following is the proper technique used to feed an infant with cleft lip?
   a. Feed the infant in an upright position
   b. Feed the infant through an nasogastric tube
   c. Feed the infant with a special spoon
   d. Feed the infant with a special cup

5. An infant is admitted for symptoms of projectile vomiting, olive-shaped mass in the left upper quadrant, and visible gastric peristalsis. Which of the following is the most likely diagnosis?
   a. Hirschsprung's disease
   b. Gastroenteritis
   c. Reflux
   d. Pyloric stenosis

6. Sara, a 16-year-old adolescent, is admitted for ulcerative colitis. You would expect to see which of the following symptoms?
   a. Severe bloody diarrhea
   b. Severe vomiting
   c. Weight gain
   d. Systemic rash

7. Sara, a child with inflammatory bowel disease, is being discharged home. In preparing for discharge teaching, which of the following would you include?

   a. Nutrition and preventing constipation

   b. Preventing the spread of the illness to others

   c. Supplements containing multivitamins, iron, and folic acid may be beneficial

   d. Decreasing participation in social activities

8. Excessive vomiting in an infant with pyloric stenosis can eventually lead to:

   a. Metabolic alkalosis

   b. Metabolic acidosis

   c. Dehydration

   d. Thrush

9. Surgery for a cleft palate usually occurs at what age?

   a. Immediately at birth

   b. At 6 months of age

   c. When the child starts solid food

   d. At 1 year of age

10. You would expect to see which of the following treatment modalities for intussusception?

   a. Nonsurgical intervention using an air enema

   b. Surgical resection

   c. Permanent colostomy

   d. Diet management

11. A father asks you to explain the difference between ulcerative colitis and Crohn's disease. Which of the following is the correct answer?

   a. Ulcerative colitis is an acute inflammation of the bowel and resolves within a few weeks.

   b. Ulcerative colitis affects primarily the colon and rectum, whereas Crohn's disease may affect the entire GI tract.

   c. Crohn's disease is usually treated surgically, whereas ulcerative colitis is not.

   d. Crohn's disease presents with severe bloody diarrhea and requires frequent blood transfusions.

ANSWERS AND RATIONALES

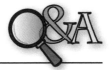

1. **The answer is b.** Rationale: Hirschsprung's disease is caused by absence of the ganglion cells in the distal portion of the colon.

2. **The answer is b.** Rationale: Intussusception causes sudden abdominal pain, irritability, and in many cases bloody mucousy stools.

3. **The answer is d.** Rationale: Oral rehydration solutions such as Pedialyte are the most effective fluid to give an infant because they contain the necessary electrolytes.

4. **The answer is a.** Rationale: Cleft lip reduces the infant's ability to suck. Feeding the infant in an upright position decreases the possibility of aspiration or formula entering the nasal cavity.

5. **The answer is d.** Rationale: Pyloric stenosis is suspected in an infant who has projectile vomiting, an olive-shaped mass, and visible peristalsis.

6. **The answer is a.** Rationale: Ulcerative colitis is characterized by mild to severe abdominal pain and bloody diarrhea.

7. **The answer is c.** Rationale: Vitamin and mineral malabsorption can occur as well as folic acid deficiencies in children with inflammatory bowel disease. Recommending multivitamins, iron, and folic acid may increase nutritional needs.

8. **The answer is a.** Rationale: Excessive vomiting in infants and children can lead to metabolic alkalosis.

9. **The answer is d.** Rationale: With advances in surgical techniques, cleft palate repair is occurring earlier, usually by 1 year of age.

10. **The answer is a.** Rationale: Treatment for intussusception is an emergency nonsurgical measure using air enemas.

11. **The answer is b.** Rationale: One of the differences between ulcerative colitis and Crohn's disease is where the location of lesions occurs. In ulcerative colitis the large intestine is involved with no skip lesions, whereas in Crohn's disease skip lesions are common anywhere in the GI tract.

XIV

Hematological Disorders

- Blood is important in the function of all body systems. A change in the blood may result in a change in several body organs or systems.

- It is important to understand the various components of blood as well as the function of each one.

- Genetic screening, follow-up, and treatment may help to improve pediatric care of these conditions.

- Over the past 20 years, states have instituted mandatory newborn screenings and newborns are now tested for hemoglobinopathies which may identify infants before the onset of symptoms.

33

Hematological Conditions of Childhood

TERMS
- ☐ Anemia
- ☐ Hemophilia
- ☐ Sickle cell anemia
- ☐ Sickle cell disease (SCD)
- ☐ Sickle cell trait
- ☐ von Willebrand disease

IRON-DEFICIENCY ANEMIA

Anemia is the most common blood disorder in children. Anemia can be defined as a reduction in the total number of erythrocytes in the circulating blood or a reduction in the quality or quantity of hemoglobin. There are two classifications for anemia based on either morphology or etiology. Morphological classification is based on size and hemoglobin content. Etiological classification is based on the premise that anemia develops because of a decrease in the production of erythrocytes or an increase in the destruction of erythrocytes. Examples of anemia with a decreased production of red blood cells are iron-deficiency anemia and aplastic anemia. Examples of anemia with an increased destruction of red blood cells are sickle cell anemia and thalassemia.

Pathophysiology

Iron-deficiency anemia is most often caused by an inadequate dietary intake of iron. Newborns have an iron reserve that lasts for up to 12 weeks. As this iron store becomes depleted, the amount of iron in formula or foods must be increased. Iron-deficiency anemia may also be caused by blood loss. In the small child this could be due to gastrointestinal lesion, parasitic infestation, or hemorrhagic disease.

Iron is required to produce hemoglobin in the body that ultimately affects the production of red blood cells. Less oxygen reaches the cells and tissues, causing tissue hypoxia and related symptoms. Symptoms in mild anemia may not be detectable to the parent until moderate anemia presents itself. Symptoms such as general irritability, decreased activity tolerance, and weakness would be signs of moderate anemia. Pallor, anorexia, tachycardia, and murmurs would be signs of severe anemia. Long-term complications of cognitive impairment have been found in children and adolescents with long-standing iron-deficiency anemia.

Levels of anemia are as follows:

Mild iron-deficiency anemia	Hemoglobin 9.5–11 g/dL
Moderate anemia	Hemoglobin 8–9.4 g/dL
Severe anemia	Hemoglobin < 8 g/dL

Treatment

The treatment for iron-deficiency anemia is aimed at correcting the underlying problem and increasing depleted iron stores. Dietary supplementation can be recommended from iron-enriched formula to foods that are high in iron. Iron supplementation may also be given orally or parenterally. Vitamin C may be added to enhance absorption.

SICKLE CELL DISEASE

Hemoglobinopathy is the umbrella term for a number of inherited disorders of the red blood cell (erythrocytes) due to the abnormalities in the protein hemoglobin. **Sickle cell disease (SCD)**, and the older term **sickle cell anemia** (Hb SS), is the most common hemoglobinopathy variant seen worldwide, is associated with severity of illness, and primarily affects people of African and southwest Asian decent. Sickle cell anemia is a homozygous condition resulting from inheriting a sickle cell gene (Hb S) from both parents. There are several hundred hemoglobin variants. Other common heterozygous hemoglobinopathy disorders include the Hb S gene interacting with Hb C, Hb D, and Hb E; α- and β-thalassemia (primarily affecting people of central and southeast Asian and Mediterranean decent), and other variant combinations. SCD is a genetic mutation of the hemoglobin β gene thought to have come about as a protection against malaria in people living in equatorial climates. The severity of the disease varies in individuals.

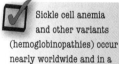

Sickle cell anemia and other variants (hemoglobinopathies) occur nearly worldwide and in a large variety of racial and ethnic groups.

Sickle cell trait (Hb AS) is the heterozygous carrier state where one receives a normal hemoglobin gene (Hb A) from one parent and an abnormal variant gene from the other parent. Sickle cell trait may be very common in many of these ethnic groups, and although patients with sickle cell trait are relatively healthy, they may show signs of disease as they age or may experience symptoms under extraordinary conditions such as exhaustion from vigorous exercise, dehydration, exposed to high altitudes, or deep-sea diving pressures.

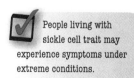

People living with sickle cell trait may experience symptoms under extreme conditions.

Pathophysiology

Fetal hemoglobin (Hb F) at birth declines after the first month of life and is replaced by normal adult hemoglobin (Hb A) during the first year in people unaffected by SCD. SCD (Hb SS) is an autosomal recessive disease where the genetic defect is a single point mutation of the sixth amino acid position on the β chain of the hemoglobin molecule, substituting valine for glutamic acid. Stressors on the body such as an infection, fever, emotional concerns, fatigue, and cold or hot weather result in red blood cell hemolysis (cell death) and, if persistent, anemia. Vasoocclusive crises or "sickling" or "sickle cell crisis" occur when the membrane of the red blood cells becomes hard, sticky, and sickle-shaped, causing clumping of the red blood cells in small vessels, blockage and interruption in blood flow, pain episodes, and progressive and irreversible cell and organ damage if not medically managed.

Hematological biochemical changes may be caused by deoxygenation of the blood, dehydration increasing intracellular hemoglobin concentrations, pH changes to acidosis, and fever. Inflammation in the endothelium of the vascular walls and overactivity of the clotting system producing fibrin clots occur during a vasoocclusive crisis, further impeding blood flow and causing tissue ischemia.

Complications from SCD and vasoocclusive events are varied and often associated with age and access to quality primary and emergency health care. Young children may present with

- Hand–foot syndrome (dactylitis)
- Infections (e.g., sepsis, meningitis)
- Splenomegaly (enlargement of the spleen) or sequestration (a life-threatening condition)
- Silent strokes or ministrokes

As people with SCD age, they are at risk for the following conditions:

- Chronic anemia
- Delayed growth and development
- Cognition problems due to brain damage
- Functional asplenia (atrophy of the spleen and its role in preventing infections)
- Pneumonia and acute chest syndrome
- Priapism (in males, > 24 hours results in erectile dysfunction)
- Menses-induced vasoocclusive events (in females)

- Pulmonary hypertension
- Gallbladder and/or liver disease
- Depression
- Vision (retinopathy) and hearing loss
- Leg ulcers
- Oral and dental health problems
- Joint/bone pain, infarctions, and/or avascular necrosis
- Chronic renal disease (nephropathy)/failure
- Mixed pain syndromes
- Iron overload syndrome (cardiac toxicity, hepatic fibrosis, and endocrine dysfunction)
- Increasing disabilities
- Acute multiorgan failure syndrome

Treatment

Newborn screening for hemoglobinopathies began in the 1980s and has become nearly universal in the United States, currently using hemoglobin electrophoresis. Early identification of people living with SCD and sickle cell trait can facilitate referral to hemoglobinopathy or genetic counselors who can provide them with information to aid them is making decisions regarding their genetic risk and pregnancy options.

SCD remains a life-threatening condition in many poor countries. Advances in medical management and the onset of new therapies and research have improved the quality of life, and the survival for many is now into middle age. Prophylactic penicillin is standard of care for infants starting at about 4 months of age to prevent infection and the sequelae of vasoocclusive crises. Chronic blood transfusions are recommended to prevent stroke in patients at risk identified with transcranial Doppler. Chelation therapy and new oral drugs are being used to prevent and decrease iron overload. Hydroxyurea is one of the drugs approved by the U.S. Food and Drug Administration for treatment that stimulates the reactivation and percentage of fetal hemoglobin in the bloodstream, reducing the frequency and severity of sickle cell crises.

Other treatments, such as bone marrow transplantation and gene therapies, are still in the research stage. Evidenced-based clinical guidelines are available for prevention of secondary conditions and acute care with algorithms for management of specific conditions. A comprehensive, community-based, and life-span approach to care is essential and includes health maintenance activities, complimentary and alternative therapeutics, acute and chronic pain management, and neuropsychological, rehabilitation, and vocational services.

Emergency management of a sickle cell crisis involves the following critical interventions:

- Increase fluids: intravenous hydration bolus followed by higher than maintenance
- Emergency individualized pain management: multimodal approach with adequate doses of parenteral agents via patient-controlled analgesia (not P.R.N. until resolved)
- Bed rest, quiet environment, complimentary and alternative therapeutics
- Transfusion when needed
- Fever indicates sepsis until proven otherwise
- Ongoing comprehensive assessment and emotional support

HEMOPHILIA

There are a number of inherited and acquired bleeding/coagulation disorders in which the clinical manifestations and treatments vary. Hemophilia A (classic/factor VIII deficiency) is seen predominantly in males (in approximately 1 in 5,000 male births) as a result of an X-linked inheritance or, in approximately one third of the cases, a mutation. Hemophilia B (factor IX deficiency) affects 10–15% of individuals with hemophilia. Diagnosis may be determined in the prenatal period by chorionic villus sampling or amniocentesis, following birth by cord blood coagulation assay, or later in life due to positive family history or unusual bleeding. Severity of **hemophilia** ranges from mild to severe, and female carriers may be mildly symptomatic. An associated disorder that tends to have a milder presentation is **von Willebrand disease**, in which there is both a prolonged bleeding time and low plasma factor VIII levels due to a defect in platelet aggregation.

Pathophysiology

Blood coagulation results from a cascade of interactions involving clotting proteins, phosphor-lipids, and calcium. However, in hemophilia there is a defect in the intrinsic hemostatic mechanism and fibrin thread

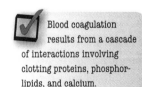

Blood coagulation results from a cascade of interactions involving clotting proteins, phosphor-lipids, and calcium.

formation. Gene deletions and point mutations are the two types of defects that underlay the cause of hemophilia. The amount of bleeding is determined by the amount of clotting factor present in the body.

A variety of blood tests confirms hemophilia, but the importance of a careful assessment should not be overlooked. Thrombin time, the time required for plasma to clot after the addition of bovine thrombin, should be evaluated, as well as prothrombin time, the time required for plasma to clot after the addition of thromboplastin and calcium. The other tests include activated partial thromboplastin time, the prothrombin consumption time, and the thromboplastin generation test, which is the most sensitive.

Treatment

Hemophilia often begins to present itself as a young child begins to move around and becomes more active. Bumps, falls, and teeth eruption often precipitate a bleed. They often experience bleeding into the joint spaces of the knees, ankles, and elbows, causing pain, limited mobility, tenderness, and swelling. Other episodes can range from serious nosebleeds to intracranial hemorrhage that can be life threatening.

Treatment options have greatly advanced in the past 50 years and currently include continuous prophylaxis to reduce the incidence of joint damage and synovitis. Current treatment for hemophilia A is a new recombinant factor concentrate that excludes proteins or raw materials derived from human or animal sources that led to complications in the past. Treatment for hemophilia B is similar except that factor IX is given instead of factor VIII. Management that is started early in the home can help to prevent disease complications.

HYPERBILIRUBINEMIA

Bilirubin is produced by a breakdown of red blood cells. When bilirubin builds up in the blood and reaches a certain level, hyperbilirubinemia occurs. Newborns and preterm infants are at risk for hyperbilirubinemia because they have more red blood cells per kilogram than adults, the lifespan of red blood cells is shorter, and as a result their liver is unable to metabolize all of the bilirubin.

Pathophysiology

There are two types of jaundice in the newborn. Physiological jaundice is normal and appears 2 to 4 days after birth and declines on days 5–7. This occurs in 60–70% of term newborns. Breast-feeding has been associated with physiological jaundice that may result from a lower caloric intake until the milk supply is well established. Pathological jaundice indicates a problem with normal bilirubin metabolism caused by neonatal sepsis, intestinal obstruction, or ABO incompatibility. In both cases, hyperbilirubinemia can become dangerous when indirect bilirubin leaves the circulation and enters the brain.

As red blood cells are destroyed, the breakdown products are released into circulation as heme and globin. The heme is converted to unconjugated bilirubin that binds to albumin. If the albumin becomes saturated, bilirubin moves into the fatty tissue where it causes jaundice. Serum bilirubin levels are measured to determine diagnosis and exceed 5 mg/dL before jaundice is present. Other factors used to determine diagnosis include the timing of presentation and the duration of symptoms.

Treatment

Therapeutic management consists primarily of phototherapy, monitoring of total serum bilirubin levels, and, if breast-feeding, monitoring of weight, wet diapers, and stooling patterns. Phototherapy consists of applying fluorescent light to the infant's skin. The purpose of the light is to reduce the amount of unconjugated bilirubin in the bloodstream by transforming it to a soluble form, thus promoting excretion through the intestines and kidneys. The side effects of phototherapy consist of skin rash, lethargy, abdominal distention, eye damage, and dehydration. When drawing total serum bilirubin levels, the lights should be turned off to avoid a false reading. Monitoring of total serum bilirubin can be done by a transcutaneous measurement device, avoiding frequent blood sticks.

 When drawing total serum bilirubin levels, the lights should be turned off to avoid a false reading.

IMMUNE THROMBOCYTOPENIC PURPURA

Immune thrombocytopenic purpura (ITP) was previously referred to as idiopathic, but with recent research advances we now know that the cause of this disorder is autoimmune. The peak incidence of ITP occurs in children between the ages of 2 and 4, with males and females affected equally. The prognosis is excellent, with 75% recovering completely in 3 months.

Pathophysiology

In most cases a viral infection such as measles, chickenpox, or rubella precedes the onset of ITP by 1–4 weeks. The child presents with bruising and a generalized petechial rash. Nosebleeds may be severe, there can be hemorrhagic blisters of the mucous membranes, and there may be bleeding on the legs and trunk.

ITP is characterized by an increased destruction of platelets in the spleen despite adequate production in the bone marrow. As the rate of platelet destruction exceeds platelet production, circulating platelets decrease and blood clotting diminishes. A platelet count of less than 20,000–30,000 mm^3/dL is often seen.

Treatment

Treatment is largely supportive, with teaching to include prevention of injury and falls and other low platelet count restrictions. Medications may include prednisone, intravenous immunoglobulin (IgG), or a newer product, anti-D, a gamma globulin fraction. Platelet administration is of little value because of the short lifespan of platelets.

SECTION XIV · REVIEW QUESTIONS

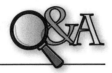

1. The most effective laboratory test for detecting sickle cell anemia in newborns and adults is:
   a. Complete blood count
   b. Solubility testing (sickle prep)
   c. Hemoglobin electrophoresis
   d. Hemoglobin and hematocrit counts

2. Daily doses of oral penicillin given to children with sickle cell anemia may prevent:
   a. Pain episodes
   b. Fatal bloodstream infections
   c. Iron overload
   d. Chronic anemia
   e. Silent strokes

3. If one parent has sickle cell trait (AS) and one has normal hemoglobin (AA), their child would have a:
   a. 25% chance of inheriting sickle cell trait
   b. 50% chance of inheriting sickle cell trait
   c. 25 % chance of inheriting normal hemoglobin
   d. 50% of inheriting sickle cell C trait

4. The effects of sickling on the body include all of the following *except:*
   a. Bleeding into joint spaces
   b. Hand–foot syndrome
   c. Priapism
   d. Ministrokes

5. The most frequent site of bleeding in hemophilia A is to the:
   a. Abdomen
   b. Chest
   c. Joint spaces
   d. Extremities

6. ITP is most often treated by:
   a. Platelet administration
   b. Blood transfusion
   c. Heparin
   d. Prednisone

7. What is an accurate description of anemia?
   a. A decrease in the oxygen-carrying capacity of the blood
   b. Red blood cells that are stiff and less able to change shape
   c. An impaired rate of hemoglobin synthesis
   d. Excessive bleeding and blood loss

8. A mother asks the nurse what foods she can feed her 6-month-old that would be rich in iron. Which of the following is the correct answer?
   a. Whole milk and baby food
   b. Formula and rice cereal fortified with iron
   c. Raisons and red meat
   d. Whole milk and rice cereal fortified with iron

9. Hyperbilirubinemia in the newborn should resolve itself by:
   a. One week
   b. One month
   c. Two weeks
   d. One year

10. John is a 9-year-old with hemophilia. He asks the nurse what would be a good sport for him to play. Which of the following should the nurse answer?
    a. Football
    b. Baseball
    c. Hockey
    d. Swimming

ANSWERS AND RATIONALES

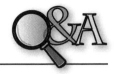

1. **The answer is c.** Rationale: Hemoglobin electrophoresis is now routinely done in most states to screen for sickle cell anemia.

2. **The answer is b.** Rationale: Penicillin may be given prophylactically to decrease the incidence of infections that may precipitate a crisis.

3. **The answer is b.** Rationale: By diagramming the genetic makeup of the two parents, one can determine that the child would have a 50% chance of having sickle cell trait (AS).

	A	A
A	AA	AA
S	AS	AS

4. **The answer is a.** Rationale: Bleeding into the joint spaces is a description of hemophilia. The other three episodes are possible in a child with sickle cell disease.

5. **The answer is c.** Rationale: The majority of bleeds for children with hemophilia are into the joint spaces of the knees, elbows, and ankles.

6. **The answer is d.** Rationale: ITP is best treated by supportive measures. Blood product administration does not help to treat ITP. If needed, prednisone is the recommended drug of choice.

7. **The answer is a.** Rationale: A decrease in the oxygen-carrying capacity of the blood caused by disease or injury best describes anemia.

8. **The answer is b.** Rationale: At 6 months of age the infant should still be on formula and might have started on cereal. Milk is not recommended until after 1 year of age. By 3–4 months, iron stores drop off and infants should have iron enriched foods.

9. **The answer is a.** Rationale: Physiological hyperbilirubinemia in the newborn resolves by day 7.

10. **The answer is d.** Rationale: Swimming is the one sport listed that has the least amount of contact and potential injury that can precipitate a bleeding episode.

XV

Human Immunodeficiency Virus

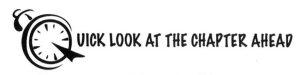

Acquired immunodeficiency syndrome (AIDS) is a chronic progressive disease affecting multiple organs. AIDS is caused by a viral infection with the **human immunodeficiency virus (HIV)** that affects the helper T lymphocytes, monocytes, and macrophages. As the virus proliferates the immune system begins to fail. HIV replicates by invading T cells and other immune system cells, thus weakening the system. Since it was first identified in 1981, HIV has reached pandemic proportions. This chapter explores the impact of HIV infection on childhood and adolescence.

34

Human Immunodeficiency Virus Infection

TERMS
- ☐ Acquired immunodeficiency syndrome (AIDS)
- ☐ Enzyme-linked immunosorbent assay (ELISA)
- ☐ Human immunodeficiency virus (HIV)
- ☐ Polymerase chain reaction (PCR)
- ☐ p24 assay
- ☐ Viral load

301

Currently, over 3 million children worldwide are infected with HIV. In the United States African-American and Latino children have higher rates of infection and death from this disease than children from other ethnic groups. HIV infection is a leading cause of death in adolescents and young adults aged 13 to 24 years. Approximately half of all new HIV cases occur in adolescents and young adults mainly due to unsafe sexual practices and intravenous drug use, although adolescents and young adults do not generally identify these activities as high risk.

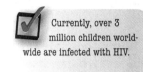

Currently, over 3 million children worldwide are infected with HIV.

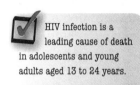

HIV infection is a leading cause of death in adolescents and young adults aged 13 to 24 years.

The signs of early HIV infection may be nonspecific in children, yet the disease often progresses more rapidly in infants and young children than it does in adults.

Children who are infected during perinatal development have an average life span of 7 to 15 years. HIV infection is suspected in high-risk children if they exhibit failure to thrive, developmental delays, and/or have frequent bacterial infections and chronic encephalopathy.

Approximately 91% of pediatric HIV transmissions occur from mother to child (vertical transmission). Virus transmission can occur through the placenta, through exposure to maternal blood and vaginal secretions during the birth process, or through breast milk. The risk of HIV infection passing from mother to infant is greatest if the mother's viral load is above 1,000 copies/mL and CD4 count is low and if there was a long period of time from rupture of the membranes to delivery. When the mother receives zidovudine and other antiretroviral therapies during pregnancy and delivery and when newborns are placed on antiretroviral therapy during the first 6 weeks of life, the risk of HIV infection in the infant is reduced. From 1992 to 2001 maternal and newborn treatment with antiretrovirals reduced perinatal HIV transmission by 83%. Newborns of HIV-infected mothers who did not have antiviral therapy during pregnancy and childbirth had a 15–30% chance of becoming infected, whereas infants born to HIV-infected mothers who were on antiretroviral therapy had only a 1–8% chance of becoming infected.

At birth, 30% of HIV-positive newborns infected while in utero have detectable levels of HIV antibodies. If the infection was acquired during the birth process, the newborn will not test positive for the infection until they are 2 to 4 weeks of age. Uninfected infants have maternal

HIV serum antibodies present for up to 18 months before seroconverting to a negative antibody titer. Blood transfusions, sexual abuse, sharing contaminated needles, and unsafe sexual practices are modes of HIV transmission (termed horizontal transmission) for children, adolescents, and young adults. Counseling concerning HIV transmission paths and diagnostic testing is vital for adolescents and young adults who engage in high-risk behavior.

Although HIV infects all age groups, children and adults are affected somewhat differently. HIV progresses more rapidly in infants and young children than in adults. Infants who do not receive antiretroviral treatment rapidly progress from an HIV-positive status to AIDS within a year and most die by age 2. This rapid progression may occur because of the high viral load passed from mother to infant. Opportunistic infections occur early and frequently in the course of the disease in children. Bacterial infections, lymphoid interstitial pneumonitis, and *Pneumocystis carinii* pneumonia may begin when the infant is only 3 months old. Because of the danger of developing *P. carinii* pneumonia, all infants born to HIV-infected mothers should receive Bactrim as a prophylaxis measure beginning at 4 to 6 weeks of age.

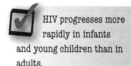 HIV progresses more rapidly in infants and young children than in adults.

PATHOPHYSIOLOGY

Two major types of the virus account for most HIV infections: HIV-1 is found in most areas of the world and HIV-2 is found primarily in West African nations.

As a retrovirus HIV carries its genetic code for reproduction in its ribonucleic acid (RNA). Once inside the CD4 cell the virus uses an enzyme called reverse transcriptase to convert its viral RNA to deoxyribonucleic acid (DNA). The viral DNA is then integrated into the CD4 cell's DNA. The virus replicates inside the CD4 cell and buds from the cell surface destroy the CD4 cell membrane, releasing millions of viral copies into the bloodstream.

The plasma **viral load,** or number of viral particles per millimeter of blood, is an indicator of clinical progression of the disease. A viral load below 10,000 copies/mm signals control of the disease and a low probability of disease progression. In contrast, a viral load above 100,000 copies/mm signals a poor prognosis and a high likelihood that the disease will progress rapidly. The aim of antiviral therapy is to reduce the viral load to a level at which the body's immune system can keep the virus in check. Treatment failure is indicated by a rising viral load even in the absence of symptoms.

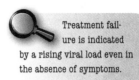

Treatment failure is indicated by a rising viral load even in the absence of symptoms.

In the acute stage of the disease process the infected child may be asymptomatic, except for short-lived (2 weeks or less), mild, flu-like symptoms. During the asymptomatic phase of the infection, which may last a few weeks or years depending on the strength of the child's immune system and the amount of virus transmitted during infection, the body's T cells are numerous enough to keep the virus in control. The virus can be transmitted to others even if no symptoms are present. During the persistent generalized lymphadenopathy stage, the child presents with several enlarged lymph nodes. Eventually, the number of viral cells will greatly outnumber healthy T cells, resulting in a weakened immune system and the development of opportunistic infections, neurological disease, and neoplasms characteristic of AIDS. Table 34-1 gives the Centers for Disease Control and Prevention classification system for disease progression.

Table 34-1 Centers for Disease Control and Prevention Classification System

Category	0–12 Months of Age	1–5 Years of Age	6–12 Years of Age
1 (no suppression) Mild signs and symptoms: lymphadenopathy, recurrent sinusitis, and recurrent otitis media	CD4 count above 1,500	CD4 count above 1,000	CD4 count above 500
2 (moderate suppression) Signs and symptoms: anemia, neutropenia, thrombocytopenia, diarrhea, fever, pneumonia, herpes simplex, and oral candidiasis	CD4 count 750–1,499	CD4 count 500–999	CD4 count 200–499
3 (severe suppression) Signs and symptoms: non-Hodgkin's lymphomas, wasting syndrome, and multiple opportunistic infections (immune system is not strong enough to kill malignant cells, bacteria, fungi, parasites, and viruses)	CD4 count below 750	CD4 count below 500	CD4 count below 200

DIAGNOSTIC TESTS

Diagnostic tests for HIV infection include serologic assays, such as **enzyme-linked immunosorbent assay (ELISA)** and Western blot, and viral detection assays, such as culture, antigen (p24) detection, and nucleic acid amplification procedures, including **polymerase chain reaction (PCR)**. The PCR method uses an in vitro replication of target nucleic acid sequences, thereby identifying specific HIV genetic information. The PCR method can detect HIV in someone newly infected.

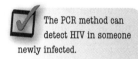

The PCR method can detect HIV in someone newly infected.

The ELISA and Western blot tests are used to detect the presence of HIV antibodies (seroconversion) in blood and blood products in children over 18 months of age. Children younger than 18 months of age may still have serum maternal antibodies to HIV, rendering these traditional tests inaccurate. HIV infection can be detected in infants as young as 1 month of age by using cultures and the PCR method. Testing is done within 48 hours of birth in high-risk infants.

Because ELISA and Western blot tests detect antibodies but not viral antigens, these tests cannot detect the earliest stage of the infection before antibody formation; however, they are sensitive enough to detect 99.5% of HIV-infected blood samples 12 weeks after initial infection. The Western blot test is used to confirm positive ELISA results because it is a more sensitive test and can detect the difference between HIV antibodies and other circulating antibodies. For those in high-risk groups, a negative ELISA should be followed by the more sensitive Western blot test. If the ELISA is negative and the Western blot is positive, the results are highly suggestive of HIV infection. False-positive results can occur because of conditions such as autoimmune disease, syphilis, leukemia, lymphoma, or alcohol abuse. False-negative tests occur before antibody formation and in the end stage of the disease.

OraQuick Advance HIV-½ Antibody test allows for intravenous testing using an oral fluid specimen or plasma. This test is highly accurate (99%), convenient, and rapid (results in 20 minutes). If someone in a high-risk group has a negative test result using an oral fluid specimen, the test is repeated or a blood sample is tested. A positive test result is generally followed up by various additional testing methods.

The immune complex–dissociated **p24 assay** is a test that detects the p24 antigen, an indication of active HIV replication, within 2 to 6 weeks of HIV infection. It is used to confirm HIV infection before seroconversion (HIV antibody production) and to monitor the effectiveness of antiretroviral therapy.

Lymphocyte immunophenotyping is a test to determine the number of serum CD4 cells. A recent viral illness and immunosuppressive drugs decrease lymphocyte counts, whereas steroids can increase the counts. Laboratories are now capable of determining HIV viral load or the number of HIV viral particles in blood. By evaluating both the CD4 count and viral load, the likelihood of appropriate antiretroviral therapy is increased.

SECTION XV · REVIEW QUESTIONS

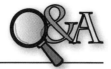

1. Which of the following statements concerning HIV/AIDS are *true* (select all that apply)?
    a. HIV infection is a leading cause of death in adolescents and young adults in the United States.
    b. The human immunodeficiency virus affects B cells.
    c. White children have the highest rate of HIV infection in the United States.
    d. Unsafe sexual practices and intravenous drug use account for 50% of new HIV cases in adolescents and young adults.

2. HIV is suspected in infants who (select all that apply):
    a. Fail to thrive
    b. Have one or two otitis media infections per year
    c. Reach developmental milestones on schedule but are in the 80% for growth
    d. Have prolonged bouts of colic

3. A vertical HIV infection can occur in which of the following ways (select all that apply)?
    a. Through breast milk
    b. Through formula prepared by an HIV-positive caregiver
    c. When mother and child share a drinking glass
    d. During a vaginal birth

4. Newborns whose HIV-positive mother did not have antiretroviral therapy during pregnancy have a(n)_____ chance of becoming infected.
    a. 83%
    b. 8%
    c. 25%
    d. 100%

5. Infants test positive for HIV:
    a. Immediately after birth if the infection was acquired during the birth process
    b. Within 10 days of birth
    c. For up to 18 months if the mother was HIV positive
    d. Within 24 hours of birth via a cesarean section

6. HIV progression in infants and young children:
   a. Is generally slower than in adults
   b. Is rapid if a high viral load was passed from mother to child
   c. Cannot be slowed by antiretroviral therapy
   d. If rapid, results in death between the ages of 8 and 10

7. Because HIV is a retrovirus it:
   a. Carries its genetic code in DNA
   b. Uses reverse transcriptase to convert its DNA to the host cell's DNA
   c. Reproduces while attached to the outside of the host cell
   d. Is able to convert its RNA to the host's DNA

8. Which of the following statements concerning viral load is correct?
   a. Viral load measures the number of viral particles needed to transmit HIV.
   b. A viral load below 50,000 copies indicates that the disease is not transmissible.
   c. If the viral load is between 75,000 and 125,000 copies, treatment has been successful.
   d. A rising viral load indicates treatment failure.

9. The polymerase chain reaction test:
   a. Can detect HIV antibodies
   b. Is less reliable than the ELISA test
   c. Identifies HIV genetic information
   d. Detects HIV if the person has been infected for a minimum of 6 months

10. In most children antibodies to HIV (seroconversion) can be detected:
    a. Within days of becoming infected
    b. By culturing blood
    c. With the use of the p24 assay
    d. Within 12 weeks of becoming infected

11. An adolescent may have a false-negative ELISA test result because they:
    a. Were infected 4–6 months earlier
    b. Have comorbidities such as leukemia or rheumatoid arthritis
    c. Are in the end stage of disease
    d. Were recently vaccinated with a flu vaccine

12. The p24 assay test is used to detect:
    a. Active HIV reproduction
    b. HIV antibodies
    c. Viral load
    d. The number of CD4 cells

ANSWERS AND RATIONALES

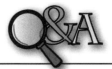

1. **The answers are a and d.** Rationale: HIV affects T cells, and African-American and Latino children have the highest rates of infection.

2. **The answer is a.** Rationale: One or two bouts of otitis media per year is not unusual in children, and colic is not a sign of HIV.

3. **The answers are a and d.** Rationale: Vertical transmission is from mother to infant, and HIV is not spread by sharing eating utensils.

4. **The answer is c.** Rationale: The rate of vertical transmission is 1–8% if the mother takes antiretroviral medications and jumps to 15–30% if she does not take the medications during pregnancy and during labor and delivery.

5. **The answer is c.** Rationale: All infants of HIV-positive mothers also test positive because the antibodies cross the placenta, infants seroconvert by 18 months of age, 30% of infants infected in utero have their own antibodies to HIV at birth, and it takes several weeks after infection for antibodies to show up on the ELISA.

6. **The answer is b.** Rationale: Children generally progress from HIV-positive status to AIDS much faster than adults and usually die within 24 months of birth.

7. **The answer is d.**

8. **The answer is d.** Rationale: Viral loads below 10,000 copies indicate treatment success and a slow disease progression, viral load measures the number of viral particles per millimeter of blood, and HIV is transmissible even with a very low viral load.

9. **The answer is c.** Rationale: ELISA and Western blot test for antibodies, and PCR identifies viral genetic information and is a very sensitive test for HIV.

10. **The answer is b.** Rationale: Cultures and PCR can detect HIV infection when the infant is 4 weeks of age, and the p24 assay detects active HIV replication not antibodies and can verify seroconversion before antibodies are produced.

11. **The answer is b.** Rationale: A false-negative ELISA can occur if the child or adolescent has an autoimmune disease or before antibodies are present in sufficient numbers to be detected.

12. **The answer is a.**

XVI

Inborn Errors of
Metabolism

Inborn errors of metabolism (IEMs), first described in 1908, are disorders caused by single faulty genes resulting in the inability of the normal metabolic pathway to function and correctly synthesize or breakdown proteins, carbohydrates, or fats. For successful metabolism to occur enzymes and transport proteins are needed. **Enzymes** are specific proteins that increase or decrease the speed of a chemical reaction but do not change themselves. The substances upon which enzymes exert their effects are called **substrates**. Once the enzyme has changed the substrate, a product is formed.

35

Inborn Errors of Metabolism

TERMS
- ☐ Carnitine
- ☐ Enzymes
- ☐ Inborn errors of metabolism (IEMs)
- ☐ Substrates

This chapter explores common pediatric inborn errors of metabolism.

A well-functioning metabolic pathway depends on many complex sequences of reactions. The child with an IEM may be missing an enzyme, leading to a buildup of substrates that may affect distant organs or may only produce a small amount of product.

Signs and symptoms of IEM may be mild or severe (Table 35-1). Treatment for IEM includes avoiding enzyme substrates in the diet, using medication to remove substrates, replacing a missing product, or providing missing enzymes. Research is focused on gene replacement therapy. Genetic counseling is recommended.

> ✓ Signs and symptoms of IEM may be mild or severe.

The newborn with an IEM may feed poorly, vomit, be lethargic or jittery, and have seizures, acidosis, and jaundice. Laboratory tests include electrolytes, ammonia level, glucose level, urine pH and ketones,

Table 35-1 Signs and Symptoms Suggesting IEMs

- Critically ill newborn
- Seizures
- Recurrent vomiting
- Mental retardation
- Liver disease
- Unusual odor
- Acidosis
- Hypoglycemia
- Cognitive regression
- Symptoms appear/worsen when the diet changes
- Food aversions
- Family history
- Alopecia
- Retinal cherry-red spot
- Retinitis pigmentosa
- Cataracts
- Enlarged liver
- Enlarged spleen
- Coarse features
- Ataxia
- Abnormal behavior
- Failure to thrive
- Short stature
- Rash
- Frequent infections

and sometimes analysis of serum/urine/cerebrospinal fluid to detect enzymes, substrates, or products. The newborn with an elevated blood ammonia level usually has acidosis, anorexia, irritability, vomiting, lethargy, seizures, and coma.

All states now screen newborns for phenylketonuria (PKU) and hypothyroidism. Most states screen for galactosemia, and some test for other IEM. Screening tests are not diagnostic, and false negatives or false positives may occur.

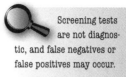
Screening tests are not diagnostic, and false negatives or false positives may occur.

EXAMPLES OF IEM

Galactosemia

Galactosemia is a disorder of carbohydrate metabolism; it is autosomal recessive and occurs in 1 in 40,000 live births. Details of this disorder with screening tests and treatment are as follows:

- *Screening:* Routine newborn screening → Beutler test (looks for enzyme deficiency in red blood cells) or by increased serum galactose.
- *Cause:* Deficiency of one of three liver enzymes needed to convert galactose to glucose→ galactose-1-phosphate uridyltransferase (GALT) → galactose and glucose result from the digestion of lactose, a sugar found in dairy products. Accumulation of galactose-1-phosphate in the eyes, liver, brain, and renal tubules causes damage to the eyes, brain, liver, and kidneys.

Galactose and glucose result from the digestion of lactose, a sugar found in dairy products.

- *Result:* Susceptibility to gram-negative sepsis, hepatic disease, mental retardation (irreversible), renal disease, cataracts, and ovarian failure.
- *Signs and symptoms:* Slow intrauterine growth, hypoglycemia, vomiting and weight loss within a few days of birth, jaundice, hepatomegaly, enlarged spleen (from portal hypertension),

cirrhosis, speech/language deficits, *Escherichia coli* sepsis, and malnutrition.

- *Treatment:* Lifelong galactose-free diet, which means no milk or milk products, garbanzo beans, cheese, sherbet, sour cream, yogurt, ice cream, and organ meats. Soy protein formula is used in place of commercial formula or breast milk.

Fatty Acid Oxidation (Breakdown of Fats) Disorders

Fatty acid oxidation disorders, among the most common of the IEMs, manifest as the inability to use fat for energy when glucose stores are low or during sleep. They are autosomal recessive. Details of this disorder with screening tests and treatment are as follows:

- *Screening:* Some states require newborn screening for a panel of acylcarnitines (essential compounds for the metabolism of fatty acids)→ blood analysis.
- *Cause:* Defect of very-long-chain acyl-CoA dehydrogenase, medium-chain acyl-CoA dehydrogenase, short-chain acyl-CoA dehydrogenase, or long-chain hydroxyacyl-CoA dehydrogenase enzymes needed for fatty acid β-oxidation. There are many variations of this disorder. Once activated, fatty acids enter the mitochondria and fatty acid oxidation occurs. **Carnitine** acts as a transport for long-chain fatty acids so they can enter the mitochondria of muscle and heart cells, resulting in energy production.
- *Result:* Inability of ingested fats to be used for energy so fatty acids build up; during pregnancy the mother may develop AFLP (acute fatty liver of pregnancy) or the syndrome of HELLP (hemolysis, elevated liver enzymes, and low platelets). Toddlers may show delays, such as in walking and so forth; learning/behavior problems; or mental retardation.
- *Signs and symptoms:* Extreme sleepiness, irritability, anorexia, hypoketotic hypoglycemia, mild hyperammonemia, hepatomegaly, encephalopathy, cardiomyopathy, coma brought on by fasting, sudden death in infancy, and lack of ketones in response to fasting.
- *Treatment:* Avoid fasting, feed infants every 2–4 hours, feed toddlers small frequent meals, carbohydrate snacks before

bedtime to prevent nighttime hypoglycemia, oral administration of carnitine, cornstarch mixed with water or milk (source of long-lasting energy), restriction of dietary long-chain fats, and riboflavin. Treatment for each of the disorders is different.

Treatment for each of the fatty acid oxidation disorders is different.

Maple Sugar Urine Disease

Maple sugar urine disease (MSUD), also called branched-chain ketoaciduria, is autosomal recessive and occurs in 1 in 200,000 live births but is as frequent as 1 per 200 newborns in some inbred populations (i.e., Mennonites in Pennsylvania). Persons afflicted with this disease are unable to break down three essential amino acids—leucine, isoleucine, and valine—because the branched-chain α-keto acid dehydrogenase enzyme is missing or defective. Details of this disorder with screening tests and treatment are as follows:

- *Screening:* Newborn screening is available for this disorder. Diagnosis is made when high levels of branched-chain amino acids are found in the blood and urine. In high-risk populations prenatal diagnosis can be made by measuring branched-chain amino acid amounts in amniotic fluid or by enzyme analysis of chorion villus cells.

  > In high-risk populations prenatal diagnosis of MSUD can be made.

- *Cause:* Deficient enzyme (branched-chain α-keto acid dehydrogenase) necessary for the breakdown of three amino acids leucine, isoleucine, and valine.
- *Result:* Toxic amounts of keto acids from leucine and isoleucine cause the characteristic maple sugar urine odor, whereas the keto acid from leucine damages the brain and nervous system. However, if treatment is begun within 10 days of birth, nearly normal growth and development is possible. If treatment is not begun soon after birth, death may occur within 1 month. There are variations in the severity of the disorder so the onset of signs and symptoms may be delayed for years; however, affected children may have developmental delays depending on the severity

of the disorder. Any event that causes increased protein catabolism, such as illness or surgery, results in metabolic decompensation.

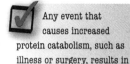

Any event that causes increased protein catabolism, such as illness or surgery, results in metabolic decompensation.

If treatment for MSUD is not begun soon after birth, death may occur within 1 month.

- *Signs and symptoms:* Characteristic sweet body fluid odor, lethargy, poor feeding, high-pitched cry, irritability, severe ketoacidosis, seizures, and coma.
- *Treatment:* Dialysis is used to remove keto acids when first diagnosed, and then formulas are used with reduced branched-chain amino acids supplemented with milk and other foods containing branched-chain amino acids so normal growth and development occurs. Blood levels of branched-chain amino acids are checked every 24–48 hours during the first month of life. Urine ketone levels are checked daily. The major dietary sources of the branched-chain amino acids include dairy products and red meat, although all protein foods contain these amino acids. Vegetables, juices, and fermented foods such as yogurt contain small amounts of the free amino acids.

All protein foods contain branched-chain amino acids.

Phenylketonuria Fatty Acid Oxidation (Breakdown of Fats) Disorders

PKU disorders are caused by a deficiency in the hepatic enzyme phenylalanine hydrolyase. They are autosomal recessive, and the incidence in whites is approximately 1 in 10,000 live births. Details of this disorder with screening tests and treatment are as follows:

- *Screening:* Guthrie heel prick test is done within 48 hours of birth; it is mandatory in all states. If done within 24 hours after birth a false negative may occur because phenylalanine has not built up to detectable levels. Recommendation is that testing occur when the newborn is at least 72 hours old, or if done within 24 hours of birth the test should be repeated within 21 days. Prenatal diagnosis uses a combination of DNA analysis, enzyme activity, and amniotic fluid metabolite levels.

If the Guthrie heel prick test is done within 24 hours after birth, a false negative may occur because phenylalanine has not built up to detectable levels.

- *Cause:* Enzyme that converts phenylalanine to tyrosine is absent so phenylalanine builds up in the bloodstream and phenyl acids are excreted in the urine. Tyrosine is one of 20 amino acids used by cells to synthesize proteins, and it is a precursor of thyroid hormones thyroxine and triiodothyronine, the pigment melanin, and catecholamines dopamine, norepinephrine, and epinephrine.
- *Result:* Toxic levels of the amino acid phenylalanine accumulate in the blood and other tissues and tyrosine production falls. High amounts of phenylalanine result in abnormal brain development in the infant, leading to mental retardation.

  High amounts of phenylalanine result in abnormal brain development.

- *Signs and symptoms:* The infant appears normal at birth, but if the PKU disorder is not detected and treated the child will not reach early developmental milestones. Mental retardation, hyperactivity, seizures, a light complexion and hair color (tyrosine is needed for the production of the pigment melanin), and eczema are characteristic of this disorder. The infant will also have a "musty" odor of skin, hair, and urine because of phenylpyruvic acid excretion. Older children may manifest bizarre behavior, such as screaming, head banging, and catatonia. If the PKU disorder is detected and treated shortly after birth, the child will have normal growth and development.

  Dietary restrictions for those with PKU disorders are lifelong.

- *Treatment:* Dietary restrictions are lifelong and limit food high in phenylalanine, including breast milk, meat, chicken, fish, nuts, cheese and other dairy products, and starchy foods such as potatoes, bread, pasta, and corn. Foods, beverages, and medications containing the sweetener aspartame are avoided because aspartame is metabolized into several chemicals, including phenylalanine.

- *Prenatal precautions:* Although a woman with a PKU disorder who becomes pregnant is not at risk for complications herself during the pregnancy, she should be advised to maintain low phenylalanine levels before and during pregnancy because phenylalanine crosses the placental barrier. If phenylalanine levels are high, birth defects such as congenital heart disease, growth retardation, microcephaly, and mental retardation may develop.

SECTION XVI · REVIEW QUESTIONS

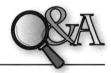

1. Which of the following statements accurately describes inborn errors of metabolism (IEMs)?
   a. IEMs are caused by a pair of autosomal dominate genes.
   b. IEMs result in the production of too much protein.
   c. IEMs disrupt the metabolic pathways.
   d. IEMs cause too much product to be produced.

2. While conducting an in-service for new graduates hired for the newborn nursery, the preceptor stresses that:
   a. Only high-risk newborns are screened for IEMs.
   b. Screening tests are not diagnostic for IEMs such as PKU.
   c. Newborns with IEMs eat more frequently than newborns without an IEM.
   d. All states now screen for 50 IEM disorders.

3. The nurse discussing galactosemia with the parents of a newborn diagnosed with the disorder correctly explains that (select all that apply):
   a. This disorder is caused by lack of a liver enzyme.
   b. Galactose is a protein in dairy products.
   c. Signs of the disorder include high serum glucose.
   d. Breast-feeding the infant is not advised.

4. Which of the following menu choices is allowed by a person with galactosemia?
   a. Garbanzo beans and spinach
   b. Fruit-free yogurt and turkey
   c. Grilled cheese sandwich and an apple
   d. Egg white omelet and orange juice

5. Which statement made by the nurse conducting an in-service about fatty acid oxidative disorders is correct?
   a. This disorder metabolizes ingested fat at a rapid rate.
   b. This disorder requires that the infant be fed every 2–4 hours around the clock.
   c. This disorder is characterized by rapid weight gain.
   d. This disorder is part of a routine screening panel in all 50 states.

6. The office nurse is reviewing nutritional requirements for Mark, a toddler with fatty acid oxidation disorder. She correctly tells the parents that:
   a. Cornstarch mixed with milk is a source of long-acting energy.
   b. Mark should have a high-protein snack at bedtime.
   c. Mark should not be given dairy products.
   d. This disorder will be corrected by the time Mark is 10 years old.

7. A child with branched-chain ketoaciduria disorder:
   a. Is unable to synthesize amino acids
   b. Usually requires treatment by the time he or she is 10 months old to prevent brain damage
   c. May decompensate metabolically when he or she is ill
   d. Has a characteristic musty body odor

8. The nurse in the prenatal clinic is explaining phenylketonuria to parents in a prenatal health education class. He correctly states that:
   a. All infants are screened within 12 hours of birth for this disorder.
   b. Left untreated, mental retardation develops.
   c. Characteristic signs of this disorder include abnormally dark skin color.
   d. It is apparent at birth if the newborn has this disorder.

9. The dietitian explaining a PKU diet to the parents of an infant with the disorder stresses that the following foods are high in phenylalanine (select all that apply):
   a. Nuts
   b. Cheese
   c. Meat
   d. Aspartame

10. What advice should a woman with PKU disorder receive before she becomes pregnant?
   a. It is important to have a very low maternal phenylalanine blood level in the third trimester of pregnancy.
   b. Phenylalanine blood levels should be low before conception and during pregnancy.
   c. Phenylalanine does not cross the placental barrier.
   d. Birth defects such as congenital cataracts may occur if maternal blood levels of phenylalanine are too high.

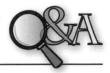

ANSWERS AND RATIONALES

1. **The answer is c.** Rationale: IEMs are the result of a single faulty gene (autosomal recessive), result in the inability to synthesize or breakdown protein, and cause a build up of substrates and little product production.

2. **The answer is b.** Rationale: All 50 states require that newborns are screened for PKU disorder and hypothyroidism, and some states require testing for additional disorders; newborns with IEM are anorexic and may vomit.

3. **The answers are a and d.** Rationale: The disorder is caused by a deficiency of a liver enzyme needed to convert galactose to glucose so hypoglycemia develops; galactose results from the digestion of lactose found in dairy products and breast milk so a special soy protein formula is required.

4. **The answer is d.** Rationale: Garbanzo beans, yogurt, and cheese all contain lactose.

5. **The answer is b.** Rationale: Fatty acid oxidative disorders result in the inability of ingested fats to be used for energy so fatty acids build up in the bloodstream, the infant will have failure to thrive, screening for this condition is required in some states but not all 50 states, and the infant must be fed every 2–4 hours around the clock because he or she needs a constant supply of glucose for energy production.

6. **The answer is a.** Rationale: Mark needs a carbohydrate snack before bed, dairy products are not restricted, and the condition is lifelong.

7. **The answer is c.** Rationale: A child with branched-chain ketoaciduria is unable to break down three essential amino acids (leucine, isoleucine, and valine), requires treatment by the time they are 10 days old to prevent nervous system damage, and has a characteristic sweet odor because of the ketoacidosis.

8. **The answer is b.** Rationale: All infants are screened before they are discharged, but not by 12 hours of age; light skin and hair color are characteristic of this disorder because of a lack of

melanin production; the newborn with PKU disorder appears normal at birth.

9. **The answers are a, b, c, and d.** Rationale: Aspartame (artificial sweetener) is metabolized into chemicals, including phenylalanine; the other foods listed naturally contain phenylalanine.

10. **The answer is b.** Rationale: Phenylalanine crosses the placental barrier and may cause birth defects such as congenital heart defects, microcephaly, and mental retardation so women with PKU disorder are advised to have low serum levels of phenylalanine before conception and during pregnancy.

XVII

Integumentary Disorders

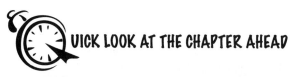

As the largest organ in the body the skin is responsible for a variety of functions, including temperature regulation, excretion, sensation, fluid balance, and protecting the internal organs from contact with potentially harmful substances such as bacteria, chemicals, ultraviolet rays, and other irritants. This chapter discuses the role skin plays in maintaining health.

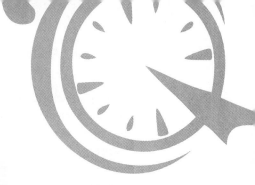

36

Anatomy and Physiology of the Integumentary System

TERMS

☐ **Apocrine glands**
☐ **Dermis**
☐ **Eccrine glands**
☐ **Epidermis**
☐ **Epithelization**
☐ **Subcutaneous tissues**

Harmless bacteria protect the skin surface from harmful bacteria, and the thin layer of fatty acids on the skin is also bactericidal. In addition to its protective properties, the skin's rich nerve supply allows it to transmit a variety of sensations such as touch, pain, temperature, pleasure, and pressure to the central nervous system. Vitamin D, a fat-soluble vitamin necessary for calcium and phosphate absorption, is manufactured when the skin is exposed to ultraviolet rays. If injury occurs the skin can quickly regenerate.

At birth the skin is immature, fragile, and thin. There is little subcutaneous tissue beneath it, making the newborn susceptible to heat loss and vulnerable to the absorption of harmful chemicals. **Eccrine glands**, which help regulate body temperature by producing sweat, do not mature until ages 2 or 3 years. These glands are found in the highest numbers in the palms, forehead, and soles of the feet. **Apocrine glands** are located in the groin area and axilla. As the fluid secreted by apocrine glands breaks down, body odor results. These glands become functional at puberty.

> At birth the skin is immature, fragile, and thin. There is little subcutaneous tissue beneath it, making the newborn susceptible to heat loss and vulnerable to the absorption of harmful chemicals.

Epithelial cells of the mucous membrane, which secrete immunoglobin A to provide protection against microorganisms that enter the mouth, do not reach maturity until ages 2 to 5. Little melanin is present at birth, resulting in a light skin color that leaves the infant susceptible to damage by ultraviolet rays.

Structure and Function

The **epidermis**, **dermis**, and **subcutaneous tissues** comprise the three major layers of the skin. The epidermis is composed of the stratum germinativum, stratum spinosum, stratum granulosum, stratum lucidum (on the palms of the hands and soles of the feet), and the stratum corneum (Table 36-1).

The dermis, or corium, is a flexible but strong and tough matrix of loose connective tissue that contains hair follicles, sweat and sebaceous glands, blood vessels, sensory nerves, and lymphatic vessels. Its main functions are to protect the internal structures from damage and provide nourishment for the living cells of the epidermis. The dermis contains three types of cells: fibroblasts, macrophages, and mast cells. Connective

Table 36-1 Layers of the Epidermis

Layer	Characteristics
Stratum germinativum (basal layer)	One cell thick Lies in contact with the dermis Basel cells attach the dermis to the epidermis Between the basal cells are melanocytes, which produce melanin and give the skin color Exposure to ultraviolet rays increases the amount of melanin produced Continuously forms new skin cells, called keratinocytes
Stratum spinosum (spinous layer)	Directly above the basal layer
Stratum granulosum (granular layer)	Two to four cells thick Allows new skin cells to mature into the scale-like cells of the epidermis
Stratum lucidum	Only found in the soles of the feel and palms of the hands Cells are dead Provides a tough layer to protect against friction, called a callous
Stratum corneum (keratin layer)	Outermost layer of skin, sheds continuously Flat cells of keratin (tough fibrous protein) Provides protection from some chemicals and damage Slows down water evaporation

tissue is made by the fibroblasts. Macrophages, a type of white blood cell, clean up dead skin cells and other debris and are an important part of the inflammatory process and wound healing. Mast cells release histamine when injury, infection, or exposure to allergens occurs. Histamine release promotes capillary permeability so that antibodies and macrophages can enter the injured area to begin the recovery process. Although the dermis is tough and flexible, prolonged stretching of the skin such as that which occurs during weight gain or pregnancy creates irreversible stretch marks or striae gravidarum.

Subcutaneous tissue, which is composed of both fat and slender elastic fibers, connects to the muscles and acts as a heat insulator, provides some shock absorption, and stores calories. Blood vessels and nerves enter the dermis through papillae in the subcutaneous tissue. Many items are found in subcutaneous tissue, including lymph vessels, hair follicle roots, portions of the sweat glands, fat, and nerve endings.

 # WOUND HEALING

There are three distinct phases of wound healing: the inflammatory stage, reconstruction stage, and maturation stage. During the initial or inflammatory stage, which lasts 3 to 5 days, the injured site is made ready for reconstruction. Platelets, red blood cells, and fibrin form a clot at the site of injury. The purpose of the clot is to protect the injured area from invasion by microorganisms and to stop bleeding. Blood vessels dilate, and white blood cells are brought to the area to begin engulfing bacteria and dead cells.

The second stage of healing lasts 4 to 14 days and is called **epithelization** or the reconstruction stage. During this stage epithelial cells grow into the injured area as capillaries establish blood flow and natural enzymes dissolve the clot or scab that has formed over the injury. Collagen is deposited at the wound site and the area fills in with new tissue. The new skin cells are very fragile.

During the final or maturation stage a mature scar forms and becomes strong. Scar tissue is never as strong as the original tissue it has replaced. The maturation stage can take months to years depending on how large the original injury was and how well the healing process was supported by adequate nutrition and so forth and whether the wound healed by primary or secondary intention. Primary intention healing occurs when little tissue is lost, the wound edges are close together and no infection has occurred. Secondary intention healing takes place when the wound is deep, wide, and open. This type of healing requires a lot of granulation tissue.

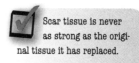
Scar tissue is never as strong as the original tissue it has replaced.

Underlying health deviations such as diabetes, low serum oxygen, and low circulating blood volume can affect wound healing. Medications like prednisone slow down healing because they inhibit the inflammatory process necessary for transporting cells to the injured area. Poor nutrition, especially low albumin levels, inhibits new collagen synthesis.

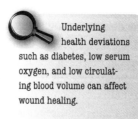
Underlying health deviations such as diabetes, low serum oxygen, and low circulating blood volume can affect wound healing.

Medications like prednisone slow down healing because they inhibit the inflammatory process necessary for transporting cells to the injured area.

Pictures of the various skin diseases discussed in the chapters of this section (Chapters 37–40) can be viewed at the following website: http://health.allrefer.com.

This chapter discusses common pediatric and adolescent skin abnormalities. An explanation of common skin assessment findings is included.

37

Skin Assessment, Birthmarks, and Acne

TERMS
☐ Acne neonatorum
☐ Capillary malformations
☐ Epstein pearls
☐ Erythema toxicum
☐ Giant pigmented nervus
☐ Hemangioma
☐ Milia
☐ Miliaria
☐ Mongolian spot
☐ Port wine stains

TRANSIENT SKIN DISEASES IN NEWBORNS

Milia occur in 40% of infants as 1-mm-diameter papules scattered over the forehead, nose, and cheeks. They are caused by superficial epidermal cysts. **Epstein pearls** are milia that occur in the oral cavity. Milia and Epstein pearls rupture spontaneously and disappear. **Acne neonatorum**, or acne in infants, may occur when the infant is 4 to 6 weeks old and may persist for 6 months to a year until spontaneous resolution occurs.

Erythema toxicum occurs in up to 50% of all full-term infants 24 to 48 hours after birth. It presents as blotchy red macules usually on the chest, back, face, or, less commonly, the extremities. Usually, the macules begin to fade in 1 to 2 days and are gone by 1 week. Although serum eosinophilia may occur, the macules are not caused by microorganisms.

Sucking blisters occur in response to vigorous sucking in the womb. They may occur on the forearms, wrists, thumbs, or upper lip and resolve on their own. **Miliaria** are caused by exposure to heat and high humidity and resolve when the infant is moved to a cooler drier environment. These eccrine sweat duct obstructions of the stratum corneum cause 1- to 2-mm grouped vesicles. Obstruction of eccrine ducts deeper in the epidermis results in grouped papules. Table 37-1 lists the skin assessment performed at birth and the meaning of the findings.

BIRTHMARKS

Birthmarks are caused by the overgrowth of skin components such as pigment cells, blood vessels, or lymph vessels.

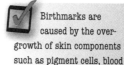
Birthmarks are caused by the overgrowth of skin components such as pigment cells, blood vessels, or lymph vessels.

Pigment Cell Birthmarks

Mongolian spot occurs in over 90% of all Native American, African-American, or Asian-American infants. It is characterized by a bluish black macule appearing on the lumbosacral area and is caused by pigment cells deep in the dermis. As the infant's skin darkens the lesion fades and blends in with the surrounding skin color.

Giant pigmented nervus is an irregular dark brown–black plaque that covers at least 5% of the body. The lesions may be large enough to cover the trunk of the body (bathing trunk nevi). Malignant changes may occur in these lesions. Large lesions may be excised followed by plastic surgery.

Table 37-1 Skin Examination at Birth

Assessment	Meaning
Bruising and/or petechiae	May be caused by forceps at delivery
Meconium staining	Sign of fetal distress during labor/birth
Jaundice	Abnormal if it presents in the first 24 hours of life
Peripheral cyanosis	Cool extremities or polycythemia
General cyanosis	Respiratory distress, cardiovascular malfunction
Pallor (in dark-skinned infants assess for pallor and cyanosis by looking at the nail beds and oral cavity)	Blood loss or acidosis
Vernix caseosa	Normal finding; whitish greasy material that covers the body and decreases in amount as term nears
Lanugo	Normal finding in preterm infants; fine hair covering the body
Dry cracking skin, superficial layers peel	Common in postterm infants
Edema	Generalized: hydrops; dorsum of the feet: Turner's syndrome
Milia	Small white cysts scattered over the cheeks, forehead, nose, and nasolabial folds
Miliaria	Blocked sweat gland ducts found on the face and scalp
Mottling	Lace-like pattern of dilated blood vessels over the extremities and trunk caused by exposure to a cool room temperature; disappears when infant warmed

Vascular Birthmarks

Capillary malformations are flat vascular birthmarks that appear either light red–orange or dark red–bluish red. Up to 50% of infants have a salmon patch, or light red macule, on the nape of the neck, upper eyelids, and the area above the eyebrows just above the nose (glabella). The eyelid lesions usually fade by the time the infant is 3 to 6 months of age, whereas those on the back of the neck fade but may last into adulthood.

The dark red–bluish red macules are called **port wine stains** and may occur anywhere on the body. The location of the port wine stain may signal syndromes. For example, port wine stains that cover one half of the face indicate possible Sturge-Weber syndrome (seizures, mental retardation, glaucoma, hemiplegia). Port wine stains over an extremity may indicate Klippel-Trenaunay syndrome (hypertrophy of the soft tissue and bone of the affected extremity). The stains may be reduced by the use of pulsed dye laser techniques.

Hemangioma is a benign tumor of capillary endothelial cells that appear red in color and rubbery with a rough surface. At birth the area affected may appear pale, but by 2 to 4 weeks of age the hemangioma appears. Ninety percent of all hemangiomas spontaneously disappear by age 9, leaving the area hypopigmented or with dilated blood vessels.

 Ninety percent of all hemangiomas spontaneously disappear by age 9, leaving the area hypopigmented or with dilated blood vessels.

 ## ACNE

Neonates may develop acne on the face, upper chest, and back at ages 4 to 6 weeks and lasting until ages 4 to 6 months in response to maternal androgens. Forty percent of children ages 8 to 10 years develop acne on the face, and 85% of all adolescents develop some form of acne, which forms in response to obstructed sebaceous follicles. The stratum corneum lining the follicles is usually one or two cells thick, but in acne the stratum corneum is overproduced in response to circulating androgens. If bacteria are present in the obstructed follicle, then inflammation occurs. External factors such as tight-fitting

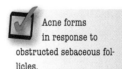 Acne forms in response to obstructed sebaceous follicles.

head bands, sport helmets, or clothing; oily cosmetics; and hairspray may cause acne. Any medication that increases plasma testosterone, such as glucocorticoids, hydantoins, and androgens, can cause acne.

Common acne treatments include topical keratolytic agents, which relieve follicular obstruction by causing a mild superficial peel of the epidermis, and topical or systemic antibiotics, which eliminate infection. Neither diet, oral vitamin A, exposure to ultraviolet light, nor drying agents have been demonstrated to effectively manage acne. Oral retinoids (Accutane) are used only for severe cystic acne because they are teratogenic (cause birth defects) and have serious side effects.

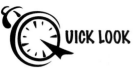

This chapter provides a close look at the etiology and treatment of two common childhood and adolescent skin disorders: dermatitis and psoriasis.

38

Dermatitis and Psoriasis

TERMS
- ☐ **Dermatitis**
- ☐ **Eczema**
- ☐ **Guttate**
- ☐ **Infantile eczema**
- ☐ **Psoriasis**

DERMATITIS

The terms **dermatitis** and **eczema** are often used interchangeably, although technically eczema denotes an acute weeping dermatosis. Dermatitis presents as an area of edema, redness, oozing, crusting, and possibly lichenification, defined as thickened skin with a shiny surface and deep skin markings caused by chronic rubbing and scratching.

Atopic Dermatitis

Atopic dermatitis (sensitive skin) is a common, chronic, superficial inflammatory disorder of the skin that causes severe dryness and itching and affects up to 20% of the population. The exact cause is unknown but has been linked to an interaction between genes, the environment, skin barrier defects, and the immune response. Irritating chemicals, temperature and humidity extremes, and fabrics such as wool may cause atopic dermatitis. Psychological stress is also associated with flare-ups because during psychological stress sweating occurs, which results in itching. Approximately 80% of children with atopic dermatitis develop asthma or allergic rhinitis, thus linking it to the antigen-antibody process.

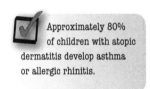
Approximately 80% of children with atopic dermatitis develop asthma or allergic rhinitis.

Pathophysiology

When the stratum corneum cannot hold water, the result is rapid evaporation along with shrinking of the stratum corneum and cracking of the epidermal barrier. This leads to irritants affecting the area, itching, and secondary skin infections. Children with atopic dermatitis are more likely to develop skin infections such as impetigo than children without atopic dermatitis.

Three clinical phases of atopic dermatitis are possible. The first phase, **infantile eczema**, begins around ages 1–4 months and ends at ages 18 to 24 months. During this phase the cheeks, scalp, trunk, and extensor surfaces of the extremities are affected and the dermatitis appears as oval patches. Two thirds of infants with infantile eczema do not progress to the second phase.

Phase 2, or flexural eczema, involves the antecubital and popliteal fossae, neck, wrists, and hands or feet. Some children have the eczema only on the soles of their feet, which will crack and become red (atopic feet). This phase lasts from age 24 months until adolescence. Two thirds of children in phase 2 do not progress to phase 3. The third phase, called adolescent eczema, mainly affects the hands and does not usually last past age 30.

Treatment

If the atopic eczema is weeping and acute, wet dressings and topical corticosteroids are frequently prescribed. Systemic antibiotics may be required if the area is infected with *Staphylococcus aureus* or another pathogen. The patient is also advised to avoid irritants and replace water lost by the stratum corneum. This is accomplished by avoiding soap, harsh shampoo, and rough clothing and applying lubrication to the skin at least three times a day or whenever the skin feels dry. Bedroom humidification is also useful in restoring water balance. If necessary, a 0.1% strength topical corticosteroid may be used.

Topical tacrolimus, a chemical produced by the *Streptomyces tsukubaensis* bacteria, is a new class of topical immunomodulators used to reduce inflammation associated with eczema. This cream is used when other methods of controlling the eczema have failed. Elidel (pimecrolimus), another topical immunosuppressive agent, is recommended for short-term use when other treatment methods have failed but is not recommended for children under 2 years of age. Cases of carcinoma have been reported in patients using Elidel, and research studies concerning its safety are ongoing.

Contact Dermatitis

Diaper Dermatitis

Primary irritant contact dermatitis peaks in about 24 hours and then disappears. Diaper dermatitis is a common form of primary irritant contact dermatitis caused by prolonged exposure to urine and feces, which contain irritating chemicals such as urea and enzymes. The affected area appears red and scaly. Infants who sleep through the night are prone to develop diaper dermatitis.

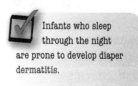
Infants who sleep through the night are prone to develop diaper dermatitis.

Frequent diaper changes and the avoidance of rubber or plastic barrier pants help to prevent diaper dermatitis.

Allergic Eczematous Contact Dermatitis

Allergic contact dermatitis is a type of delayed hypersensitivity reaction (cell-mediated) that may be caused by ingesting foods such as eggs, peanuts, milk, and wheat or by contact with substances such as certain plants, including poison ivy, poison sumac, and poison oak. Breast-fed babies prone to develop allergic contact dermatitis may do so if the mother eats foods such as peanuts, eggs, and fish. Allergic contact dermatitis usually peaks 2 to 3 days after exposure to the antigen and lasts 2 to 3 weeks even if exposure to the antigen is eliminated.

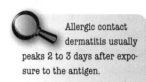

Allergic contact dermatitis usually peaks 2 to 3 days after exposure to the antigen.

Pathophysiology

The release of inflammatory mediators after exposure to the offending substance is responsible for the manifestations of allergic dermatitis. Immunoglobulin E antibodies signal mast cells to release histamine and other cytokines that, in turn, cause edema, vesicular lesions, skin breakdown, and pruritus. The affected area appears red, excessively dry, very itchy, and scaly.

Treatment

The first line of treatment involves removing contact with the offending antigen. Avoiding strong soaps, temperature extremes, and psychological stress is recommended. Emollients, systemic antihistamines, and topical corticosteroids are also used. Antibiotics are prescribed if a secondary infection occurs.

PAPULOSQUAMOUS ERUPTIONS

Papulosquamous eruptions are characterized by papules or plaques with various degrees of scaling. **Psoriasis,** a type of papulosquamous eruption, presents as red papules covered by thick white scales. Children may develop **guttate** (Latin for drop-like) psoriasis 2 to 3 weeks after they have had a streptococcal pharyngitis or URI. The child presents with small red dots that quickly become covered with thick white scales occurring mainly over the trunk.

Psoriasis vulgaris, or common psoriasis, is a chronic, persistent, or relapsing skin disorder with no known cause and is characterized by thick, large, red patches covered by silvery scales on the elbows, knees, and scalp. The rapid turnover of epidermal cells every 3 to 4 days instead of the usual 28 days results in the excessive production of stratum corneum. Usually, skin cells shed, but in psoriasis the cells pile up and form plaque (lesions).

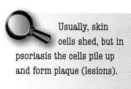 Usually, skin cells shed, but in psoriasis the cells pile up and form plaque (lesions).

Treatment

The focus of therapy is to slow epidermal turnover time and plaque formation. Common drugs used include Tazorac, a vitamin A derivative (topical retinoid); fluocinonide (Lidex, 0.05%), a topical steroid; calcipotriene (Dovonex), a vitamin D analogue that also flattens lesions and removes scale; and Anthralin, a synthetic substitute for Goa powder from the bark of the araroba tree of South America. Coal tar therapy slows cell growth and also reduces inflammation, itching, and scaling. Salicylic acid helps remove scales and is often combined with other topical medications.

Use of artificial light, including ultraviolet B, penetrates the skin and slows rapid cell growth. Psoralen, a light-sensitizing medication, is combined with ultraviolet A, a type of ultraviolet light, to slow cell reproduction. Pulsed dye lasers are used to eliminate tiny blood vessels that feed the epidermal cells responsible for rapid cell turnover.

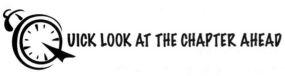

This chapter discusses common bacterial and viral skin infections common to children and adolescents. The etiology and treatment plan for each infection is described.

39

Skin Infections

TERMS
☐ Bullous impetigo (impetigo neonatorum)
☐ Dermatophytes
☐ Herpes labialis
☐ HSV-1 infections
☐ HSV-2 infections
☐ Impetigo contagiosa
☐ Plantar warts
☐ Tinea
☐ Tinea capitis
☐ Tinea cruris
☐ Tinea pedis
☐ Warts
☐ Wood lamp

BACTERIAL INFECTIONS

Impetigo

Impetigo presents as a red rash with many small blisters that may be itchy and break easily. Once the blisters rupture they are covered by honey-colored crusts.

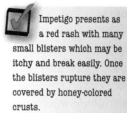
Impetigo presents as a red rash with many small blisters which may be itchy and break easily. Once the blisters rupture they are covered by honey-colored crusts.

Bullous impetigo (impetigo neonatorum) is a superficial skin infection of neonates that usually affects the buttocks, perineum, trunk, face, and extremities. The blisters form in response to toxins produced by the bacteria, are filled with fluid, and rupture easily within 24 to 48 hours. Little crust formation occurs after rupture. Oral and topical antibiotics are used to treat the infection. Because bullous impetigo is highly contagious, the infant should be isolated in the nursery to prevent spread to other infants.

Impetigo contagiosa is a common, highly contagious, superficial skin infection caused by the staphylococci (*Staphylococcus aureus*) and/or streptococci (*Streptococcus pyogenes*) bacteria. The face, arms, and legs are the most often affected. It is most common in the summer, and children with poor hygiene or those in daycare settings are especially susceptible to developing impetigo. The infected child's washcloths,

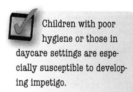
Children with poor hygiene or those in daycare settings are especially susceptible to developing impetigo.

towels, drinking glass, clothing, and bed linen should not be shared to prevent infecting others.

Pathophysiology

Any skin abrasion, cut, insect bite, or burn creates a method of entry for the bacteria. *Staphylococcus aureus* is normally found on the skin and mucous membranes, especially in the nose and throat. The bacteria can enter a break in the skin if the child touches his or her nose and then the skin.

Treatment

Impetigo is treated with oral or topical antibiotics for 7 to 10 days. A serious complication of impetigo is the development of glomerulonephritis, whether or not the child received antibiotic therapy. Scarring may result if a secondary bacterial infection takes place.

FUNGAL INFECTIONS

Tinea

Tinea infections are also called ringworm because of the red rings that appear on the affected area. **Tinea capitis** affects the scalp, producing bald spots, and is more common in African-American children than in other groups. **Tinea cruris** (jock itch) affects the inner thighs, inguinal creases, or perianal area; tinea corporis affects the body; and **tinea pedis** (athlete's foot) affects the webbed areas of the toes and feet. Tinea infections are spread by direct skin-to-skin contact with an infected person or pet or by contact with personal objects, such as towels, hats, hairbrushes, bed linen, shower stalls, or furniture used by someone with the infection.

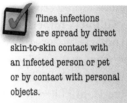

Tinea infections are spread by direct skin-to-skin contact with an infected person or pet or by contact with personal objects.

Children with allergies are most susceptible to developing the infection. A depressed immune system resulting from use of immunosuppressants, antineoplastic drugs, or corticosteroids also increases the likelihood of developing a tinea infection. Treatment with a potent antibiotic or diabetes, poor hygiene, warm moist skin folds, and skin irritation are additional factors that produce an environment conducive to tinea infections.

Tinea infections are diagnosed by culture, microscopic examination of skin scrapings, or by looking at the skin with an ultraviolet light, also called a **Wood lamp**.

Pathophysiology

Tinea infections are caused by a type of fungi called **dermatophytes** that require keratin found in the stratum corneum, hair, and nails to flourish. The itchy, contagious, red, scaly lesions with well-defined margins typical of tinea infections are the result of a superficial infection of the dead keratin layers of the epidermis, nails, and hair that does not penetrate to the lower epidermis or dermis. The dermatophytes live on, not in, the skin. The fungi produce an enzyme that dissolves and digests keratin.

Treatment

Tinea infections are treated with topical antifungal agents for approximately 6 weeks. Systemic antifungals are used if the infection affects the hair or nails. Approximately 20% of those affected develop a chronic infection.

 # VIRAL INFECTIONS

Herpes Simplex

In infants, herpes simplex type 1, **HSV-1**, infections generally involve the gingival, lips, and/or the periorbital region or the thumb in children who suck their thumbs. **Herpes labialis** is commonly called "cold sores" or "fever blisters" and is caused by HSV-1. Only 15% of HSV-1 infections produce symptoms.

Herpes simplex type 2, **HSV-2**, infections are usually found in the genital area and are primarily sexually transmitted infections; however, type 1 and type 2 infections can occur anywhere on the skin. Laboratory tests can distinguish between type 1 and type 2 herpes viruses.

HSV-1 can be transmitted to new-borns during vaginal delivery and is life-threatening. Vesicles, if they develop, present when the newborn is 6 to 10 days old. The infected infant may have a variety of signs and symptoms, including lethargy, irritability, poor feeding, vomiting, seizures, 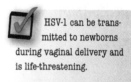 HSV-1 can be transmitted to newborns during vaginal delivery and is life-threatening.

respiratory distress, and coma. It is estimated that up to 50% of children have been infected with HSV-1 by the time they are 5 years of age.

HSV-2 is rare in children before the age of 14, and such cases suggest child abuse and should be investigated. In teenagers, HSV-2 infections are generally found on the genitalia and mouth. Lesions present as clumps of clear fluid-filled vesicles that crust once the vesicles break; it can be painful. Outbreaks generally last 2 to 6 weeks. Once the lesions form a crust healing occurs in 8 to 10 days.

Pathophysiology

The first phase or primary infection occurs after contact with an infected person when the virus enters the skin. There is a 2- to 30-day incubation period during this phase before symptom development. The virus initially affects epithelial cells, which subsequently die, releasing clear fluid intradermally, which forms vesicles. The virus then invades the nerve ganglion, innervating the original site of infection and becomes dormant.

The lifelong second phase of infection involves reactivation of the dormant virus. Once reactivated, the virus travels up the neuron back to the epithelium, where it reproduces causing another outbreak. Before the appearance of the vesicles the child may complain of a burning sensation, increased sensitivity of the area, or numbness and tingling. Herpes simplex viruses are very contagious if there is skin-to-skin contact during viral shedding, which can occur at any time, even when no vesicles are present. Reactivation of the virus is linked to fatigue, menstruation, skin irritation, fever, other infections, and exposure to ultraviolet light. The role stress plays in reactivation is under debate.

Treatment

Treatment consists of either topical or systemic antiviral agents. Vaccines to prevent herpes infections are under development.

VIRUS-INDUCED TUMORS

Warts

Warts are intraepidermal tumors caused by infection with the human papillomavirus that has entered the body through a break in the skin. The result is an overgrowth of epidermal cells forming a flesh-colored papule with an irregular surface. Warts commonly form on the upper surface of the hands, the fingers, feet, and genitalia. Flat warts appear on the face and are smoother and smaller that other warts.

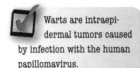

Warts are intraepidermal tumors caused by infection with the human papillomavirus.

Plantar warts appear on the bottom (sole) of the foot. They can be very painful and tender. Standing and walking push the warts flat and as a result they grow up into the skin. Plantar warts resemble a callus, but the warts have a tiny black dot (capillary blood vessel) in the center. A callus does not contain capillaries and forms only on weight-bearing areas. Approximately 1 in 10 teens has a plantar wart. Warm moist environments, such as locker rooms and sweaty socks and shoes, harbor the virus.

Treatment includes freezing the wart with liquid nitrogen. Approximately 30% of warts reappear after treatment.

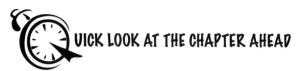

Insect infestations of the skin are common in children. This chapter explains the etiology and treatment plan for scabies and lice.

40

Insect Infestations

TERMS
☐ Scabies

SCABIES

Scabies is a superficial skin infestation caused by *Sarcoptes scabiei,* a parasitic mite, and is most common in children younger than 2 years of age. The mite, which needs contact with human skin to survive, burrows into the stratum corneum, especially near the wrists, ankles, finger webs, areolas, anterior axillary folds, genitalia, or the face in infants. This widespread contagious condition is transmitted by close personal contact with an infected person or by contact with infected bedding and clothing.

Pathophysiology

It takes approximately 45 minutes for the female mite to burrow into the outer layer of the epidermis (stratum corneum) where she lays eggs every 14 to 17 days. The eggs hatch in 3 to 5 days, and then the larvae migrate to the skin surface where they mature. After 4 to 5 weeks the female dies.

Itching is severe, especially at night, and is an inflammatory reaction to the mites, the mite eggs, and mite excrement. Generally, itching starts about 21 days after the first infestation begins as the child becomes sensitized to the mite and mite excrement and the inflammatory response is initiated. In subsequent exposures, because the child has already become sensitized, itching begins within 48 hours of infestation.

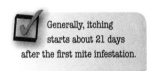

Generally, itching starts about 21 days after the first mite infestation.

Mites and eggs are collected under fingernails when an infected area is scratched. When the child then touches another part of the body, the mites and eggs are transferred to that area. A complication of scabies is a secondary infection, such as impetigo.

Infants who have scabies may present as irritable because they are tired from lack of sleep, and they may rub their hands and feet together. Water blisters may occur on the palms of their hands and soles of their feet.

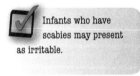

Infants who have scabies may present as irritable.

Burrows appear as fine threadlike lines and can be hard to detect.

Treatment

Topically applied permethrin or lindane cream is used to treat the infestation. Lindane should not be used in children younger than 2 years of age due to its neurotoxicity danger. All members of the household should be treated at the same time to help prevent reinfestation. Benadryl is used to help control itching, which may last up to 2 weeks after treatment. Antibiotics are used to treat secondary infections that occur in response to scratching.

 Lindane should not be used in children younger than 2 years of age due to its neurotoxicity danger.

The affected child's bedding and clothing should be washed daily in hot water and ironed before use. Items such as toys that cannot be washed should be placed in a sealed plastic bag for a week. Removing human contact with scabies for at least 3 consecutive days kills the mite.

 Removing human contact with scabies for at least 3 consecutive days kills the mite.

PEDICULOSES (LOUSE)

Infestation with the human louse, a blood-sucking parasite, occurs in all age and socioeconomic groups. It causes severe itching, especially at night, which in turns leads to excoriated papules, pustules, and secondary infections. Itching is caused by a reaction to louse saliva deposited into the skin as they feed several times a day. The higher the number of lice present and subsequent bites, the more severe the itching. The lesions produced at the feeding sites are flat, pinpoint, and red. Excoriations and bloody crusts are caused by scratching. The louse may be seen in clothing seams, on scalp hair presenting as gelatinous nits, in the pubic area, and on the eyelashes of newborns born to a mother with pediculoses. The female louse produces hundreds of nits every 14 days. Body lice (*Pediculus corporis*) live mainly in clothing, moving to the body to feed, whereas head and pubic lice live attached to the hair shaft.

Body lice (*Pediculus corporis*) live mainly in clothing, moving to the body to feed, whereas head and pubic lice live attached to the hair shaft.

Head lice (*Pediculus capitis*) and body lice can live up to 72 hours on clothing, combs, and so forth; are most common in school-aged children; and are highly contagious if the child comes into contact with personal items such as pillows and combs used by an actively infested person. Transmission may also occur via sharing headphones, hair clips, clothing, or blankets. The lice may look like common dandruff flakes but are not easily brushed away. Using a Wood lamp (ultraviolet light) allows the nits to be seen as a fluorescent spot. The occipital region, nape of the neck, and above the ears are common sites of infestation. The oval hair shaft shape of African-Americans makes it difficult for the parasite to cling, thus African-Americans have a lower incidence of head lice than do other ethnic groups.

Pubic lice (*Phthirus pubis*) resemble a crab, and therefore the infection is commonly called "crabs." Common sites of infestation in addition to pubic hairs include eyelashes, mustache, beard, and axillary hair. Young children should be screened for infestations on their eyelashes and eyebrows. These lice are easily detected by using a magnifying glass and looking for reddish-brown specks in the pubic area. They can only live 24 hours without a blood supply and are easily spread.

Treatment

Treatment for head lice includes shampooing with lindane (Kwell) or 1% permethrin and then combing with a fine-tooth comb to remove nits, boiling clothing for 10 minutes, and ironing clothing seams for body lice; lindane cream is applied to the pubic area for pubic lice. If the hair is matted and cannot be separated for proper treatment, it may need to be cut. Pregnant or lactating women or infants are advised not to use lindane because of possible neurotoxicity associated with the product. Infants and children may use permethrin 1% (Nix). RID, a combination of pyrethrin, piperonyl butoxide, and petroleum distillate, should not be used if the child has a contact allergy to ragweed, chrysanthemums, or turpentine. If the child has head lice, combing the hair with a nit comb daily is recommended until no more nits are found.

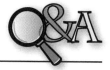

SECTION XVII • REVIEW QUESTIONS

1. The skin performs each of the following functions *except:*
   a. Producing vitamin C
   b. Acting as a bactericidal barrier
   c. Transmitting sensations
   d. Maintaining fluid balance

2. When assessing a newborn's skin the nurse can expect:
   a. Very dark skin color on an African-American newborn
   b. Subcutaneous fat pads under the newborn's skin
   c. Sweat droplets on the newborn's brow if the room is very warm
   d. Small white cysts scattered over the cheeks, forehead, and nose

3. The nurse documents correctly when she notes that a wound is:
   a. Healing by primary intention, wound open, moderate yellow/green drainage
   b. Healing by secondary intention, wound edges approximated
   c. Healing by primary intention, no drainage noted, wound edges approximated
   d. Healing well by secondary intention, wound edges pale

4. The delivery room temperature is set at 68 degrees. The nurse assisting with the delivery of a full-term infant would expect to assess which of the following (select all that apply)?
   a. Vernix caseosa
   b. Dry cracking skin
   c. Mottling
   d. Peripheral cyanosis

5. The nurse practitioner notes that the infant has miliaria. The nurse knows that this condition is caused by:
   a. Blocked tear ducts
   b. Exposure to heat and high humidity
   c. *Staphylococcus* organism
   d. A high eosinophil count

6. Infant Thomas has a Mongolian spot. The nurse explains to the parents that this discoloration:
   a. May become malignant and should be checked every 6 months
   b. Is common in white infants
   c. Is the result of an overgrowth of blood vessels
   d. Will fade as the infant ages

7. Infant Keisha has a hemangioma. The nurse explains to the parents that a hemangioma:
   a. Will probably disappear by the time Keisha is 9 years old
   b. Will become darker as Keisha ages
   c. Is the result of a maternal infection during pregnancy
   d. Will require laser removal when Keisha is older

8. Baby Carl is being treated for infantile eczema. The parents should be taught that:
   a. It is likely that Carl will have eczema into adulthood.
   b. Applying lubrication frequently to Carl's skin will help replace skin moisture.
   c. Topical immunosuppressants are safe to use on infants.
   d. Carl's skin is thicker than usual.

9. Porsha, a 16-year-old, has psoriasis. The nurse explains that psoriasis is:
   a. A common occurrence after a *Staphylococcus* infection
   b. The result of slow epidermal cell turnover
   c. Treated by a variety of methods, including ultraviolet light and pulsed dye lasers
   d. Definitely caused by a genetic mutation

10. The nurse is conducting a health education session for daycare center personnel. When asked about impetigo contagiosa the nurse correctly responds:
    a. Impetigo is caused by a virus called *Staphylococcus aureus*.
    b. Towels and drinking glasses used by a child with impetigo are not considered contaminated objects.
    c. The child with impetigo will be on oral antibiotics for 7–10 days.
    d. Once the blisters break, the child is no longer contagious.

11. The school nurse has been asked to be the featured speaker at a PTA meeting. Tinea is the topic selected for discussion. The school nurse correctly tells the program participants that tinea:
    a. Is caused by a dermatophyte that lives on the skin
    b. Is also called ringworm and is caused by a parasite
    c. Lesions are generally nonitchy, red, and scaly
    d. Treatment includes systemic and/or topical antibiotics

12. A community health nurse is making a home visit to a mother and her newborn infant who was born by a vaginal delivery. When assessing for HSV-1 (herpes simplex virus-1) the nurse knows that:
    a. This type of infection is usually mild in newborns.
    b. Vesicles develop when the infant is 6–10 days old.
    c. If the infant has HSV-1, a high fever will be present.
    d. HSV-1 infection is associated with child abuse.

13. Damian, age 15, visits the nurse practitioner because of a herpes simplex virus infection. The nurse practitioner correctly explains that:
    a. The virus enters the body by way of the respiratory tract.
    b. Each outbreak of blisters indicates a new infection.
    c. The virus can be spread only when blisters are present.
    d. The virus invades a nerve ganglion and remains dormant for varying amounts of time.

14. Select all of the following statements about warts that are correct.
    a. Plantar warts usually appear on the palms of the hands.
    b. Warts are caused by the human papillomavirus.
    c. Warts are the result of an overgrowth of dermal cells.
    d. Plantar warts have a tiny black dot in their center.

15. Which of the following statements concerning scabies is *true*?
    a. The female mite burrows into the dermis where she lives for about a month.
    b. The female mite lays eggs approximately every 14 days.
    c. Infants who have scabies often have blisters on the trunk and face.
    d. Burrows created by mites are easy to detect.

16. The nurse is explaining a louse infestation to teachers. Which statement made by the nurse is correct?
    a. Louse infestations cause severe itching during the day.
    b. Itching from lice is caused by the lice burrowing into the skin.
    c. Body lice live mainly on clothing.
    d. Head lice are more common in African-American children than in other ethnic groups.

ANSWERS AND RATIONALES

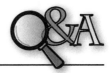

1. **The answer is a.** Rationale: The skin manufactures vitamin D, not vitamin C.

2. **The answer is d.** Rationale: Milia, small white cysts, are common in newborns; until melanin production increases dark-skinned infants have a light skin color; at birth newborns have little subcutaneous fat; sweat glands do not mature until the infant is 24–36 months of age.

3. **The answer is c.** Rationale: Wounds that are small, shallow, noninfected, and have approximated (touching) wound edges heal by primary intention.

4. **The answers are a and c.** Rationale: Vernix caseosa is a normal finding in full-term newborns as is mottling when the newborn is exposed to cold.

5. **The answer is b.** Rationale: Miliaria is caused by blocked sweat gland ducts and occurs most frequently in hot, humid weather.

6. **The answer is d.** Rationale: Mongolian spots are most common in Native American, African-American, and Asian-American infants. As the infant's skin darkens the spot fades.

7. **The answer is a.** Rationale: Ninety percent of hemangiomas spontaneously disappear by age 9. They are not caused by a maternal infection.

8. **The answer is b.** Rationale: Infantile eczema is caused by an inflammatory reaction and results in dry skin so parents/caregivers are encouraged to apply moisturizing lotion several times a day.

9. **The answer is c.** Rationale: Psoriasis is the result of rapid cell turnover and is treated by a variety of methods, including ultraviolet light and pulsed dye lasers.

10. **The answer is c.** Rationale: Impetigo, which is caused by bacteria, is treated with antibiotic therapy; the child is contagious until the lesions are gone; impetigo is highly contagious and can be spread by sharing eating implements and personal items.

11. **The answer is a.** Rationale: Tinea is caused by a type of fungi (dermatophytes) that lives on the skin, the lesions itch, and antibiotics are not used to treat a fungal infection.

12. **The answer is b.** Rationale: A newborn may acquire an HSV-1 infection during a vaginal birth if the mother has the infection. It is life-threatening in newborns, and blisters characteristic of the infection appear 6–10 days after delivery.

13. **The answer is d.** Rationale: Herpes simplex infections have periods of remission and exacerbations; the virus enters the body by direct contact, not via the respiratory tract; it can be spread even when no lesions are present.

14. **The answers are b and d.** Rationale: Warts are caused by the human papillomavirus and resemble a callus, but warts have a black dot (capillary blood vessel) in the center; plantar warts usually appear on the sole of the foot; overgrowth of epidermal cells results in warts.

15. **The answer is b.** Rationale: The female mite burrows into the outer layer of skin (epidermis) where she lays eggs every 7–14 days, the burrows are hard to detect, and watery blisters often appear on the palms of the hands and soles of the feet.

16. **The answer is c.** Rationale: A louse infection (parasite) causes itching at night, due to a reaction to louse saliva; body lice live mainly on clothing, moving to the body to feed.

XVIII

Liver and Pancreas Disorders

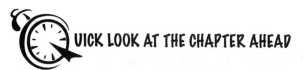

This chapter covers liver disorders, including jaundice, hyperbilirubinemia, bilirubin encephalopathy, biliary atresia, and viral hepatitis. Signs and symptoms and treatments are also included.

41

Liver Disorders

TERMS
- ☐ Colostrum
- ☐ Glucuronyl transferase
- ☐ Hyperbilirubinemia

BILIRUBIN PRODUCTION

Hemolysis of red blood cells → release of heme and globin (protein)→ heme is broken down into iron (conserved) and carbon monoxide (exhaled), and biliverdin → biliverdin is metabolized to bilirubin (yellow pigment) → free bilirubin (unconjugated, fat soluble, and indirect) and then binds to albumin and is carried to the liver → in the liver it is conjugated (made water soluble, direct) → conjugated bilirubin is excreted as part of bile into the intestine → bacteria in the intestine further metabolizes bilirubin into urobilinogen and this end product is excreted in stool, giving it a characteristic brown color, and urine, giving it a characteristic yellow color.

Blood tests can measure the amount of conjugated (direct) and unconjugated (indirect) bilirubin. When certain dyes are added to a blood sample, conjugated (water soluble) bilirubin acts directly with the dyes so it is called "direct bilirubin." Unconjugated (fat-soluble) bilirubin does not react to the dyes until alcohol is added to the solution, so it is called "indirect bilirubin."

ICTERUS NEONATORUM

Jaundice, a yellow discoloration of the skin, sclera, body fluids, and mucous membranes, normally develops in approximately 65% of full-term newborns and 80% of preterm newborns beginning after the infant is 24 hours old. This is a mild self-limiting condition and is not associated with disease pathology. Clinical jaundice appears at a bilirubin level of 5 mg/dl and begins on the head and then travels down the chest and abdomen to the distal extremities. Pathology is suspected if jaundice is present within the first 24 hours after birth, if the total serum bilirubin level rises by more than 5 mg/dl per day, or if signs and symptoms of disease pathology are present. A normal bilirubin level is between 0.2 and 1.4 mg/dl. Table 41-1 presents the differences between physiological and pathological jaundice.

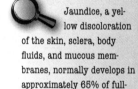

Jaundice, a yellow discoloration of the skin, sclera, body fluids, and mucous membranes, normally develops in approximately 65% of full-term newborns and 80% of preterm newborns.

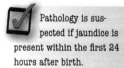

Pathology is suspected if jaundice is present within the first 24 hours after birth.

Table 41-1 Physiological Versus Pathological Jaundice

Physiological	Pathological
Appears *after* 24 hours of age, usually by day 2 or 3 in 50–60% of newborns	Appears *before* 24 hours of age
Peak bilirubin level of 5–6 mg/dl occurs by days 3–5	Total bilirubin level rises more than 5 mg/dl a day
Jaundice resolved by day 14 in full-term infants and after 2–4 weeks in premature infants	Total bilirubin level higher than 12 mg/dl in a full-term infant
Total bilirubin rises less than 5 mg/dl a day	Total bilirubin level higher than 10–14 mg/dl in a premature newborn
	High bilirubin level remains longer than 2 weeks

HYPERBILIRUBINEMIA

Excess bilirubin in the blood is called **hyperbilirubinemia**. By the time a full-term infant is 72 hours old his or her bilirubin level may reach 6 mg/dl. This level decreases to 2–3 mg/dl by the time the infant is 5 days old and remains at this level for up to 14 days.

Hyperbilirubinemia develops because of more rapid red blood cell destruction in the newborn, lower levels of **glucuronyl transferase** (the enzyme used to conjugate bilirubin), and low albumin levels. Slow intestinal motility and low gut bacteria also play a role because conjugated bilirubin stays in the intestine longer, where it then becomes unconjugated and is reabsorbed. Feeding the infant encourages the passage of meconium, which is rich in bilirubin, increases intestinal bacteria, and stimulates peristalsis, thereby decreasing the amount of unconjugated bilirubin that is reabsorbed.

Unconjugated hyperbilirubinemia may also develop because of rapid red blood cell destruction due to maternal antibodies, as occurs in Rh incompatibility, abnormal red blood cell shape, sepsis, prematurity, bile duct obstruction, or abnormal red blood cell enzymes. The rate of conjugation may be dramatically slowed due to low levels or complete absence of the enzyme that adds sugar to fat-soluble bilirubin so that it becomes water soluble (UDP-glucuronosyltransferase). Premature infants, infants of Asian race, and infants born at high altitudes are at higher risk of hyperbilirubinemia than are full-term white or black infants or infants born at sea level.

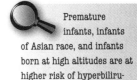

Premature infants, infants of Asian race, and infants born at high altitudes are at higher risk of hyperbilirubinemia.

BILIRUBIN ENCEPHALOPATHY

Free bilirubin, which is neurologically toxic, is deposited in brain cells if serum unconjugated bilirubin levels exceed the binding capacity of albumin. Bilirubin bound to albumin can also cross the blood–brain barrier if the infant has acidosis, hypoxia, hypoperfusion, hyperosmolality, or

 Free bilirubin is neurologically toxic.

sepsis. The administration of sodium bicarbonate to correct acidosis has been implicated in brain damage caused by high bilirubin levels. Signs of bilirubin encephalopathy (kernicterus) include lethargy, hypotonia, poor sucking, and a high pitched cry. Left untreated, the infant may develop cerebral palsy, deafness, severe muscle spasms, mental retardation, and seizures. Serum bilirubin levels do not indicate how much of a risk the infant with hyperbilirubinemia faces.

 Serum bilirubin levels do not indicate how much of a risk the infant with hyperbilirubinemia faces.

BREASTFEEDING AND JAUNDICE

Colostrum, a form of breast milk produced during the first 48–72 hours of breastfeeding, is a natural laxative that encourages the passage of meconium, which is high in bilirubin. Breast-fed infants may develop early-onset or late-onset jaundice. Early-onset jaundice (breastfeeding jaundice) develops in 13–25% of breast-fed infants between 2 and 7 days of age and may be triggered by a low fluid intake secondary to low breast milk production or poor feeding by the infant. Signs that inadequate breast milk is being produced or consumed

 Early-onset jaundice (breastfeeding jaundice) develops in 13–25% of breast-fed infants between 2 and 7 days of age.

include a weight loss of approximately 10% since birth, less than six wet diapers per day, fewer than four bowel movements per day, and nursing fewer than eight times per day for at least 10 minutes each time. Treatment is aimed at increasing the infant's intake of breast milk or formula. Sugar water supplements do not reduce bilirubin levels.

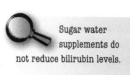

Sugar water supplements do not reduce bilirubin levels.

Late-onset jaundice (breast milk jaundice) develops in approximately 10–30% of breast-fed infants. The etiology of this type of jaundice is unknown. It is thought to occur because of high free fatty acid levels in the breast milk, which may hinder bilirubin conjugation. The serum bilirubin level may rise as high as 20 mg/dl, although it is usually in the 5- to 10-mg/dl range.

TREATMENT

Hyperbilirubinemia may be treated by fluorescent light phototherapy (bililight), fiberoptic blanket therapy (Bil-iBed® with Bilicombi Blanket™), or exchange transfusion. Bilirubin absorbs light (blue or white spectrum) and converts to a water-soluble substance that is excreted in the bile. With traditional phototherapy, increasing the amount of skin exposed to the light and moving the light closer to the infant increases its effectiveness. The infant's eyes should be covered during phototherapy to prevent retinal damage.

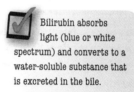

Bilirubin absorbs light (blue or white spectrum) and converts to a water-soluble substance that is excreted in the bile.

Placing the infant on a fiberoptic blanket allows for home therapy, increases parent–infant bonding, and has been shown to be as effective as traditional phototherapy when used correctly. The fiberoptic blanket must be used at all times, even during feeding. The infant's eyes do not need to be covered during this therapy, and the infant can wear clothing.

Various phases of clinical trials to determine the effectiveness and safety of the drug tin-mesoporphyrin to prevent hyperbilirubinemia have been completed. The drug shows promise as a replacement treatment for phototherapy but has not yet been approved for use in the United States. This drug inhibits the enzyme heme oxygenase, which is responsible for the metabolism of heme into its components, thereby reducing bilirubin production.

An infant rarely requires an exchange transfusion. This procedure may result in sudden death, thrombocytopenia (platelets are removed), hypoglycemia, necrotizing enterocolitis, infection, and electrolyte imbalance (hypocalcemia).

BILIARY ATRESIA

Biliary atresia, a progressive fibroinflammatory disorder of the intrahepatic and extrahepatic biliary tree, affects 1 in 10,000 to 15,000 infants, with Asian-Americans having a higher rate of the disorder than other ethnic groups. Symptoms of biliary atresia usually present before the infant is 12 weeks old and may be perinatal (80% of cases) or fetal–embryonic (20% of cases) in origin (Table 41-2). The bile ducts are destroyed by 4 months of age as a result of this inflammatory process. An infant with perinatal biliary atresia has normal-looking stool, which means that bile is able to pass into the intestine initially. The role viruses, toxins, and chemicals play in the development of perinatal biliary atresia is being studied.

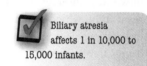

Biliary atresia affects 1 in 10,000 to 15,000 infants.

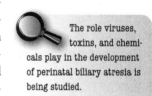

The role viruses, toxins, and chemicals play in the development of perinatal biliary atresia is being studied.

Table 41-2 Signs and Symptoms of Biliary Atresia

- Jaundice lasting longer than 2–3 weeks
- Bile-stained urine on diapers
- Pale yellow, buff-colored, or gray stools
- Hepatomegaly
- Firm liver
- Splenomegaly
- Pruritus
- Digital clubbing
- Poor weight gain by 2–6 months of age
- Ascites
- Bleeding
- Elevated levels of aminotransferase, alkaline phosphatase, and gamma glutamyl transpeptidase

In contrast to perinatal biliary atresia, the infant with fetal–embryonic biliary atresia has an abnormally developed bile duct and other nonhepatic congenital abnormalities. The infant with biliary atresia eventually develops malnutrition and failure to thrive (because fat and fat-soluble vitamins cannot be absorbed), cirrhosis, portal hypertension, and liver failure.

Surgical correction (liver transplant) is necessary or the infant will develop hepatic failure and die by 2 years of age. While waiting to find a suitable donor, the infant or child may have a Kasai procedure (hepatic portoenterostomy), which creates a bile duct from part of the small intestine. Although this procedure is usually successful and buys the child time, up to 90% of children who have the procedure develop progressive cirrhosis requiring a liver transplant. Table 41-3 lists metabolic liver functions.

 # VIRAL HEPATITIS

Viral hepatitis is an inflammatory process of the liver caused by a viral infection. It may result in either acute or chronic liver disease (Table 41-4).

Table 41-3 Metabolic Liver Functions

- Produces bile
- Metabolizes steroid hormones—sex hormones, glucocorticoids, aldosterone
- Metabolizes drugs
- Synthesizes protein such as albumin
- Synthesizes glucose from amino acids, glycerol, and lactic acid
- Synthesizes clotting factors: fibrinogen, prothrombin, factors V, VII, IX, X
- Stores vitamins A, D, B_{12}, K
- Stores iron
- Changes ammonia into urea
- Converts fatty acids to ketones
- Degrades extra nutrients
- Builds carbohydrates from proteins
- Converts extra sugar to fat for storage
- Stores excess glucose as glycogen
- Converts excess carbohydrates as triglycerides for storage in adipose tissue
- Produces bile salts from cholesterol
- Eliminates bilirubin
- Forms lipoproteins
- Synthesizes, recycles, and eliminates cholesterol
- Filters blood to remove bacteria and other waste products
- Forms urea from ammonia

Hepatitis viral agents are identified by letters. Approximately 46,000 children acquire hepatitis each year. Once the virus invades the liver the inflammatory process begins, and liver cells die and are removed by macrophages. As the inflammatory process continues bile ducts are swollen and blocked, resulting in icterus. The liver usually recovers in 12 weeks, but some children rapidly develop widespread liver necrosis (acute fulminating hepatitis) and require a liver transplant for survival. Symptoms include anorexia, nausea, vomiting, headache, fatigue, abdominal pain, and irritability followed by the icteric phase, during which they experience a change in the color of their skin, sclera, mucous membranes, urine, and stool.

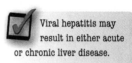 Viral hepatitis may result in either acute or chronic liver disease.

Table 41-4 Viral Hepatitis

Type	Transmission	Incubation	Mortality	Carrier	Vaccine	Symptoms
A	Fecal–oral from contaminated food/water or food handlers, day care settings Highly contagious virus can live on surfaces for 1 month	15–40 days	0.1–0.2%	No	Yes	66% of children are asymptomatic May not have jaundice Lifelong immunity after infection
B	Transmission from mother to fetus, body fluids, blood products, shared needles, skin piercing, tattoos	50–135 days	0.5–2%	Yes	Yes— recommended for all infants and adolescents	Slight fever, mild gastrointetsinal upset, jaundice

Type	Transmission	Incubation	Mortality	Carrier	Vaccine	Symptoms
C	30% unknown cause, transmission from mother to fetus, blood products, body piercing	30–150 days	1–2%	Yes	No	Many are asymptomatic, flu-like symptoms 70–80% progress to chronic hepatitis, may develop cirrhosis and/or liver cancer
D	Sexual contact, blood—only occurs when there is also a type B infection, rare in United States	20–90 days	2–20%	Yes	No	Chronic hepatitis and liver failure may develop
E	Fecal–oral, rare in United States	14–65 days	1–2%	No	No	

SECTION XVIII • REVIEW QUESTIONS

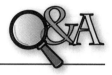

1. The nurse suspects icterus neonatorum when she reviews a newborn's history and finds that the newborn:
   a. Developed jaundice when she was 12 hours old
   b. Has had a 5-mg/dl rise in her bilirubin level every day for 3 days
   c. Had a peak bilirubin level of 6 mg/dl on day 4
   d. Is bottle fed

2. When teaching students about blood bilirubin production, the nurse stresses that a normal bilirubin level is _____ mg/dl.
   a. 0.0
   b. 0.8
   c. 1.8
   d. 2.0

3. Direct bilirubin is:
   a. Water soluble
   b. Fat soluble
   c. Unconjugated
   d. Unreactive to lab dyes until alcohol is added to the solution

4. Newborns are likely to develop hyperbilirubinemia because they have (select all that apply):
   a. Low levels of intestinal bacteria
   b. Low levels of glucuronyl transferase
   c. Rapid intestinal motility
   d. Slow red blood cell turnover

5. The byproducts of heme break down are (select all that apply):
   a. Iron
   b. Carbon dioxide
   c. Biliverdin
   d. Indirect bilirubin

6. A child with bilirubin encephalopathy may develop _____ if the encephalopathy is not treated promptly.
   a. Hypoxia
   b. Acidosis
   c. Hyperexcitability
   d. Cerebral palsy

7. Early-onset breast-feeding jaundice:
   a. Is an indication that breast milk production is low
   b. Can be offset by offering the infant sugar water every 2 hours
   c. Results in diarrhea
   d. Develops in approximately 75% of breast-fed infants

8. Kenisha, a 3-day-old full-term infant with hyperbilirubinemia, is brought back to the hospital for treatment. The nurse explains to her parents that Kenisha will be treated by:
   a. Placing her on a BiliBed® for 6 hours a day for 2 days
   b. Using a bililight and covering her eyes during its use
   c. An exchange transfusion
   d. One dose of tin-mesoporphyrin

9. When teaching a breast-feeding class to expectant mothers, the nurse explains that late-onset breast milk jaundice
   a. Signals dehydration
   b. Results from low colostrum levels
   c. Is a sign that liver disease is present
   d. Occurs in up to one third of breast-fed infants

10. Biliary atresia (select all that apply):
    a. Is more common in black infants than infants of other races
    b. Causes clay-colored stools within 72 hours after birth
    c. Is a progressive inflammatory disorder of the biliary tree
    d. Shows signs and symptoms before the infant is 3 months of age

11. Signs/symptoms of biliary atresia include:
    a. Boggy liver
    b. Bruising
    c. Low gamma glutamyl transpeptidase levels
    d. Greenish stools

12. Metabolic liver functions include (select all that apply):
    a. Storage of vitamins E and C
    b. Production of ammonia from protein metabolism
    c. Storage of iron
    d. Metabolism of glucocorticoids

13. When conducting a community health class at a teen center, the nurse stresses that:
    a. Hepatitis A is transmitted via contaminated blood
    b. Hepatitis D occurs when cirrhosis is present
    c. The process of tattooing can transmit hepatitis B
    d. Sexual contact can transmit hepatitis E

ANSWERS AND RATIONALES

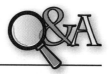

1. **The answer is c.** Rationale: Icterus neonatorum develops 24 hours after birth, rises less than 5 mg/dl per day, and is common in infants regardless of the feeding method; jaundice that develops sooner than 24 hours after birth or rises more than 5 mg/dl per day is pathological in nature.

2. **The answer is b.** Rationale: The normal bilirubin level is between 0.2 and 1.4 mg/dl.

3. **The answer is a.** Rationale: Direct bilirubin is water soluble, conjugated, and does not require alcohol to react to lab dyes.

4. **The answers are a and b.** Rationale: Newborns have slow intestinal motility and rapid red blood cell turnover.

5. **The answers are a and c.** Rationale: Heme breaks down into iron, which is saved; carbon monoxide, which is exhaled; and biliverdin. Indirect bilirubin is a byproduct of biliverdin metabolism.

6. **The answer is d.** Rationale: Bilirubin encephalopathy may result in seizures, mental retardation, cerebral palsy, deafness, and severe muscle spasms.

7. **The answer is a.** Rationale: Early-onset breast-feeding jaundice develops in 13–25% of breast-fed infants and may be triggered by low breast milk production or poor feeding by the infant. Sugar water supplements do not lower bilirubin levels.

8. **The answer is b.** Rationale: Tin-mesoporphyrin has not yet been approved for use in the United States, an exchange transfusion is rarely needed, and the infant is placed on the BiliBed for longer than 6 hours at a time.

9. **The answer is d.** Rationale: Early-onset breast milk jaundice signals dehydration, and the cause of late-onset breast milk jaundice is unknown.

10. **The answers are c and d.** Rationale: Biliary atresia is more common in Asian children, and an infant with this disorder has brown stools until the bile ducts are destroyed.

11. **The answer is b.** Rationale: The infant with biliary atresia has a firm liver; pale yellow, buff-colored, or gray stool; an elevated gamma glutamyl transpeptidase level; and bruising due to a bleeding tendency.

12. **The answers are c and d.** Rationale: The liver stores vitamins A, D, B_{12}, and K, and it produces urea from ammonia.

13. **The answer is c.** Rationale: Hepatitis A and E are spread by the fecal–oral route, and hepatitis D occurs in conjunction with hepatitis B.

XIX

Neurological and
Muscular Disorders

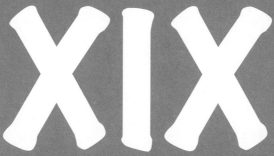

- Children with neuromuscular and neurological disease require a thorough assessment and monitoring of all systems.

- Head injuries can be described as mild, moderate and severe and are often assessed using the Glasgow Coma Scale.

- Hydrocephalus is caused by an obstruction of cerebrospinal fluid or impaired absorption of cerebrospinal fluid.

- Children with neuromuscular conditions require collaboration of several disciplines such as physical therapy, occupational therapy, speech, and social work in order to maximize their growth and development.

42

Pediatric Neurological and Neuromuscular Conditions

TERMS
☐ Autonomic dysreflexia
☐ Central nervous system (CNS)
☐ Cerebral palsy
☐ Hydrocephalus
☐ Seizures
☐ Spina bifida

There are two basic assumptions of neurodevelopment in children:

1. Early identification leads to better outcomes.
2. Comprehensive, multidisciplinary, and continuity of therapeutic services are important components for reaching potential development.

Table 42-1 lists the developmental, health, and psychosocial considerations to apply in the following pediatric neurological and neuromuscular conditions.

Table 42-1 Developmental, Health, and Psychosocial Considerations

General Considerations	Assessments and Needs	Health Promotion and Illness Prevention
Perinatal history impact vs. acquired or progressive degenerative disorder	Prematurity or low birth weight Teratogenic exposure Genetic condition Anoxia/hypoxia or trauma to CNS Infection (local or systemic) tumor/mass; capsulated or invasive cancerous, fatty (lipoma), or arteriovenous malformation (AVM)	Comprehensive patient and family history Ongoing laboratory, diagnostic imaging, and multidisciplinary assessments Coordinated primary, specialty, and rehabilitative care
Sensory manifestations	Cranial nerve involvement Deficits in any of the 5 senses (sight, hearing, smell, taste, touch) Impairments in speech or language communication	Vision, auditory, and speech and language screenings at developmental milestones and primary care visits Therapeutic and adaptive equipment intervention
Muscle tone and motor control abnormalities	Muscle tone strength, weakness, paralysis, or dyskinesia of movement (i.e., spasticity, ataxia, choreiform) Deep tendon, primitive and pathological reflexes (tonic neck, Babinski, etc.) Range of motion Coordination Delays in milestones Head, trunk, limb control Postural control and alignment	Low or high muscle tone at risk for developmental delays, deformities, and injury Postural and limb supports Positioning and prevention of deformities 24/7 Adapted equipment for ADLs, seating, and sleeping Degree of personal support and equipment needs may vary depending on the environment (household or community) and level of endurance

General Considerations	Assessments and Needs	Health Promotion and Illness Prevention
Anomalies/other congenital defects	Associated anomalies or comorbid conditions	Comprehensive and coordinated management for promoting health and functional status
Alterations in physical growth and sexual development	Identify adjusted growth charts for diagnoses (Down's syndrome) if available	Assessments, interventions, and psychosocial supports for growth delays, short stature, precocious puberty
Behavior/emotional Intellectual/educational Vocational	At risk for lower self-concept and isolation, inappropriate behaviors Attention deficits (heightened or lower) disorders Mood or psychiatric disorder Sleep disorders Cognitive delays due to localized or generalized CNS deficits	Psychological and neuropsychological evaluations and interventions Peer activities: support groups, camps, and recreational opportunities
Nutritional needs	Adequate fluid intake Timing and frequency Special dietary needs Augmented feeding; assistance, parenteral, gastrostomy Gastroesophageal reflux disease evaluation	Promotion of growth and development Dietary/nutrition consultation Supplementary feeding program Exercise and weight management program
ADLs; toileting and hygiene	Bowel and bladder programs that include behavioral, pharmacological, and dietary components Personal care assistance needs Personal care during menses	Habilitative/rehabilitative programs for incontinence Age-appropriate self-management training in personal care Reinforcement of privacy and confidentiality
Alteration in sexual health care needs	Alterations in sex organs or development Risk for precocious or delayed puberty Incontinence, infertility, and/or impotency issues Pregnancy risks for fetus or mother	Evaluation of sexual functioning and fertility Reinforcement and support for risk of sexual abuse Encourage social supports and circle of friends that can build an environment of trust, empowerment, and freedom of expression

Table 42-1 Developmental, Health, and Psychosocial Considerations (continued)

General Considerations	Assessments and Needs	Health Promotion and Illness Prevention
Adaptive equipment; recreational, educational, and vocational	Need for communication aids; orthotics, trunk, or limb braces; ambulation aids or wheelchairs; adaptive seating	Assessments of needs at different developmental, educational, and societal milestones with identification of resources and suppliers
Comfort, safety, and emergency measures	Altered status of consciousness Breathing difficulties due to positioning, obstruction, and/or chronicity Skin breakdown Muscular skeletal trauma or falls Risk for abuse or neglect Allergies and toxicities Poor progressive prognosis, DNR needs	Ongoing assessment and priority of comfort and safety across environments of care

ADLs, activities of daily living; DNR, do not resuscitate.

ACQUIRED BRAIN INJURY

An acquired brain injury (ABI) is defined as an insult to the **central nervous system (CNS)** that impedes function most often due to hypoxia or anoxia (reduced oxygen to the brain due obstructed airway, near drowning, electrocution, etc.), a traumatic event such as blunt trauma to the head or speed-associated injury (motor vehicle or fall), or CNS cell damage from a tumor, mass (arterial venous malformation), or bleed. The encephalopathy event occurs after the age of 2 years or is most often classified as cerebral palsy (below). ABI often impacts development and requires various acute and/or chronic treatments and rehabilitation programs.

Pathophysiology

The ABI event and the impact of decreased blood flow, oxygenation to the tissues of the brain, and resulting inflammatory effects may cause damage to cell tissues and scarring that are localized or diffuse and global. Sequelae may be mild to severe and may include the following associated disorders:

- Trauma to the scalp or face (laceration) or cranium (skull fracture)
- Period of loss of consciousness, concussion, and/or comatose state (Table 42-2)
- Period of increased intracranial pressure
- Seizure disorder
- Cognitive, learning, and/or vocational deficits
- Sensory deficits (vision, hearing, taste/smell)
- Language and/or communication deficits (aphasia, dysphagia)
- Behavioral or mental health disorders
- Sensory–motor–movement disorder (e.g., emiplegia/paresis, ataxia, etc.)

Treatment

There are three phases of treatment:

1. Emergency and critical care: Focus is on preserving brain homeostasis and managing intracranial pressure and any other injuries.
2. Acute rehabilitation (usually the first 2 months after the event): Focus is on preventing complications, orienting the patient, patient/family teaching and support, and safety measures.
3. Long-term rehabilitation and multidisciplinary follow-up.

 ## CEREBRAL PALSY

Cerebral palsy (CP) is an umbrella term for a group of CNS conditions that occur pre- or perinatally or early in life (often classified as CP if diag-

Table 42-2 Glasgow Coma Scale to Assess Level of Consciousness

Eye opening
  Spontaneous opening (4), to loud noise (3), to pain (2), no response (1)
Verbal response
  Smiles, uses words (5), irritable, confused (4), inappropriate crying or words (3), grunts, incomprehensible sounds (2), none (1)
Motor response
  Spontaneous movement (6), withdraws to touch (5), withdraws to pain (4), abnormal flexion (3), abnormal extension (2), none (1)

nosed before 2 years of age). Conditions may be mild to severe, and further classifications of CP are complex and definitions have varied worldwide. Classifications of CP include severity (mild, moderate, or severe), type of movement (spastic, athetoid, or other dyskinesia), and the parts of the body involved (quadriplegic/paresis, hemiplegic/paresis, or paraplegic/paresis). Dysarthria is the impaired, stammering, or slurred speech pattern and dysphagia is the swallowing difficulty resulting in drooling that may be associated with CP.

Pathophysiology

The underlying etiology is not progressive (although sequelae may be due to growth factors and associated conditions) and includes the following:

- Maternal factors during pregnancy (high parity, thyroid disorder, history of pregnancy loss, teratogen/substance abuse exposure)
- Congenital viral infections
- Intraventricular bleed in premature neonates
- Low birth weight
- Birth asphyxia
- Hypoxic episode or ABI during infancy

Neuroimaging (static and dynamic) is critical to identify the extent and location of brain damage and presence or absence of anomalies. Neurodevelopmental evaluations, electrophysiological studies, and multidisciplinary comprehensive assessment are essential during infancy, performed as needed in early childhood, and used for long-term follow-up to rule out genetic or progressive disorders and support treatment programs.

Treatment

The extent of brain injury (local or generalized), type, and severity dictate treatment needs and are predictors of outcomes. Sequelae are similar to those associated with ABI. Early intervention programs and comprehensive rehabilitation follow-up in collaboration with primary care and educational programs are critical for healthy outcomes, optimal functioning, and quality of life.

MENINGITIS

Meningitis is an inflammation of the membranes of the brain or spinal cord at the level of the lining (meninges) caused by an infectious process. Meningitis is often secondary to a respiratory illness but may be transmitted from other foci from the blood, lymphatic system, or after trauma to the adjacent sinus or mastoid. Bacteria are the most common cause; however, viruses may also be a contributory agent. Infants and young children are at great risk for bacterial meningitis, with boys affected more often than girls.

Pathophysiology

In most cases when an infection precedes the incidence of meningitis, bacteremia spreads the infectious agent to the CNS. As an inflammatory response occurs, white blood cells collect, covering the surface of the brain with a purulent exudate. A classic symptom of nuchal rigidity and headache occur as inflammation of the spinal nerves takes place. Resulting complications that can occur are increased intracranial pressure, hydrocephalus, and even hearing loss, blindness, and developmental disabilities.

Treatment

Diagnostic testing includes blood cultures, lumbar puncture, and computed tomography. Antibiotics are started as soon as possible for bacterial meningitis and may continue for up to 21 days. If a diagnosis of viral meningitis is confirmed, treatment becomes more palliative. Intravenous fluids are started, and corticosteroids may be given to reduce the risk of severe neurological impairment. The child should be carefully monitored to avoid any potential complications.

 # MUSCULAR DYSTROPHIES

There are a variety of diseases in this category, each having different manifestations. Some conditions are fairly static in pathology, whereas others are progressive and degenerative, in particular Duchenne's muscular dystrophy and spinal muscular atrophy. Duchenne's muscular dystrophy is an X-linked recessive inherited disorder affecting 1 in 3,600 live male births. Symptoms start to present around 5 years of age. These include tripping, toe walking, and weakness in lower extremities. Improvements in care have increased the quality of life and life expectancy for many with these conditions.

Pathophysiology

The muscle groups targeted and the etiology and progression of degeneration of muscles cells and/or motor neurons depends on the type of muscular dystrophy. The specific genes that program cell development during embryology and growth and function of muscle cells during life may be impaired, causing atrophy or pseudohypertrophy of muscle groups. Symptoms may be present at birth or hypotonia may present later in life, ensuing in limitations in motor function and risk for deforming forces on limbs during growth periods and safety issues due to postural instability and respiratory compromise. An increased risk for malignant hyperthermia, a complication of anesthesia, occurs in Duchenne's muscular dystrophy and other muscular dystrophies.

Treatment

An interdisciplinary approach to the therapeutic management is needed to ensure the health and development of children and adults with muscular dystrophy. Most people living with muscular dystrophy have normal intelligence and can be productive members of society, but they are also at risk for a shortened life span due to potential respiratory compromise and other mortality and morbidity conditions associated with disability.

 SEIZURE DISORDERS

Also called epilepsy, **seizures** are a disorder where abnormal electrical discharges from the brain trigger alterations or interruptions in sensory, motor, and/or cognition systems. Depending on individual differences and etiologies, seizures may vary in location or may be generalized with different time frequencies and durations (Table 42-3).

Table 42-3 Seizures, Manifestations, and Considerations

Seizure Type	Manifestations	Diagnosis
Neonatal seizure	Seen birth to 1 month old Atypical limpness or sudden posturing, with or without mild apnea, nystagmus, cry, lip smacking, or twitching Due to intracranial insult, metabolic imbalance, or drug withdrawal	LP to rule out viral infection Blood work Ultrasonography or computed tomography for intraventricular bleed or structural anomaly
Infantile spasms	Generalized clonic-tonic or focal twitching beginning in infancy up to 4 years Due to hypoxic or ischemic brain damage; biochemical, infectious, or degenerative factors; and idiopathic in approximately one third of the cases	Funduscopic and skin examinations, metabolic workup, neuroradiographic imaging scanning, genetic testing
Febrile convulsions	Most common childhood seizure Seen in ages 3 months to 5 years Usually generalized lasting < 15 minutes during febrile illness > 39°C and with positive family history	Electroencephalogram (within 10 days of Seizure) LP to rule out meningitis
Absence	More prevalent in females 4 years to adolescence when they start to disappear Brief loss of consciousness, staring No aura Slight increase or loss of muscle tone	Possible genetic link
Partial complex	3 years to adolescence Aura frequently present Posturing, staring, abdominal pain	Check for brain lesions, birth or traumatic injury, tumor
Simple partial	Postseizure amnesia, confusion No loss of consciousness No aura Occurs many times a day Motor and sensory involvement May have hallucinations, buzzing sound, or feel anxious	Check for tumors, lesions, abscess, AVM
Generalized; tonic-clonic or grand mal	Strong familial incidence Child falls to ground, jaw clenches shut, compromised airway, body becomes rigid Urinary or bowel incontinence afterward Postictal state afterward	Check for genetic link Metabolic or neuromuscular disorders

LP, lumbar puncture.

Treatment

Pharmacological treatment is often started with one drug selected for the clinical situation and begun at a low dose and titrated to a maximum dose for age and weight and side effects. If seizures are not controlled, the drug is changed to a new class or a second class is added and titrated under observation. There is a need to assess for interactions, toxicity, and indications for adult life choices (e.g., driving, pregnancy, etc.)

Counseling and education are provided for child, parents, and school community personnel as needed on medication administration and adherence, safety, supervision, and emergency management. Support should be provided for optimal development and quality of life with transition plan to adulthood.

Ketogenic (limited intake of protein and carbohydrate) and other diets have been recommended with seizure conditions not responsive to drugs or in lieu of pharmaceutical treatment with varying outcomes. Diets may be expensive and difficult to adhere to.

Seizures that are intractable and of an apparently focal origin may be responsive to neurosurgical incisions to remove the damaged area. The more common CNS procedures have included corticectomy, temporal lobectomy, and hemispherectomy. A peripheral approach, the implant of a vagal nerve stimulator that can be intermittently turned on by an external magnetic wand, has been shown to be effective in some individuals with prolonged intractable seizures.

Follow-up and long-term management with a multidisciplinary approach include periodic assessments and a life plan approach to care in place. Ongoing laboratory (e.g., liver function studies) and diagnostic analyses (i.e., magnetic resonance imaging) and neurological–psychological–habilitation–vocational assessments are preformed as needed.

HYDROCEPHALUS

Hydrocephalus is either caused by a congenital anomaly or occurs after a traumatic or acquired encephalopathy (inflammation, neoplasm, or bleed) that disrupts the anatomy or physiology of the CNS and the balance between the formation and absorption of the cerebrospinal fluid. The partial or full occlusion of the flow of cerebrospinal fluid requires the surgical placement of a shunt to reroute and drain off the buildup of cerebrospinal fluid and prevent brain damage or sequelae.

Pathophysiology

Most of the cerebrospinal fluid is made daily in the choroid plexus of the large lateral ventricles of the brain and circulates throughout the third and fourth ventricles; a small amount is made in the extracellular space around the brain and down the central canal of the spinal cord. The pathophysiology of hydrocephalus is varied due to age at onset and associated anatomical anomalies. Suggested terminology or classification of hydrocephalus includes (1) site of blockage to cerebrospinal fluid circulation, (2) etiology, and (3) dynamic status (progressive or arrested).

Agenesis and/or thinning of the cerebral mantel of the corpus callosum may be associated with hydrocephalus and results in learning disabilities, primarily in directionality and in spatial relationships. Seizure disorders and mental retardations are associated in cases where multiple shunt malfunctions and delayed treatment of shunt infections have occurred.

Treatment

Signs of hydrocephalus vary according to the age of the child. In the infant they include increasing head circumference and frontal bossing (pronounced forehead), "sunset eyes" or inability to gaze upward, with late signs including a shrill high-pitched cry, difficulty feeding, and vomiting. In the older child signs include irritability, lethargy, poor appetite, headache, papilledema, personality changes, and altered level of consciousness. Subtle signs of intermittent or chronic shunt malfunction include the above as well as hand-writing deterioration, upper extremity function changes, and slow progression of vision loss.

Cranial ultrasonography, computed tomography, magnetic resonance imaging, or other diagnostic scans are performed to determine the extent of hydrocephalus and location of blockage or narrowing. Surgical placement of the shunt is usually located from the lateral, third, or fourth ventricle to the peritoneal cavity or at times the right atrium. Families and community care teams should be educated to the signs and symptoms of malfunctioning or infected shunts and emergency management plans.

SPINA BIFIDA

Spina bifida is a term that is often synonymous with myelomeningocele, myelodysplasia, or neural tube defect. This birth defect occurs during the 21st to 28th day of embryonic development and is considered a multi-factorial birth defect (having both genetic and environmental contributing factors). In spina bifida there is a bony and often neurological birth defect that occurs anywhere along the spinal cord. At times there is a fatty mass associated with the bony or nervous system lesion called a lipoma or lipomeningocele. There are many variations and differences in the severity of the lesion due to the location on the spinal cord and if the spinal cord is completely or only partially involved or damaged at the area of the defect. Hydrocephalus or other anomalies such as club foot, limb deficiency, or renal defects may be associated with spina bifida.

The incidence of neural tube defects is 0.7–1 per 1,000 live births. The incidence has decreased over the years because folic acid has been strongly recommended for young women and foods enriched with folate have been mandated by the U.S. Food and Drug Administration.

Pathophysiology

During fetal development the neural tube, consisting of the brain and spinal cord, develop during the first trimester. Historically, the neural tube was assumed to close in a cephalocaudal (head to sacrum) "zipper-like" manner in the first month of fetal development. However, recent studies indicate that the development is more complex and closure is more fragmented, resulting in birth defects that occur in a variety of places from the crown of the head and down the cervical, thoracic, lumbar, or sacral spine. The amount of spinal bone and spinal cord damage varies widely in each individual. Tethering cord syndrome, the adherence of the nervous tissue to the bones from scar formation, can occur prenatally or after surgical closure and attempts at repair of the meningocele or defect. Tethering and the presence of a syrinx (narrowing of the spinal canal which causes pressure on the spinal canal) may result in an increase in symptoms or loss in function, especially at times of the individual's growth spurts.

Symptoms associated with spina bifida include loss or decrease in sensation or motor function below the level of injury, neurogenic bowel and bladder problems and incontinence, deformation of the lower extremities that may increase during growth spurts, developmental delays, alterations in sexual health/functioning, and other problems due to associated conditions (see Hydrocephalus, above). Arnold-Chiari II malformation is a congenital malformation of the hindbrain associated with hydrocephalus in persons with spina bifida resulting in varying degrees of cranial nerve, upper extremity, and respiratory disorders.

Treatment

Early closure of the spinal defect is usually done in the first 48 hours after birth, and there are new attempts to improve outcomes with interuterine fetal surgery. Diligent and coordinated follow-up and interventions by neurosurgical, orthopedic, urologic, nursing, rehabilitation specialist, and primary care providers are needed to promote development, quality of life, and integration into educational, recreational, social, and vocational programs. People with spina bifida or congenital genitourinary anomalies are at risk for latex allergies and need to avoid exposure to latex products and to be prepared for an allergic reaction.

> People with spina bifida or congenital genitourinary anomalies are at risk for latex allergies and need to avoid exposure to latex products and to be prepared for an allergic reaction.

SPINAL CORD INJURY (PEDIATRIC ACQUIRED)

Pediatric spinal cord injury occurs at birth through age 15 years due to trauma (birth delivery, falls, sports, violence, motor vehicle accidents), abnormality to blood flow (arterial-venous malformation), a tumor or mass (benign or cancer), or inflammation/infection to the neurons of the spinal cord or their peripheral nerve tracts. The level and extent of lesion may vary as well as the amount (complete or incomplete) of loss to motor function and sensation. In most cases the area of loss in motor, sensation, position sense, bowel, bladder, and sexual functions is below the level of injury. In central cord syndrome the injury or edema is usually in the cervical spine and the upper extremities are more affected by motor and sensory deficits than the lower extremities.

Pathophysiology

In traumatic spinal cord injury the amount and type of force is a predictor of the injury and of outcome. However, in all etiologies the length of time and the resulting inflammation and ischemia at the time of onset and secondary throughout the initial course of management are critical to the outcomes. Surgical intervention may be necessary to remove pressure and support blood flow, and steroids and other pharmaceuticals may be needed to decrease inflammation. Maintaining vertebral alignment, postural trunk support, pulmonary functioning, and routine elimination of bowel and bladder; decreasing muscle spasticity; and self-care for activity of daily living during growth and development are paramount. Ongoing comprehensive rehabilitative programs and social/recreational activities are essential to living well with a spinal cord injury.

Treatment

There are three phases to treatment:

1. Emergency and critical care: Focus is on corticosteroids for inflammation, decompression and/or surgical fixation, and managing respiratory and life-sustaining functions.
2. Acute rehabilitation (1–2 months): Focus is on preventing complications, patient/family teaching, and support.
3. Long-term rehabilitation and multidisciplinary follow-up.

   Autonomic dysreflexia or hyperreflexia is a life-threatening complication of spinal cord injury. Warning signs and symptoms include:

- Flushing and diaphoresis (sweating) above the level of injury
- Headache
- Elevated blood pressure

Actions and emergency interventions are as follows:

- Remove the precipitating stimulus, the painful environmental trigger, pinching or pressure item in area loss of sensation (e.g., sharp object, loosen shoes or braces)
- Transfer and change position but keep the head elevated
- Monitor blood pressure
- Catheterize if bladder is distended

- Empty bowel, use Xylocaine jelly if disimpacting or on a suppository
- Administer antihypertensive agent if hypertension persists and at risk of a stroke
- Provide emotional support to decrease anxiety
- Emergency referral

SECTION XIX · REVIEW QUESTIONS

1. The Glasgow coma scale consists of all of the following areas of assessment *except:*
   a. Verbal response
   b. Motor response
   c. Eye opening
   d. Sensory response

2. A fixed and dilated pupil is indicative of:
   a. Late sign of increased intracranial pressure
   b. Hydrocephalus
   c. Grand mal seizure
   d. Brain tumor

3. Sam has just been diagnosed with Duchenne's muscular dystrophy. An early sign that the parents might have noticed would be:
   a. Difficulty breathing
   b. Tripping, toe walking
   c. Frequent falls down stairs
   d. Difficulty voiding

4. Early signs of hydrocephalus in the infant include all of the following *except:*
   a. Increased head circumference
   b. Frontal bossing
   c. Headache
   d. Sunset eyes

5. Factors that contribute to cerebral palsy include all of the following *except:*
   a. Prematurity
   b. Birth trauma
   c. Infantile seizures
   d. Intrauterine infection

6. Febrile seizures are most often seen in children of what age?
    a. 12–24 months
    b. 17–24 months
    c. Birth to 5 years of age
    d. Birth to adolescence

7. Suzy had a shunt placed for hydrocephalus. Signs of an infected shunt are similar to:
    a. Meningitis
    b. Seizure
    c. Increased intracranial pressure
    d. Headache

8. The incidence of neural tube defects has decreased over the past 10 years as:
    a. Prenatal genetic testing has improved
    b. Foods enriched with folate have been mandated
    c. Herbal remedies have gained popularity
    d. Birth trauma rates have decreased

9. Meningitis is most often characterized by symptoms of:
    a. Fever and seizures
    b. Septic shock
    c. Loss of consciousness
    d. Headache and nuchal rigidity

10. Absence seizures are characterized by all of the following *except:*
    a. No aura
    b. Brief loss of consciousness
    c. Bowel and bladder incontinence
    d. Staring

ANSWERS AND RATIONALES

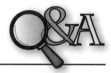

1. **The answer is d.** Rationale: The Glasgow coma scale measures motor response, verbal response, and eye opening for individuals to assess level of consciousness.

2. **The answer is a.** Rationale: As increased intracranial pressure increases, fixed and dilated pupils are a neurosurgical emergency indicative of brainstem herniation.

3. **The answer is b.** Rationale: Duchenne's muscular dystrophy is often diagnosed around 5 years of age as the child progresses through gross motor development and is seen to be tripping and toe walking.

4. **The answer is c.** Rationale: Early signs of hydrocephalus in the infant are increased head circumference, frontal bossing, and sunset eyes. Headache is seen in the older child.

5. **The answer is c.** Rationale: There are many factors that contribute to cerebral palsy, but infantile seizure is not one of them.

6. **The answer is c.** Rationale: Febrile seizures are most often seen in young children between birth and 5 years and are the most common childhood seizure.

7. **The answer is a.** Rationale: Shunt infections can be caused by sepsis and wound infection or may be present at the time of shunt placement. Monitoring for symptoms similar to meningitis include elevated temperature, local inflammation, vomiting, and nuchal rigidity.

8. **The answer is b.** Rationale: The incidence of neural tube defects has decreased over the years as women have been counseled to start on folate if considering pregnancy and foods enriched with folate have been mandated by the U.S. Food and Drug Administration.

9. **The answer is d.** Rationale: Headache and nuchal rigidity best describe the symptoms seen in meningitis.

10. **The answer is c.** Rationale: Bowel and bladder incontinence is seen most often in generalized or tonic-clonic seizures.

XX

Orthopedic Disorders

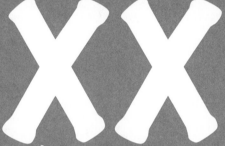

- Developmental milestones can be affected in children with musculoskeletal disorders.

- Orthopedic injuries in children are often caused by sports or recreation related activities.

- Immobilization related to an orthopedic injury can impact psych-social, intellectual, and physical development in a child.

- Injury to epiphyseal growth plates can arrest further growth in bones.

- Infections in the bone can be difficult to treat and eradicate.

43

Orthodpedic Disorders

TERMS
- ☐ Closed fracture
- ☐ Dislocatable hip
- ☐ Dislocated hip
- ☐ Greenstick fracture
- ☐ Idiopathic scoliosis
- ☐ Kyphosis
- ☐ Lordosis
- ☐ Oblique fracture
- ☐ Open fracture
- ☐ Osteomyelitis
- ☐ Scoliosis
- ☐ Spiral fracture
- ☐ Subluxated hip
- ☐ Transverse fracture

395

DEVELOPMENTAL DYSPLASIA OF THE HIP

In the past the common term for a child born with a hip condition was congenital hip dysplasia. The current term of developmental dysplasia of the hip encompasses three conditions that may affect an infant at birth or shortly thereafter with dislocation, subluxation, or dysplasia of the hip (Figure 43-1). A dislocated hip occurs in 1 in 1,000 births, is usually unilateral, and occurs most often in females. The left hip is involved in 60% of cases.

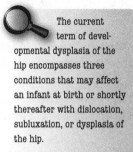

The current term of developmental dysplasia of the hip encompasses three conditions that may affect an infant at birth or shortly thereafter with dislocation, subluxation, or dysplasia of the hip.

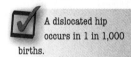

A dislocated hip occurs in 1 in 1,000 births.

Pathophysiology

Several factors influence the incidence of developmental dysplasia of the hip. Many hip dysplasias occur during the second or third trimester as a

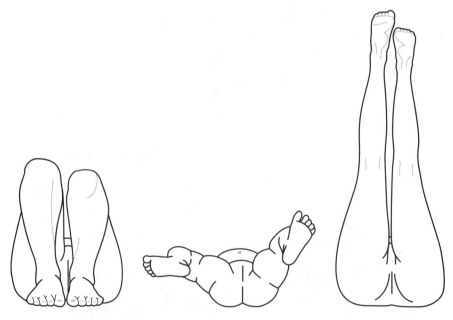

Figure 43-1 Developmental dysplasia of the hip.

result of fetal positioning. The left hip is involved more often because of intrauterine positioning of the fetus against the mother's sacrum. Girls are more affected because it is thought that maternal levels of estrogen influence ligamentous laxity that females respond to differently. Developmental dysplasia of the hip is also more common in infants born in the breech position.

A **dislocated hip** is one that is characterized by a complete loss of contact of the femoral head with the acetabulum, a **dislocatable hip** is one that can be manually displaced but returns to the acetabulum with release of pressure, and a **subluxated hip** is one where the femoral head remains in the acetabulum but comes partially out of the joint with manipulation.

In the infant two tests that may be done are the Barlow maneuver and the Ortolani test. These tests are most reliable within the first month of life. In the Barlow maneuver slight pressure is applied with the thumb on the medial side of the thigh as the thigh is adducted. A jerk is elicited as the hip dislocates. In the Ortolani test both hips are flexed and 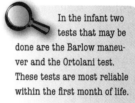 In the infant two tests that may be done are the Barlow maneuver and the Ortolani test. These tests are most reliable within the first month of life.

gently abducted and externally rotated. A click is heard as the dislocated head reduces into the acetabulum. There are several cardinal signs and symptoms that indicate an infant may have developmental dysplasia of the hip. They differ for the infant and older child (Table 43-1).

Treatment

Early detection and treatment are important to ensure that hip function is optimized. Treatment varies depending on age and extent of involvement. In the infant positional 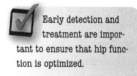 Early detection and treatment are important to ensure that hip function is optimized.

Table 43-1 Differences in Clinical Manifestations of Developmental Dysplasia of the Hip

Infant	Older Child
Unequal leg length	Gait abnormalities
Asymmetry of thigh and gluteal folds	Unequal level of pelvis
Limited hip abduction	Positive Trendelenburg sign
Positive Ortolani sign	Apparent short leg

casting, skin traction, or the Pavlik harness may be used. In the older child casting and traction may be tried initially to gently stretch the ligaments and tissue before a closed reduction being attempted. An open reduction may be necessary to correct the deformity, with a hip spica cast applied postoperatively.

CURVATURE OF THE SPINE

The three common pediatric curvatures of the spine are **kyphosis**, which is an increased convex curve, normally in the thoracic region; **lordosis**, which is an increased concave curve, normally in the lumbar region; and **scoliosis**, which is a lateral curvature of the spine. Each of these disorders may be classified as congenital, neuromuscular, or idiopathic. Many states now mandate school screening for curvatures of the spine in an effort to identify children early on and get treatment started. **Idiopathic scoliosis** occurs most often in girls and often presents during the pre-adolescent growth spurt. Young girls diagnosed with scoliosis are at an increased risk for osteopenia as they age. Curvatures of the spine may be associated with other pediatric chronic disorders such as spina bifida, cerebral palsy, and muscle diseases classified as neuromuscular.

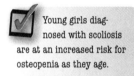

Young girls diagnosed with scoliosis are at an increased risk for osteopenia as they age.

Pathophysiology

New research has hypothesized that adolescents with idiopathic scoliosis have an abnormality in the function of the posterior columns of the spinal cord. Others have found an abnormality of the central nervous system involving the balance mechanism in the midbrain. In scoliosis, as the vertebral curve increases the ribs and spine rotate toward the convex portion of the curve. A compensatory curve results as the child attempts to maintain erect posture. Respiratory function may be impacted as the thoracic curve increases.

Kyphosis may be postural, congenital, or secondary to other disorders. Postural kyphosis tends to occur during the adolescent years when teens are self-conscious about their height, breast development, or size. Congenital kyphosis is often referred to as Scheuermann's kyphosis, which involves wedging of the vertebra, causing curves greater than 45 degrees.

Kyphosis may also be associated with chronic diseases such as muscle disease, cerebral palsy, and spinal muscle atrophy.

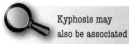

Kyphosis may also be associated with chronic diseases such as muscle disease, cerebral palsy, and spinal muscle atrophy.

With lordosis the muscles of the spine are unable to support themselves in an erect position. This may often cause lower back pain and fatigue.

Figure 43-2 demonstrates the screening process for curvature of the spine. Stand behind the individual and instruct him or her to keep the feet together and arms at the side. Look for the following:

- One shoulder higher than the other
- Uneven hips
- Prominent scapula
- Asymmetry of waist line

Next, have the child bend over, hanging his or her arms together in front. Look for the following:

- Rib hump
- Visible curvature

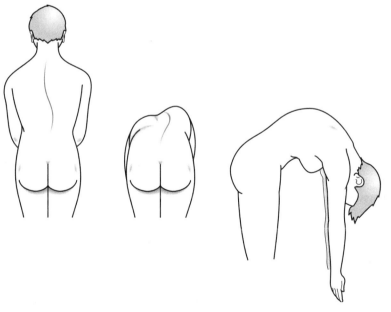

Figure 43-2 Screening process for curvature of the spine.

Treatment

Treatment depends on the degree of curvature and the type of curve. Kyphosis and lordosis may be treated with exercises and/or bracing. As the curve progresses in scoliosis bracing may be used, with a spinal fusion reserved for severe curves. Bracing for kyphosis or scoliosis usually involves a Milwaukee brace, Boston brace, or Charleston brace. A spinal fusion involves rods, hooks, and wires along with bone grafting to correct the curvature.

OSTEOMYELITIS

Osteomyelitis, an infection in the bone, occurs most often in the lower extremities. It may occur after trauma or puncture to an infected area (exogenous), after surgery, or by spread of infection to the bone through the bloodstream from elsewhere in the body (hematogenous). Hematogenous osteomyelitis is seen most often in infants and very young children.

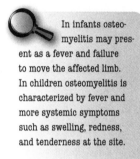

In infants osteomyelitis may present as a fever and failure to move the affected limb. In children osteomyelitis is characterized by fever and more systemic symptoms such as swelling, redness, and tenderness at the site.

Pathophysiology

Osteomyelitis may begin as a bloody abscess in the metaphysis of the bone. The usual causative agent is *Staphylococcus aureus* that travels from the local site of infection to the small end arteries in the bone. Inflammation, edema, and local bone destruction can occur along with abscess formation. Pressure increases as the pus collects, causing localized pain, swelling, and heat and eventually leading to bone necrosis. In infants osteomyelitis may present as a fever and failure to move the affected limb. In children osteomyelitis is characterized by fever and more systemic symptoms such as swelling, redness, and tenderness at the site.

Treatment

Positive blood cultures, an elevated erythrocyte sedimentation rate, and C-reactive protein tests confirm diagnosis. The white blood cell count may also be elevated. Bone scans in infants and young children aid in diagnosis and determination of whether multiple sites are involved.

When treatment is started promptly prognosis is excellent. Antibiotics should be started as soon as the diagnosis is made. Antibiotics are usually given intravenously for 3–6 weeks to obtain and maintain high concentrations in the blood. In some cases debridement and surgical drainage may be necessary.

FRACTURES

Fractures are a very common occurrence in children due to falls, sports injuries and other mishaps, and child abuse. Because of the porous nature of immature bones and open growth plates, fractures during childhood can lead to long-term complications such as shortened limbs or angular deformities. A fracture may be open or closed and may be classified by the type of break (Figure 43-3). An **open fracture** is one that breaks through the skin, whereas a **closed fracture** has no contact outside the skin surface. A **transverse fracture** is one in which the fracture occurs on the shaft of the bone, breaking straight across. In a **spiral fracture** the fracture line circles around the bone; this type of fracture is often seen in child abuse. A partial break in the bone with bending on the opposite side is a **greenstick fracture**. When the fracture line is diagonal across the long bone it is referred to as an **oblique fracture**.

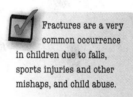

Fractures are a very common occurrence in children due to falls, sports injuries and other mishaps, and child abuse.

Pathophysiology

There are several unique characteristics of fractures in children. The first is the presence of open growth plates and the risk of damaging them with a fracture. The second feature is the presence of thicker and more elastic periosteum. This helps to partially stabilize the bone in a fracture, providing more opportunities for a closed reduction and casting rather than surgery. Children's bones are more vascular and have a decreased mineral content, allowing bones to be more flexible and to bow or bend rather than break completely. Because of increased blood flow in children, fractures heal more quickly and a nonunion is less common.

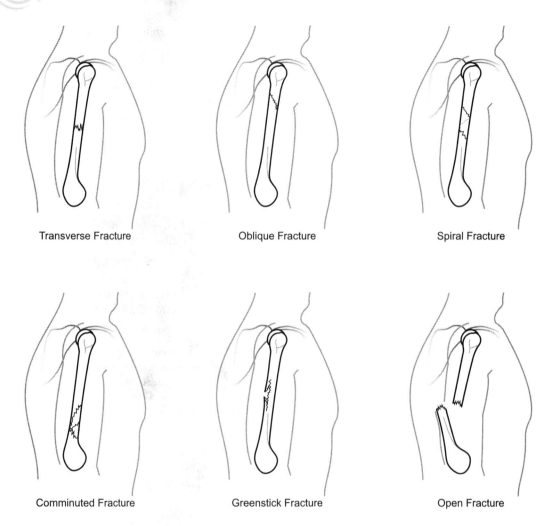

Transverse Fracture   Oblique Fracture   Spiral Fracture

Comminuted Fracture   Greenstick Fracture   Open Fracture

Figure 43-3 Types of fractures.

After a fracture occurs there are several things that happen. In stage one, within 48 hours a hematoma forms as blood leaks between and around the fragments of bone, causing a decrease of perfusion to the bone tissue. An inflammatory response occurs characterized by vasodilation, exudation of plasma and leukocytes, and infiltration of inflammatory leukocytes and mast cells. In stage two cellular proliferation occurs within 24 hours and lasts 2–3 days. During this time blood supply increases, the hematoma becomes granulation tissue, and fibroblasts convert to osteoblasts. During the third to fourth week the callus forms. Fibroblasts and new capillaries form a bridge between fracture ends; osteoblasts migrate to the area, forming collagen that leads to callus formation; and cartilage differentiates to bone tissue. During the third phase ossification occurs as mature bone replaces the callus, stabilizing the fracture. It may be safe to remove a cast at this point. This stage usually occurs about 10 weeks after fracture. In the last phase remodeling occurs as bone continues to thicken and become stronger in response to use and function. Remodeling and total bone healing usually takes up to 9 months.

Treatment

Diagnosis is confirmed by history, symptoms, and x-ray. Treatment is determined by type and location of fracture. Reduction and then immobilization are the standard order of care. Reduction may be open or closed. In children most fractures can be managed by closed reduction (manual manipulation without surgery). Immobilization may be by cast, traction, or external fixator. Immobilization allows for the bone to remain aligned, decreases pain, and prevents rotation at the fracture site. In children the ability to promote involvement in normal activities, while maintaining proper alignment, is important to the child's growth and development.

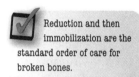

Reduction and then immobilization are the standard order of care for broken bones.

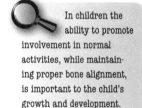

In children the ability to promote involvement in normal activities, while maintaining proper bone alignment, is important to the child's growth and development.

SECTION XX REVIEW QUESTIONS

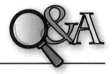

1. 1. The five "P"s of a fracture include all of the following *except*:
    a. Pallor
    b. Pain
    c. Paralysis
    d. Paresthesia
    e. Pulse loss
    f. Pressure

2. When assessing an infant for developmental hip dysplasia, what test can be relied on for confirmation of diagnosis?
    a. Homen's test
    b. Ortolani test
    c. Trendelenburg test
    d. Electromyogram

3. As a school nurse performing an assessment of a child for scoliosis, the nurse should expect to find which positive finding?
    a. Distended abdomen
    b. Asymmetry of the thigh folds
    c. Convex curve in the lumbar spine
    d. Asymmetry of the shoulders and waist

4. Which of the following terms is used to describe a type of fracture that breaks through the skin?
    a. Comminuted
    b. Open
    c. Closed
    d. Compound

5. If an infant is suspected of having osteomyelitis, which of the following symptoms would be present?
    a. Fever
    b. Inflamed reddened area
    c. Irritability, poor feeding
    d. Bone pain

6. In children with suspected child abuse, the most common type of fracture is a:
   a. Greenstick
   b. Spiral
   c. Comminuted
   d. Oblique

7. Young adolescents diagnosed with lumbar scoliosis are most often treated with:
   a. Surgery
   b. Brace
   c. Physical therapy
   d. Exercises

8. Why should a fracture that involves the growth plate be managed carefully?
   a. Avascular necrosis can occur.
   b. Compartment syndrome can occur.
   c. Limb length discrepancies can occur.
   d. Amputation may be necessary.

9. Treatment for osteomyelitis usually involves:
   a. Steroids
   b. Intravenous antibiotics
   c. Incision and drainage
   d. Casting

10. Initial treatment for developmental hip dysplasia includes:
    a. Traction
    b. Pavlik harness
    c. Casting
    d. Triple diapers
    e. a, b, and c only

11. In which stage of bone healing would it be safe to remove the cast?
    a. Inflammatory stage
    b. Reparative stage
    c. Ossification stage
    d. Remodeling stage

12. What is the organism most frequently associated with osteomy-
    elitis?
    a. *Salmonella*
    b. *Streptococcus pneumoniae*
    c. *Staphylococcus aureus*
    d. *Escherichia coli*

13. The callus that develops at a fracture site is important because it
    provides for:
    a. Adequate blood supply to the site
    b. Protection from infection
    c. Support for weight bearing
    d. Means for holding bone fragments together

14. A convex angulation in the curvature of the spine is called:
    a. Scoliosis
    b. Lordosis
    c. Kyphosis
    d. Ankylosis

ANSWERS AND RATIONALES

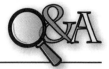

1. **The answer is f.** Rationale: Pressure is not a common finding in a child with a fracture.

2. **The answer is b.** Rationale: The Ortolani test or Barlow maneuver are the only tests used to test for developmental dysplasia of the hip in an infant.

3. **The answer is d.** Rationale: Asymmetry of the shoulders and waist are findings indicative of scoliosis.

4. **The answer is b.** Rationale: An open fracture breaks through the skin, whereas a closed fracture does not.

5. **The answer is c.** Rationale: The typical signs and symptoms of osteomyelitis are different from an infant to a child. For an infant irritability and poor feeding are more common than pain or inflammation at the site.

6. **The answer is b.** Rationale: Spiral fractures are the most common in children suspected of child abuse because the child may be pulled or yanked, causing twisting around the bone shaft.

7. **The answer is d.** Rationale: Lumbar scoliosis usually responds well to exercise and does not require bracing or surgery.

8. **The answer is c.** Rationale: Damage to the growth plate can arrest growth of the bone, especially long bones, causing limb length discrepancies.

9. **The answer is b.** Rationale: Osteomyelitis is usually caused by bacteria and responds well to antibiotic treatment.

10. **The answer is e.** Rationale: Depending on the type of hip dysplasia, skin traction, Pavlik harness, or casting may be used.

11. **The answer is c.** Rationale: Bone healing occurs quickly in children because of the thickened periosteum and generous blood supply; casts may be removed in 6 to 8 weeks once the callus has formed bone.

12. **The answer is c.** Rationale: *Staphylococcus aureus* is the most common causative microorganism in osteomyelitis for both infants and children.

13. **The answer is d.** Rationale: The callus that forms at the fracture site is important because it is a means for holding bone fragments together and provides stability.

14. **The answer is c.** Rationale: Kyphosis is an abnormally increased convex curvature in the thoracic spine.

XXI

Renal Disorders

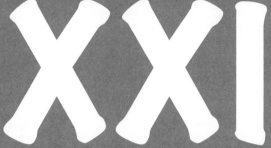

This chapter discusses renal function and structure. By 35 weeks' gestation the renal system is fully developed, although the kidneys do not fully function until several days after birth. The kidneys continue to grow until adolescence when overall body growth stops. The regulation of fluid volume, blood pressure, excretion of metabolic waste products, and drug metabolites are the primary functions of the renal system. The kidneys are also responsible for conversion of vitamin D to its active form, serum pH regulation, and synthesis of hormones, such as erythropoietin and renin.

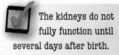

The kidneys do not fully function until several days after birth.

44

Anatomy and Physiology of the Renal System

TERMS
- ☐ Atrial natriuretic peptide
- ☐ Erythropoietin
- ☐ Glomerulus
- ☐ Nephrons

411

Atrial natriuretic peptide, a hormone discovered in 1981, is released from muscle cells in the atria when the atrial walls are stretched. This hormone causes the vasodilation of afferent arterioles, which lead into the glomerulus, and efferent arterioles, which lead out of the glomerulus, resulting in an increased glomerular filtration rate. Atrial natriuretic peptide also inhibits aldosterone secretion and sodium reabsorption from the collecting tubules. All these actions result in increased urine production and a reduction in blood volume.

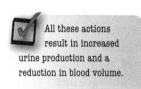

All these actions result in increased urine production and a reduction in blood volume.

The hormone **erythropoietin** stimulates the bone marrow to produce red blood cells in response to hypoxia from conditions such as anemia or from cardiac and/or pulmonary disease. If iron stores are adequate, an increase in red blood cells results in added oxygen-carrying capacity and reduced tissue hypoxia. As renal insufficiency progresses to renal failure, the kidneys' ability to produce erythropoietin declines, causing one form of anemia.

Blood pressure and blood volume are partially under the control of the renin-angiotensin-aldosterone regulatory cascade (Figure 44-1). A drop in renal blood flow stimulates the kidneys to release renin, which in turn converts angiotensinogen to angiotensin I. Angiotensin I enters the bloodstream and circulates through lung tissue where the angiotensin-converting enzyme converts angiotensin I to angiotensin II, a powerful vasoconstrictor. Angiotensin II also causes the kidneys to reduce sodium and water excretion and stimulates aldosterone release, which increases sodium retention. These actions increase blood pressure, blood volume, and renal blood flow.

Vitamin D, in an inactive form, is either produced by the action of ultraviolet rays on cholesterol in the skin or is ingested. The inactive form of vitamin D is converted to the active form by the kidneys. Active vitamin D, necessary for calcium and phosphate absorption from the small intestine, helps maintain strong bone formation. Children with renal disease cannot convert vitamin D to its active form.

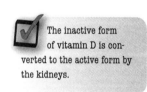

The inactive form of vitamin D is converted to the active form by the kidneys.

The kidneys either conserve bicarbonate, a base, or eliminate hydrogen ions, an acid, from the blood to help maintain serum pH. Buffers in the urine that combine with hydrogen ions so they can be eliminated include bicarbonate, phosphate, and ammonia.

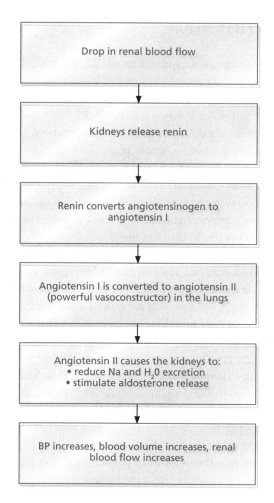

Figure 44-1 Renin-aldosterone-angiotensin system.

 RENAL PERFUSION

The renal blood flow rate averages 20% to 25% of cardiac output each minute. Adequate blood flow to the kidneys is required to produce a sufficient glomerular filtration rate and urine production. When the sympathetic nervous system is stimulated, such as occurs in a stress response, both the afferent and efferent renal arterioles constrict, producing a decrease in renal blood flow.

GLOMERULAR FILTRATION

The glomerular filtration rate is approximately 20 ml/min in full-term newborns and 10–13 ml/min in infants born at 28–30 weeks' gestation. It reaches adult levels by ages 12–24 months. Until then the kidneys are unable to fully maintain water balance and to filter solutes and medications out of the bloodstream. Any fluid that is not returned to the circulation becomes a component of urine. It is expected that the neonate produces urine and voids within 12–24 hours after birth. Daily urine production is approximately 1–3 ml/kg/h (200–300 ml), producing approximately six wet diapers per day by the time the neonate is 4 days old.

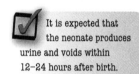

It is expected that the neonate produces urine and voids within 12–24 hours after birth.

Nephrons are the functional units of the kidneys, and each kidney has approximately 1.2 million nephrons. Although infants are born with the same number of nephrons they will have as an adult, their nephrons are immature and do not fully function. In each tubular-shaped nephron is a plasma-filtering capillary tuft created by the efferent and afferent arterioles called a **glomerulus**, which deposits its filtrate into a thin double-walled capsule called Bowman's capsule. From Bowman's capsule the filtrate travels through the proximal convoluted tubule, the loop of Henle, the distal convoluted tubule, and finally the collecting tubule. The collecting tubules empty into the renal pelvis, which is drained by the ureters. The ureters then empty into the bladder.

The role of the glomerulus is to filter plasma, and this filtering capability is controlled by capillary pressure, colloidal osmotic pressure, and capillary permeability. The proximal convoluted tubules are responsible for approximately 65% of the reabsorption and secretion functions of the tubular system. In the proximal tubules reabsorption of essential substances such as Na, Cl, HCO_3, phosphate, glucose, amino acids, and water and the secretion of H^+ ions and waste products, including drug metabolites, take place. The loop of Henle is primarily concerned with reabsorbing water, some Na and Cl, and calcium. Because the loop is short in the newborn, sodium and water are not efficiently absorbed, producing a dilute urine.

The distal convoluted tubule reabsorbs Na, K, Cl, bicarbonate, urea, and water and secretes H^+ ions and K. The collecting duct either reabsorbs or secretes Na, K, H$^+$ ions, and ammonia depending on the body's requirements. By 3 months of age the tubules are able to concentrate urine at the same efficiency as a mature kidney.

Children up to 12 months of age are in danger of developing severe metabolic acidosis because of several factors, including a reduced renal hydrogen ion excretion rate and a low plasma bicarbonate level. They are also prone to fluid overload because their kidneys do not respond to excess serum water in the same way a more mature kidney responds. Table 44-1 lists renal function tests and their related physiology.

By 3 months of age the tubules are able to concentrate urine at the same efficiency as a mature kidney.

Children up to 12 months of age are in danger of developing severe metabolic acidosis.

Table 44-1 Renal Function Tests

Test	Related Physiology	Levels
Serum blood urea nitrogen (BUN)	The end product of protein metabolism by the liver is urea, which is excreted entirely by the kidneys; therefore the BUN is an indication of liver and kidney function.	0 to 6 months of age, 4–15 mg/dl; 6 months to 24 months of age, 5–15 mg/dl; and 24 months of age to adulthood, 5–25 mg/dl are considered within normal limits.
Serum creatinine	When creatinine phosphate is used in skeletal muscle contractions creatinine is formed, which is entirely excreted by the kidneys; therefore the serum creatinine level is an indication of renal function. The creatinine level is not affected by hepatic function so it is a more precise indication of renal function than is the BUN. A 50% reduction in glomerular filtration rate doubles the creatinine level.	Creatinine levels at birth reflect the mother's level. The level should drop during the first month of life from 0.8 to 0.3 for a full-term newborn. If the level rises it is considered abnormal and requires immediate investigation.
24-hr urine collection for creatinine clearance	Measures glomerular filtration rate and depends on renal artery perfusion and glomerular filtration.	By 6 days of age the creatinine clearance rate should be 15–90 ml/min/1.73 m^2 compared with an adult value of 75–125 ml/min/1.73 m^2.

Table 44-1 Renal Function Tests (continued)

Test	Related Physiology	Levels
Urinalysis	Cloudy, foul smelling, white blood cell counts → urinary tract infection Dark yellow → dehydration Acetone odor → diabetic ketoacidosis Presence of protein → injured glomerular membrane Glucose → diabetes mellitus Ketones → fatty acid metabolism Crystals → renal stone formation possible many hyaline casts → proteinuria Cellular casts → nephrotic syndrome	Up to age 12 months the infant may normally spill small amounts of protein in the urine. Glucose should be less than 5 mg/dl. The newborn may excrete urate crystals, which give the urine a pink tinge.

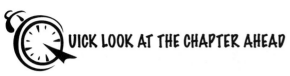

QUICK LOOK AT THE CHAPTER AHEAD

This chapter discusses the pathophysiology concerning voiding and incontinence.

45

Micturition and Incontinence

TERMS

- ☐ Diurnal enuresis
- ☐ Enuresis
- ☐ Overflow incontinence
- ☐ Reflex incontinence
- ☐ Secondary enuresis
- ☐ Stress incontinence
- ☐ Urge incontinence

MICTURITION

By the age of 3 most children learn to recognize the signals indicating the urge to void, and bladder training can begin (Figure 45-1). Enuresis, or bed wetting, may last until late childhood. Children who sleep deeply may not notice the urge to void, and thus bedwetting occurs. Transient incontinence can be caused by medications such as diuretics, by caffeinated beverages, or by a urinary tract infection, which causes bladder and urethral irritation.

Transient incontinence can be caused by medications such as diuretics, by caffeinated beverages, or by a urinary tract infection, which causes bladder and urethral irritation.

Pathophysiology

As the bladder fills to between 150 and 300 cc, stretch receptors in the bladder walls are activated, creating the sensation of the need to void. Parasympathetic pelvic nerves transmit this signal to the detrusor muscle, initiating bladder contractions. The higher the amount of urine in the bladder, the stronger the impulse to micturate. Sympathetic nerve innervation of the detrusor muscle and internal sphincter prevent premature parasympathetic stimulation and maintain the muscle tone of the internal sphincter. Higher level motor impulses inhibit the voiding reflex by constricting the urethral sphincter and delaying voiding. Generally, ignoring the urge to void prevents release of the external sphincter and neuron fatigue delays further stimulation of the voiding reflex arc for a few minutes to 1 hour. If the urge to void continues to be ignored, eventually bladder reflex contractions take over and cause involuntary voiding. Although micturition is generally under voluntary control, an overfilled or irritated bladder results in incontinence or the involuntary passage of urine.

Enuresis

By age 9 most children no longer experience **enuresis**, a condition during which the child has either voluntary or involuntary wetting either at night or during the day. Primary nocturnal enuresis (PNE), the most common type of enuresis, affects 5–7 million children over age 5 and occurs dur-

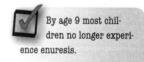

By age 9 most children no longer experience enuresis.

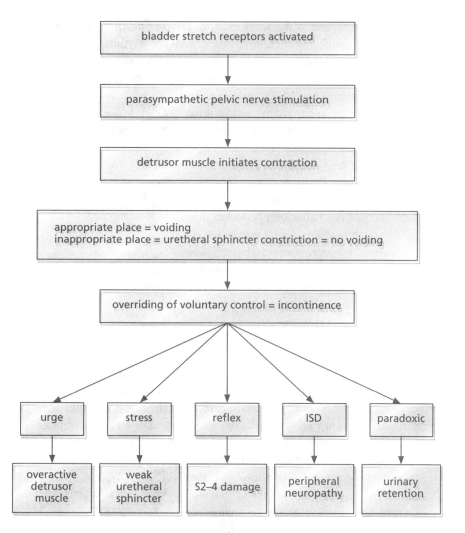

Figure 45-1 Micturition.

ing deep sleep cycles with the child never having a sustained period of dryness at night. This type of enuresis is often due to a developmental lag, small bladder capacity, and possible sleep apnea and/or night time vasopressin deficiency. Three times more boys than girls experience PNE, which may have a familial link. The familial risk factor for developing PNE is as follows: a 77% risk if both parents had PNE, a 44% risk if one parent had PNE, and a 15% risk if neither parent had PNE.

Diurnal enuresis is the term used to describe daytime wetting. At age 5 approximately 8% of children still experience daytime wetting, but by the age of 6 the vast majority of children are able to stay dry during the daytime. Some young adolescents may experience a short period of diurnal enuresis at age 12. Diurnal enuresis is more common in shy children or in those with attention deficit hyperactivity disorder and may signal the onset of diabetes mellitus. Boys and girls are affected equally, and 60–80% also have PNE.

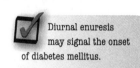

Diurnal enuresis may signal the onset of diabetes mellitus.

Secondary enuresis describes wetting after the child has had a long period of time during which bladder control was achieved. It is associated with stress and regression such as may occur with the birth of a sibling or illness requiring hospitalization. Diurnal enuresis and secondary enuresis account for 10% of all cases of enuresis.

Secondary enuresis is associated with stress and regression such as may occur with the birth of a sibling or illness requiring hospitalization.

Enuresis may also occur in response to a urinary tract infection, pinworm infestation, diuretic therapy, diabetes mellitus, distraction and delaying voiding during playtime, sexual abuse, inappropriate toilet training, reluctance to use public or school restrooms, seizures, or structural abnormalities of the urinary tract. Regardless of the cause, the child often feels shame and low self-esteem. They may be taunted by peers, siblings, and other family members. Some children become shy and reluctant to make friends and avoid sleep-over activities because of their inability to remain dry. Parents or caregivers who do not understand enuresis may punish or try to shame the child into staying dry, which only increases anxiety and low self-esteem.

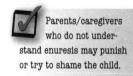

Parents/caregivers who do not understand enuresis may punish or try to shame the child.

Management

PNE is often caused by a developmental delay, and the child will outgrow this condition without any special intervention. To help minimize PNE the child should not drink caffeinated beverages, and fluids should be limited after dinnertime. Bladder and sphincter exercises such as stopping urine midstream when using the toilet or trying to delay daytime voiding to increase bladder capacity may help. The child is also encouraged to get up and use the bathroom if he or she awakes during the night.

Approximately 40% of children with PNE are helped by limiting fluid, bladder/sphincter exercises, and caffeine avoidance. There are devices that attach to nighttime garments or bed sheets that vibrate to wake the child if wetting starts, which is sometimes helpful in controlling PNE in children over 7 years of age. Desmopressin acetate (DDAVP) nasal spray, a form of vasopressin, reduces urine volume by promoting water reabsorption and is an effective treatment for 50% of children with PNE. Children with diurnal enuresis and/or secondary enuresis may benefit from counseling techniques that explore language as a means to express emotions and feelings.

INCONTINENCE

Although incontinence is generally associated with elders, children and adolescents can also experience incontinence not associated with bladder/sphincter maturational delays, behavioral problems, or unresolved emotional issues discussed previously. **Urge incontinence**, also called instability incontinence or detrusor hyperreflexia, is a type of chronic incontinence that is caused by inappropriate, repetitive, strong contractions of the detrusor muscle, which eventually overcomes urethral sphincter control. This type of incontinence has numerous etiologies, such as a hyperactive detrusor muscle, nervous system disease, or brain tumors. When the detrusor muscle becomes overactive the bladder contracts when the urge to void is felt, and the ability to postpone voiding is lost. A feeling of urgency precedes the passage of large amounts of urine, thus the name urge incontinence.

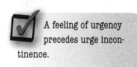

A feeling of urgency precedes urge incontinence.

Reflex incontinence is caused by trauma or damage to the nervous system, as seen in spinal cord injury above S2-4 or with diabetes mellitus. Detrusor hyperreflexia occurs even though there is no sensation of the need to void. These conditions do not result in a feeling of urgency before the incontinence.

Urinary retention causes **overflow incontinence** (paradoxic incontinence) and involves a deficient detrusor muscle or bladder outlet obstruction. In this type of incontinence the bladder does not empty completely because of detrusor muscle malfunction, as occurs with multiple sclerosis, or from blockage of the bladder outlet, from conditions such as a urethral stricture. Diabetes mellitus may result in overflow incontinence because of damage to the parasympathetic innervation of the detrusor muscle. Symptoms associated with overflow incontinence may include urgency, frequency, nocturia,

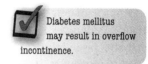

Diabetes mellitus may result in overflow incontinence.

dribbling, and an intermittent urinary stream or a lack of urgency if nerve damage is present.

Stress incontinence involves a weak urethral sphincter, in contrast to urge incontinence and overflow incontinence, which involve the detrusor muscle. An adolescent with stress incontinence experiences leakage of urine with any activity that increases intraabdominal pressure, such as coughing, sneezing, or exercises such as running. Pelvic floor relaxation, which results in the descent of pelvic organs associated with obesity, has also been implicated as a cause of stress incontinence because it causes the urethra to move out of its normal position. As a result the urethral sphincter does not sense the sudden increase in intraabdominal pressure; thus when bladder pressure exceeds urethral closure pressure the urethral sphincter does not close and leaking of urine occurs.

Intrinsic sphincter deficiency (ISD) is another cause of stress incontinence. Intrinsic sphincter deficiency occurs when there is damage to the neuromuscular components of the proximal urethra or pelvic floor muscles. Conditions such as peripheral neuropathy associated with diabetes mellitus may result in intrinsic sphincter deficiency.

Diagnostic studies that identify the cause of incontinence include voiding cystourethrogram, urodynamic testing, cystoscopy, and urine culture.

This chapter discusses the pathophysiology and management of urinary tract infections (UTIs). A UTI is a bacterial infection that affects any part of the urinary tract. They are further classified as upper or lower UTIs. When bacteria get into the bladder or kidney and multiply in the urine, they cause a UTI.

Types of UTIs include urethritis and cystitis. Hemolytic-uremic syndrome is also covered.

46

Urinary Tract Infection

TERMS
☐ Cystitis
☐ Urethritis
☐ Urinary tract infection (UTI)

URINARY TRACT INFECTION

Urinary tract infection (UTI), defined as significant amounts of bacteria in the urinary tract, are classified as lower or upper tract infections. Upper UTIs involve the ureters and kidneys, whereas lower UTIs involve the urethra and bladder. **Urethritis** is the inflammation of the urethra, whereas **cystitis** indicates inflammation of the bladder. In newborns UTIs may develop when bacteria in the bloodstream attach to the kidneys and proliferate. Approximately 3–8% of girls and 1–2% of boys develop a UTI during childhood. Uncircumcised boys younger than 3 months of age develop UTIs more often than do girls in that age group, whereas by 6 months of age girls develop UTIs more frequently than do boys. Girls are most likely to develop a UTI at ages 7 to 11.

> ✓ Approximately 3–8% of girls and 1–2% of boys develop a UTI during childhood.

As a rule UTIs are caused by gram-negative bacteria common in the intestine, especially *Escherichia coli* (80% of cases). UTIs caused by *Klebsiella* and *Proteus* usually occur because of abnormal urinary tract structure or after catheterization.

Pathophysiology

Normally, UTI is prevented by acidic urine, complete bladder emptying, a competent ureterovesical junction to prevent urine backflow, and bacteriostatic properties of the urethra and bladder. The urinary tract above the urethra is sterile; therefore if bacteria ascends the urethra and colonizes in the bladder, an inflammatory process is initiated. The process of voiding routinely cleanses the bladder and urethra. Thus anything that interferes with this process, such as outflow obstruction, postponement of voiding, low fluid intake, vesicoureteral reflux, or diabetes mellitus, increases the risk of developing a UTI. Other causes of a UTI include catheterization, constipation (inhibits complete bladder emptying), poor perineal hygiene, and a neurogenic bladder. Sexually active adolescent girls are also prone to develop UTIs.

 Sexually active adolescent girls are prone to develop UTIs.

The catheterization procedure may introduce bacteria into the bladder because the process of catheterization causes irritation and minute scraping of the urethra, creating a portal for bacterial entry. Additionally, an indwelling catheter prevents normal flushing of the urethra by urine, and bacteria may travel to the bladder through the catheter itself or via the exudate that collects between the outside of the catheter and the urethral walls. As bacteria adhere to the catheter, they produce a protective film that covers the surface of the catheter and protects the bacteria against antibiotic action, making eradication of the infection difficult.

Newborns and infants may exhibit non-specific signs of a UTI, such as irritability, reluctance to feed, failure to thrive, and vomiting. Other signs and symptoms of a UTI commonly include an offensive urine odor and cloudy urine (pyuria). Toddlers and older children may complain of abdominal pain, frequency, urgency, and burning upon void-

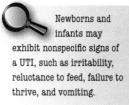
Newborns and infants may exhibit nonspecific signs of a UTI, such as irritability, reluctance to feed, failure to thrive, and vomiting.

ing because the inflamed lining of the urinary tract creates irritation that triggers the micturition reflex.

Diagnostic tests that confirm a UTI include urinalysis and midstream clean-catch urine sample for bacteriuria. To obtain a reliable urine sample, infants and young children require catheterization. Bagged urine samples are difficult to obtain and are often contaminated. Older children who are toilet trained can generally cooperate in obtaining a clean-catch urine sample. Girls should straddle the toilet seat (this position normally separates the labia), and boys who are not circumcised should retract the foreskin. Collecting the sample midstream helps to avoid contamination.

If multiple organisms are cultured from the sample, it usually means that the sample was contaminated. Children may have white blood cells in the urine because of a UTI, contamination of the specimen, or a systemic infection. Nitrites found by dipstick analysis indicated pyuria. Bacteria require several hours to convert ingested nitrates to nitrites, but because most young children empty their bladders frequently nitrites are not usually detected unless a first voided morning specimen is collected.

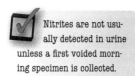
Nitrites are not usually detected in urine unless a first voided morning specimen is collected.

Management

Reduction of controllable risk factors is the primary way to prevent UTIs. Cranberry juice has been used as a home remedy to prevent UTIs for many years. The benefit of drinking cranberry juice daily lies in its ability to acidify urine, which decreases the bacteria's ability to adhere to bladder walls. For sexually active adolescent girls, having their partner use a condom and increasing fluid intake before sexual activity can also lessen the likelihood of developing a UTI because voiding immediately after intercourse removes bacteria from the bladder outlet. Other preventative measures include wiping from front to back after a bowel movement; wearing cotton, not synthetic, underwear; avoiding tight clothing, including diapers, jeans, and pants; avoiding bubble baths (irritates urinary system); and changing sanitary pads often during menstruation.

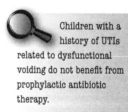 Cranberry juice has been used as a home remedy to prevent UTIs for many years. The benefit of drinking cranberry juice daily lies in its ability to acidify urine, which decreases the bacteria's ability to adhere to bladder walls.

Infants younger than 3 months of age and those who are dehydrated or septic require hospitalization and intravenous antibiotic therapy. Older infants and children who are not dehydrated or septic can be treated at home with a 7- to 10-day course of oral antibiotics. Adolescents with cystitis may only require a 3-day course of treatment. Left untreated UTIs may progress to pyelonephritis, hypertension, and renal failure.

 Left untreated UTIs may progress to pyelonephritis, hypertension, and renal failure.

Controversy continues related to the efficacy of giving children prophylactic antibiotics because of the possible development of resistant strains of bacteria. If the child has a structural abnormality such as vesicourethral reflex, however, prophylactic antibiotics to prevent UTIs may be used in place of surgery. Children with a history of UTIs related to dysfunctional voiding do not benefit from prophylactic antibiotic therapy.

Children with a history of UTIs related to dysfunctional voiding do not benefit from prophylactic antibiotic therapy.

 ## HEMOLYTIC-UREMIC SYNDROME

Hemolytic-uremic syndrome (HUS) causes endothelial damage and coagulopathy of the kidneys, gastrointestinal system, and central nervous system; hemolytic anemia; and thrombocytopenia. HUS is the most common cause of acute renal failure in children younger than age 5 years. Nonepidemic HUS is associated with nephrotoxic drugs (cyclosporine A), viruses (human immunodeficiency virus), or genetic factors (factor H deficiency), although the exact cause is often unclear.

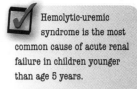

Hemolytic-uremic syndrome is the most common cause of acute renal failure in children younger than age 5 years.

In contrast to noninfectious HUS, the epidemic form of HUS has an infectious etiology and is transmitted through food and person-to-person contact. Although *Salmonella typhimurium, Shigella dysenteriae,* and *Campylobacter* are associated with HUS, the most common causative organism related to HUS outbreaks is Shiga's toxin-producing strains of *Escherichia coli,* which is usually transmitted via contaminated ground beef, unpasteurized milk or apple juice, alfalfa sprouts, unwashed raw vegetables, cheese, and public swimming pools.

Initially, most children have an acute gastrointestinal system infection (Figure 46-1). The bacteria attach to the intestinal lining and proliferate. They then produce a toxin that binds to endothelial cells of the capillary walls, triggering the inflammatory process. Occlusion of arterioles and prevention of protein synthesis leads to cellular death. Lipopolysaccharides produced by *E. coli* also cause the activation of the coagulation cascade, using up available platelets and putting down a fibrin network in the kidneys. As red blood cells pass through this fibrin network and occluded arterioles, they are hemolyzed.

Signs and symptoms of HUS include diarrhea, which may be bloody; vomiting; electrolyte imbalance; thrombocytopenia; hematuria; hemolytic anemia; hypertension; renal failure; anorexia; seizures; and fluid overload (Figure 46-1). Children usually recover from HUS in 2–3 weeks, although approximately one third continue to show signs of hypertension and 15% will have end-stage renal failure. Mortality (3–5%) is generally caused by central nervous system complications.

Management

Avoidance of undercooked beef, unpasteurized dairy products, and people with HUS is the primary mode of prevention. Treatment includes blood transfusions, fluid and electrolyte replacement, and dialysis if needed. Antibiotics that cause *E. coli* cell death result in additional release of toxins and are avoided, as are antimotility medications.

Antibiotics that cause *E. coli* cell death result in additional release of toxins and are avoided, as are antimotility medications.

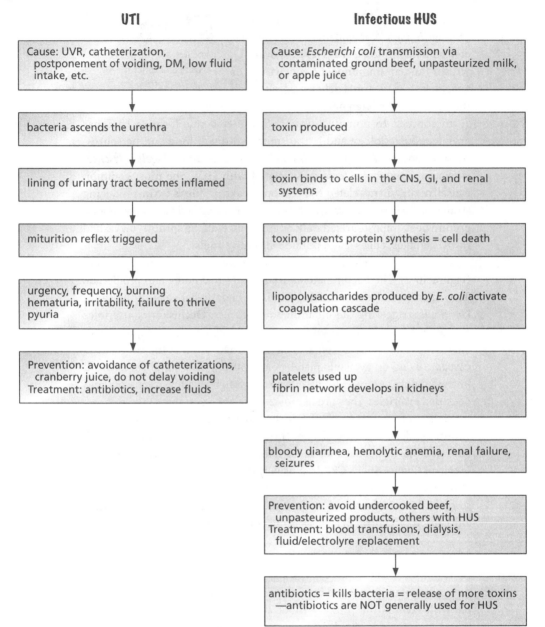

Figure 46-1 UTIs versus infectious HUS.

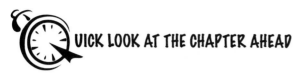

QUICK LOOK AT THE CHAPTER AHEAD

This chapter discusses the etiology of **renal failure** defined as the inability to concentrate water, balance electrolytes, and remove waste products. Renal failure is classified as either acute or chronic. Acute renal failure begins abruptly and is generally reversible. Chronic renal failure has an eventual mortality rate of 100% (without dialysis and/or renal transplantation), is irreversible, and results in a slow steady decline of renal function.

47

Renal Failure

TERMS
- ☐ Azotemia
- ☐ Intrarenal ARF
- ☐ Postrenal or obstructive ARF
- ☐ Prerenal factors
- ☐ Renal failure
- ☐ Renal insufficiency
- ☐ Renal osteodystrophy
- ☐ Uremia

ACUTE RENAL FAILURE

The most common causes of acute renal failure (ARF) in children are hemolytic-uremic syndrome and dehydration. Prevention of ARF depends in part on limiting the child's exposure to nephrotoxic agents, eliminating exposure to unpasteurized products and undercooked meat, and prevention and prompt treatment of dehydration and shock.

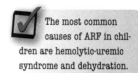

The most common causes of ARF in children are hemolytic-uremic syndrome and dehydration.

In ARF the glomerular filtration rate (GFR) is greatly reduced, the blood urea nitrogen level rises, and sodium is not efficiently reabsorbed from the proximal tubule. Because the distal tubule has a high amount of sodium the renin-angiotensin system is activated, which causes constriction of the afferent arteriole, thereby further reducing the GFR and continuing the cycle (Figure 47-1).

Pathophysiology

Prerenal, intrarenal, and postrenal factors may cause ARF. **Prerenal factors** (factors that occur before blood being filtered by the kidneys) may be caused by anything that promotes renal hypoperfusion. Prerenal factors include shock, congestive heart failure, volume depletion from vomiting/diarrhea, or diabetic acidosis. The most common cause of decreased renal perfusion in children is dehydration. In prerenal ARF urine osmolality is high (50 mOsm/kg higher than plasma osmolality), urine sodium is low (below 10 mEq/l), and specific gravity is less than 1.020. Although renal per-

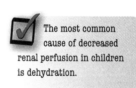

The most common cause of decreased renal perfusion in children is dehydration.

fusion is greatly decreased, renal tubular function is normal. Children may exhibit nonspecific symptoms such as fever, dehydration, and tachycardia.

Intrarenal ARF (intrinsic) results from injury to the kidney itself. This type of ARF may be caused by hemolytic-uremic syndrome, nephrotoxins such as contrast dye, ingestion of poison, glomerulonephritis, acute tubular necrosis, severe infection, liver failure, and chemotherapy, resulting in large amounts of calcium and uric acid excretion. Because of glomerular damage sodium cannot be conserved and urine cannot be concentrated. The child may present with nausea/vomiting, hypertension, and oliguria.

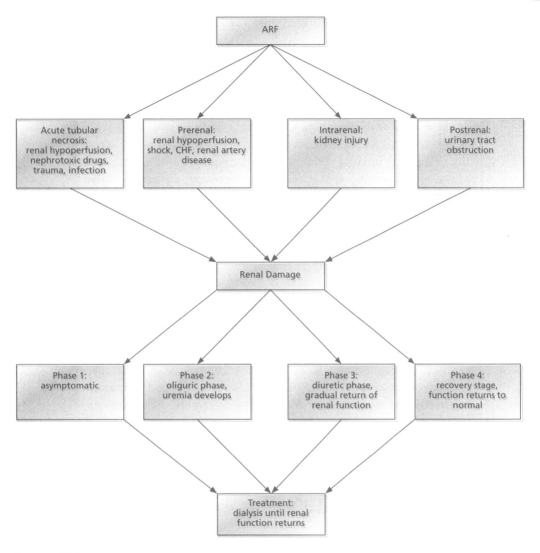

Figure 47-1 Acute renal failure.

Postrenal or obstructive ARF results from urinary tract outflow obstruction by renal calculi, tumors, trauma resulting in hematoma, neurogenic bladder, or structural abnormalities such as ureterovesical junction stricture. Newborn delayed voiding after birth, electrolyte imbalance, a poor urinary stream, and/or abdominal mass suggests a structural abnormality and should be investigated promptly. Urine osmolality and sodium levels are usually unaffected.

ARF has four phases. In the initial phase, although renal damage is occurring, the child may be asymptomatic. During the second, or oliguric, phase less than 1 mL/kg/hr of urine is produced. This stage usually lasts from 10 days to several weeks. Impaired glomerular filtration causes solute and water reabsorption, urine output declines, and serum waste products cannot be removed. As the child becomes symptomatic, a condition known as uremia (urine in the blood) develops. Neurotoxicity from uremia causes an altered mental status and altered peripheral sensation. Electrolyte imbalance causes dysrhythmias, water retention may lead to congestive heart failure and hypertension, and metabolic acidosis may develop because of the kidney's inability to excrete hydrogen ions. In addition to anemia caused by decreased erythropoietin production, blood loss may be caused by gastrointestinal bleeding secondary to platelet and protein anticoagulant dysfunction.

During the third phase, or the diuretic phase, which lasts days to weeks, there is a gradual return of renal function due to cellular regeneration and healing. Excessive urine output leading to dehydration and electrolyte imbalance may occur during this stage as a result of incompetent tubular transport of water and solutes. The fourth and final phase is the recovery stage during which glomerular function gradually returns to normal. The recovery stage may take several months. If left untreated ARF can result in fluid overload, electrolyte imbalance, metabolic acidosis, uremia, and coma. ARF is treated by supportive care, including volume restoration, diuretic administration, and/or dialysis.

CHRONIC RENAL FAILURE

Chronic renal failure (CRF) in children is rare and most commonly develops because of abnormal renal and urinary tract structure. CRF in children younger than 5 years of age may develop because of uncorrected urinary tract structural abnormalities. Children ages 5 to 15 may develop CRF because of chronic renal infections and heredity disorders such as polycystic kidney disease (Figure 47-2). Long-term uncontrolled hypertension and/or diabetes mellitus can lead to CRF in young adults.

> CRF in children younger than 5 years of age may develop because of uncorrected urinary tract structural abnormalities.

In some children the kidneys do not develop (agenesis), whereas in others development is poor (dysgenesis). Untreated severe vesicoureteral reflux, chronic glomerulonephritis, diabetes, lupus, and polycystic disease may also lead to CRF. Renal function steadily declines as nephrons are replaced with scar tissue. **Renal**

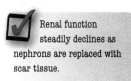

Renal function steadily declines as nephrons are replaced with scar tissue.

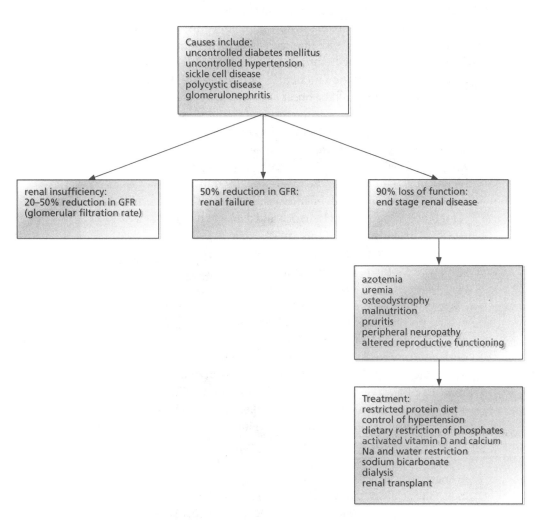

Causes include:
uncontrolled diabetes mellitus
uncontrolled hypertension
sickle cell disease
polycystic disease
glomerulonephritis

renal insufficiency:
20–50% reduction in GFR
(glomerular filtration rate)

50% reduction in GFR:
renal failure

90% loss of function:
end stage renal disease

azotemia
uremia
osteodystrophy
malnutrition
pruritis
peripheral neuropathy
altered reproductive functioning

Treatment:
restricted protein diet
control of hypertension
dietary restriction of phosphates
activated vitamin D and calcium
Na and water restriction
sodium bicarbonate
dialysis
renal transplant

Figure 47-2 Chronic renal failure.

insufficiency denotes a 20% to 50% reduction in the GFR. When renal function in each kidney is reduced by 50%, signs and symptoms of mild **azotemia** (buildup of nitrogenous waste products in the blood), polyuria, nocturia, hypertension, and anemia become apparent. As the GFR drops to 20–25% of normal, the term renal failure is used.

Pathophysiology

During renal failure **uremia** (symptom complex indicating a toxic condition resulting from azotemia involving multiple organ system dysfunction) is apparent along with fluid and electrolyte imbalances. When the GFR drops to less than 15 ml/min/1.73 m^2 the kidney's loss of ability to maintain its homeostatic functions occurs, denoting the destruction of 90% of the nephrons and the onset of end-stage renal disease.

End-stage renal disease is the result of glomerulosclerosis, tubulointerstitial injury, and/or vascular injury. Glomerulosclerosis is the progressive hardening of the glomerular capillaries. This process of epithelial and endothelial injury results in protein spilling into the urine. Tubulointerstitial injury causes the loss of tubular transport functions as the tubules become inflamed, edematous, and necrotic. Vascular injury to renal blood vessels causes ischemia and damage to renal tissue.

Clinical signs and symptoms of CRF occur as compensatory mechanisms fail. Early in the course of the disease the child will appear pale and have headaches, nausea, and fatigue. If the child is of school age teachers may report that the child cannot concentrate well and is not alert. If the child's kidneys are

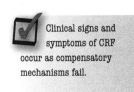

Clinical signs and symptoms of CRF occur as compensatory mechanisms fail.

unable to concentrate urine, polyuria, dehydration, and salt loss occur. Some children in end-stage renal disease continue to produce large amounts of poor quality urine. Children whose CRF is caused by renal injury or damaged glomeruli retain sodium and water, possibly leading to hypertension and congestive heart failure. Children may also develop metabolic acidosis and failure to thrive or grow.

Additional effects of long-term uremia include renal osteodystrophy, malnutrition, pruritus, peripheral neuropathy, uremic pericarditis, and metabolic acidosis. Growth is delayed because of altered calcium, phosphorus, and vitamin D metabolism; metabolic acidosis; and osteodystrophy. **Renal osteodystrophy**, demineralization of bone, has three major causes. First, the kidneys lose their ability to activate vitamin D, which results in decreased absorption of calcium from food. Second, there is a decreased excretion of parathyroid hormone, which leads to demineralization of bones and teeth. Third, there is retention of phosphate, which leads to increased renal excretion of calcium.

Malnutrition occurs because of anorexia, malaise, dietary protein restriction, and proteinuria. Dietary protein is restricted in an attempt to reduce the protein load on the kidneys. Hypoalbuminemia causes fragile capillaries, poor wound healing, and decreased immune system function, which increases susceptibility to infections.

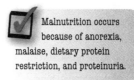 Malnutrition occurs because of anorexia, malaise, dietary protein restriction, and proteinuria.

Retained serum toxins cause a dermal inflammatory process and pruritus. The skin may have a grayish-yellowish cast because of the buildup of urinary pigments.

Uremic frost occurs when the body attempts to rid itself of uric acid and other toxins through sweat.

Restless leg syndrome (spontaneous movement of the feet and legs), altered sensation, weakness, and diminished deep tendon reflexes occur because of neurotoxicity caused by uremia. Children may also exhibit central nervous system symptoms such as confusion, lethargy, seizures, and apathy. In adolescent girls an alteration in hormone levels causes a lack of ovulation and menstruation, whereas adolescent boys experience impotence and decreased sperm counts.

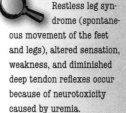 Restless leg syndrome (spontaneous movement of the feet and legs), altered sensation, weakness, and diminished deep tendon reflexes occur because of neurotoxicity caused by uremia.

Management

Treatment for ARF includes dialysis until renal function returns. CRF is treated by conservative management of renal insufficiency and then by dialysis or renal transplantation as needed. Conservative management aimed at retaining as much renal function as possible includes utilization of a protein-restricted diet and control of hypertension, acidosis, and electrolyte imbalance. Anemia has been successfully treated with recombinant human erythropoietin (Epogen). Human recombinant growth hormone has helped some children achieve greater growth potential. Dietary restriction of phosphates and the administration of phosphate-binding antacids and activated vitamin D and calcium have been shown to reduce osteodystrophy. Metabolic acidosis is treated with sodium bicarbonate. Salt and water restriction, along with antihypertensives, may be necessary to control hypertension.

Small children benefit from peritoneal dialysis, with hemodialysis being more appropriate for the older child. Pediatric hemodialysis centers are available in many large dialysis centers. Renal transplantation, if available, affords the child a more normal life span and growth pattern. The best chance for a successful transplant occurs in infants who weigh at least 15 kg and who have a living related donor. Children, parents/caregivers, and family members should have access to psychological counseling. The emotional stress associated with ARF/CRF for the child and family should not be overlooked. Education related to treatment modalities can help to improve the child/family's acceptance and adherence to treatment plans.

SECTION XXI · REVIEW QUESTIONS

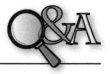

1. Which of the following statements concerning renal function is *correct*?
   a. The kidneys are fully functional at birth.
   b. By age 10 the kidneys have reached their full size.
   c. At 35 weeks' gestation the renal system is fully developed.
   d. Vitamin C is converted to an active form by kidneys.

2. The function of atrial natriuretic peptide is to:
   a. Help regulate fluid volume
   b. Increase red blood cell production
   c. Decrease the glomerular filtration rate
   d. Decrease bicarbonate excretion

3. The kidneys are responsible for (select all that apply):
   a. Conserving bicarbonate
   b. Eliminating hydrogen ions
   c. Manufacturing atrial natriuretic peptide
   d. Maintaining red blood cell function

4. The nursery RN expects that full-term newborn Timmy will:
   a. Manufacture 0.5 ml/kg/hr by day 1
   b. Produce at least six wet diapers per day by day 4
   c. Void within 5 hours of birth
   d. Produce 10–12 wet diapers per day

5. The nurse explains to Sasha, mom to 5-year-old David, that enuresis (select all that apply):
   a. Can be caused by medications
   b. May last until late childhood
   c. Is uncommon
   d. May be caused by deep sleep

6. When explaining diurnal enuresis to a parent, the preschool nurse correctly states that:
   a. By age 4 almost all children are able to stay dry during the day.
   b. More boys than girls experience diurnal enuresis.
   c. Diurnal enuresis disappears by age 10.
   d. Children who are shy are more likely to have diurnal enuresis than children who are not shy.

7. The clinic nurse providing a community education program explains that secondary enuresis:
   a. Is caused by a small bladder
   b. Signifies enuresis that occurs during toilet training
   c. May occur after the birth of a sibling
   d. Accounts for 45% of all cases of enuresis

8. The school nurse conducting a health program explains to teachers that enuresis may be (select all that apply):
   a. A sign of child abuse
   b. Caused by seizure activity
   c. A symptom of a urinary tract infection
   d. Caused by a reluctance to stop playing

9. The pediatric neurological nurse explains to nursing students that incontinence (select all that apply):
   a. Does not occur in children/adolescents
   b. May be caused by a complication of diabetes mellitus
   c. May be associated with obesity
   d. Is caused exclusively by behavioral problems

10. Which statement concerning UTI is correct?
    a. Urine with a base pH discourages bacteria growth and UTI.
    b. Protective bacteria colonize the ureters and bladder and help prevent UTIs.
    c. Constipation can lead to a UTI.
    d. UTIs are more common in adolescent boys than in adolescent girls.

11. The nurse is explaining the association between UTI and catheterization to a student nurse working on a pediatric unit. Which of the following statements are true? (Select all that apply.)
    a. Insertion of a catheter helps prevent a UTI by emptying the bladder.
    b. Bacteria on a catheter produce a protective film that protects the bacteria from destruction by antibiotics.
    c. Dipstick urinalysis is the most effective way to detect nitrites in the urine of young children.
    d. Infants with a UTI may present as irritable.

12. Hemolytic-uremic syndrome (epidemic form) is:
    a. A common cause of chronic renal failure in young children
    b. Commonly caused by the staphylococcus bacteria
    c. Associated with a factor H deficiency, which is genetically transmitted
    d. Transmitted through food and/or person-to-person contact

13. The pathophysiologic process of HUS includes (select all that apply):
    a. The inflammatory process produced by toxin damage to endothelial cells in the kidneys
    b. Activation of the anticoagulation process
    c. Rapid bacterial reproduction in the intestine
    d. Vasodilation of arterioles, leading to hypotension

14. Common causes of chronic renal failure in young adults include:
    a. Dehydration
    b. Hemolytic-uremic syndrome
    c. Diabetes mellitus
    d. Nephrotoxic drugs

15. Prerenal factors that may lead to acute renal failure include:
    a. Congestive heart failure
    b. Contrast dyes
    c. Chemotherapy
    d. Neurogenic bladder

16. When explaining acute renal failure to the student caring for Sasha, a 3-year-old who developed ARF as the result of HUS, the nurse stresses that:
    a. Symptoms develop immediately.
    b. Urine output is generally less than 1 ml/kg/hr.
    c. Metabolic alkalosis results from excess hydrogen ion excretion.
    d. The oliguric phase usually lasts 48–72 hours.

17. The parents of Kenny, a 16-year-old with polycystic disease, ask the nurse to explain the term *renal insufficiency* to them. The nurse correctly replies that renal insufficiency means that:
    a. Nitrogen waste products are building up in the bloodstream.
    b. There has been an 80% drop in the kidneys' ability to filter the blood.
    c. A toxic condition is developing.
    d. The kidneys are still able to filter the blood but at a reduced capacity.

18. A child with CRF will develop renal osteodystrophy because:
    a. Renal activation of calcium is diminished.
    b. Excessive parathyroid hormone is excreted.
    c. Excessive calcium is absorbed.
    d. Phosphate is retained.

19. The nurse assessing Lennie's skin (a child in end-stage renal disease) can expect to find (select all that apply):

a. Orange-brown discoloration

b. Itching

c. Frost-like crystals

d. Flushing

20. Treatment plans for a child in CRF includes (select all that apply):

a. Protein-restricted diet

b. Recombinant human erythropoietin

c. Recombinant growth hormone

d. Phosphate-binding antacids

ANSWERS AND RATIONALES

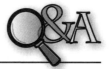

1. **The answer is c.** Rationale: The kidneys are not fully functional until the infant is several days old; they reach their full size when body growth stops, usually in late adolescences; and vitamin D is converted to its active form in the kidneys.

2. **The answer is a.** Rationale: Erythropoietin increases red blood cell production.

3. **The answers are a and b.** Rationale: Muscle cells in the atria produce atrial natriuretic peptide.

4. **The answer is b.** Rationale: By the time the newborn is 4 days old, she or he will produce six wet diapers a day or 1–3 ml/kg/day; voiding is expected by the time the newborn is 12–24 hours old.

5. **The answers are a, b, and d.** Rationale: Primary nocturnal enuresis is a common problem affecting approximately 5–7 million children over age 5.

6. **The answer is d.** Rationale: Boys and girls are equally affected, 8% of children experience diurnal enuresis at age 5, and diurnal enuresis may occur for a short time during early adolescence.

7. **The answer is c.** Rationale: Secondary enuresis is associated with stress, such as occurs during the birth of a sibling, illness, and so forth; it is not associated with a small bladder and accounts for less that 10% of all cases of enuresis.

8. **The answers are a, b, c, and d.**

9. **The answers are b and c.** Rationale: Behavioral problems are not the sole cause of incontinence in children/adolescence (neurological disease and diabetes mellitus are two additional causes).

10. **The answer is c.** Rationale: Acidic urine helps prevent UTI, the renal system is sterile, adolescent girls are more prone to develop a UTI than are adolescent boys, and constipation inhibits bladder emptying and stasis of urine can lead to a UTI.

11. **The answers are b and d.** Rationale: Insertion of a catheter causes irritation to the urethra and is a common cause of UTI, and nitrites are most easily detected in the first morning void.

12. **The answer is d.** Rationale: Epidemic HUS is the most common cause of acute renal failure in young children, and it is commonly caused by *E. coli*; nonepidemic HUS may be the result of a genetic mutation; and epidemic HUS can be transmitted by eating contaminated foods or by direct contact (swimming pools).

13. **The answer is c.** Rationale: HUS causes damage to the endothelial cells of the intestine, the inflammatory process activates the coagulation cascade, and arterioles constrict.

14. **The answer is c.** Rationale: Uncontrolled or poorly controlled diabetes mellitus or hypertension are common causes of chronic renal failure in young adults; acute renal failure is caused by HUS, nephrotoxic drugs, and dehydration.

15. **The answer is a.** Rationale: Prerenal causes of ARF include any conditions that reduce blood flow to the kidneys, such as congestive heart failure.

16. **The answer is b.** Rationale: During the initial stage of ARF the child is asymptomatic even though the kidneys are damaged, the oliguric phase lasts 10 days to weeks, and metabolic acidosis develops because hydrogen ions cannot be excreted.

17. **The answer is d.** Rationale: During renal insufficiency the kidneys ability to filter blood is diminished by 20–50% but is still functional, azotemia denotes nitrogen waste product buildup in the blood, and uremia denotes toxemia.

18. **The answer is d.** Rationale: Retention of phosphate results in excretion of calcium, which demineralizes bones; renal activation of vitamin D is lost; and decreased excretion of parathyroid hormone occurs, which also leads to bone demineralization.

19. **The answers are b and c.** Rationale: Uremic frost is the result of uric acid crystals and toxins deposited on the skin, it causes the skin to itch, and the skin takes on a grayish-yellow color.

20. **The answers are a, b, c, and d.** Rationale: All treatments are indicated for a child in CRF.

XXII

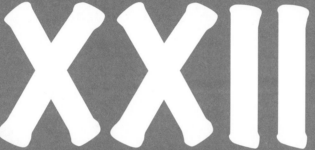

Respiratory
Disorders

The functions of the respiratory system are to provide oxygen to cells during inhalation; to remove carbon dioxide, a byproduct of cell metabolism, during exhalation; and to help regulate serum pH. Oxygen is needed to produce ATP (adenosine triphosphate, a nucleic acid) that, in turn, powers cellular activity. Cellular activity produces carbon dioxide, which must be removed to prevent a buildup of carbonic acid (carbon dioxide + water = carbonic acid) in the bloodstream, which would lower blood pH to life-threatening levels. Although the term *respiration* is frequently used to denote respiratory activity, ventilation and respiration are more precise descriptors. **Ventilation** means the movement of air and thus denotes inhalation and exhalation, whereas **respiration** denotes the exchange of oxygen and carbon dioxide between cells, the alveoli, and environment.

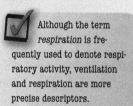 Although the term *respiration* is frequently used to denote respiratory activity, ventilation and respiration are more precise descriptors.

48

Anatomy and Physiology of the Respiratory System

TERMS
- [ ] **Accessory muscles**
- [ ] **Carbonic anhydrase**
- [ ] **Parietal pleura**
- [ ] **Pleural effusion**
- [ ] **Respiration**
- [ ] **Surfactant**
- [ ] **Turbinates**
- [ ] **Ventilation**
- [ ] **Visceral pleura**

FUNCTIONAL ANATOMY

The pulmonary system consists of the airways (nasal passages, mouth, nasopharynx, larynx, and trachea), lungs (two lobes on the left, three on the right), diaphragm, and pulmonary blood vessels. **Turbinates** are tissue protrusions in each nostril that create air turbulence. Large pollutants, such as dust, are trapped by nasal hairs, whereas the tiny capillaries of the nares warm and humidify the air. Stimulation of nasal irritant receptors by triggers such as pollen activates the sneeze reflex and clears the nares. Insensible water loss of approximately 1 pint per day occurs as we provide humidity to the air we breathe. The frontal, maxillary, and ethmoid sinuses are air-filled spaces that provide resonance to the voice. The larynx contains the vocal cords. Aspiration is prevented by the epiglottis, a tissue flap that closes over the tracheal opening during swallowing.

The trachea branches into the right and left bronchus and then further divides 16 times, finally ending in terminal bronchioles. Mucus and cilia, which line the airway, trap and remove inspired foreign particles by an escalator motion. When the mucus reaches the pharynx it is either swallowed or expectorated. If tracheal or large airway irritant sensors are triggered, the cough reflex is activated and the lower airways are cleared. The ability to clean and humidify the airway and prevent an environment where bacteria can flourish is impaired by anything that damages the mucociliary system, such as dehydration, smoking, dry air, mouth breathing, or a tracheostomy that bypasses the nares.

There is a double-layered membrane that lines the inside of the thoracic cavity (**parietal pleura**) and outside of the lungs (**visceral pleura**) so that the lungs slide up and down easily during inspiration and expiration. A thin layer of serous fluid lubricates the pleura and reduces friction associated with ventilation. Accumulation of excess pleural fluid is called **pleural effusion** and results in lung tissue compression and inadequate ventilation.

Table 48-1 explains lung development in the womb. At birth the gas exchange function of the placenta is taken over by the respiratory system. The medulla oblongata in the lower brainstem contains "pacemaker" cells that stimulate autonomic ventilation. The phrenic nerve, which innervates the diaphragm and internal intercostal muscles, transmits neural impulses that trigger inspiration. Stimulation of the apneustic center in the pons triggers gasping ventilation when the higher respiratory center is damaged by trauma.

Table 48-1 Lung Development

Gestational Age	Structure	Possible Abnormalities
3–7 weeks	Conducting airway development begins Large pulmonary arteries and veins develop	Lung aplasia Tracheoesophageal fistula Pulmonary cysts
5–17 weeks	Bronchi and bronchioles completed Airway epithelium differentiates Cartilage, smooth muscle, mucous glands develop Pleuroperitoneal cavity divides into two parts	Diaphragmatic hernia
16–26 weeks	Alveolar type II cells develop Pulmonary capillary system develops	Lung hypoplasia Neonatal respiratory distress syndrome
26–36 weeks	Alveolar development begins Fusion of type I alveolar cells to the basement membrane At 35 weeks surfactant is produced	
36 weeks to 3–8 years of age	Secondary septal formation Capillary network continues to spread True alveoli develop	Lung hypoplasia Bronchopulmonary dysplasia

Chemoreceptors located in the carotid and aortic bodies, brainstem, stretch and irritant receptors in the airways, and motion receptors in the joints and muscles also help regulate the rate and depth of ventilation. If additional oxygen is required, such as occurs during crying, the ventilatory rate and volume increases. Although ventilation is mainly an involuntary process controlled by the brainstem, the rate and depth of breathing can be consciously altered by a child. If a child decides to hold his or her breath, during a temper tantrum for example, lack of oxygen to the brain causes unconsciousness, at which time the child automatically resumes breathing.

When peripheral chemoreceptors in the carotid and aortic bodies sense a rise in the level of arterial carbon dioxide, decrease in arterial oxygen, or serum pH the respiratory center is stimulated to increase the ventilatory rate and depth. When the central chemoreceptors located near the respiratory center sense a drop in cerebrospinal fluid pH, which closely mirrors serum pH, the respiratory center is again stimulated, resulting in a deeper and faster rate of ventilation to blow off carbon dioxide and lower carbonic acid production.

During inhalation the diaphragm and external intercostal muscles contract, causing an enlarged chest wall and decreased pressure in the lungs, enabling air to enter. **Accessory muscles** are used during dyspnea to assist in ventilation and include the sternocleidomastoid and scalenus muscles in the neck and possibly facial muscles.

Airway diameter plays an important role in successful ventilation. Bronchodilation occurs because of sympathetic nerve stimulation in an attempt to increase the body's oxygen supply during times of stress. Irritant receptors in the pharynx, trachea, and bronchus when stimulated by cold air, secretions, or pollutants, such as pollen, dust, and tobacco smoke, cause bronchoconstriction and/or coughing and sneezing. If bronchoconstriction continues, the ventilatory effort increases, resulting in dyspnea.

The differences between an adult and pediatric airway are the larger head and tongue of the infant/child, a larynx that is more anterior, a long floppy epiglottis, and a short trachea and neck. Recent research indicates that lung abnormalities that develop during fetal and neonatal growth periods may lead to lifelong respiratory problems such as asthma and an increased risk of other chronic airway limitation disorders.

 Recent research indicates that lung abnormalities that develop during fetal and neonatal growth periods may lead to lifelong respiratory problems such as asthma and an increased risk of other chronic airway limitation disorders.

OXYGEN AND CARBON DIOXIDE

Alveoli contain macrophages on the inner surface to fight bacteria, chemicals, and other irritants. A fluid called **surfactant** coats the inner surface of each alveolus and allows it to remain partially opened during exhalation. If an infant is delivered before 35 weeks' gestation when surfactant production begins, she or he has immediate respiratory distress and possible long-term lung disease.

 If an infant is delivered before 35 weeks' gestation when surfactant production begins, she or he has immediate respiratory distress and possible long-term lung disease.

The pulmonary artery, which receives deoxygenated blood from the right ventricle, divides into arterioles and finally pulmonary capillaries, which are composed of capillary endothelium and a basement membrane. These pulmonary capillaries surround the alveoli. Each surfactant-coated alveolar wall consists of epithelial cells and a basement membrane. A very thin layer of interstitial fluid separates the pulmonary capillary basement membrane from the alveolar basement membrane. Oxygen and carbon dioxide diffuse across this alveolar–capillary respiratory membrane. A thick or damaged respiratory membrane impairs this diffusion process.

Hemoglobin, a protein contained in red blood cells, is responsible for transporting 99% of dissolved oxygen to the cells, with 1% transported in plasma. Oxygen and hemoglobin combine in the lungs to form oxyhemoglobin. At the cellular level the oxygen is released, a process called hemoglobin desaturation. Acidosis, hypercapnia, high altitude, heart failure, and anemia cause the oxygen–hemoglobin bond to weaken, thereby easily releasing oxygen to the cells. In contrast, alkalosis or a subnormal body temperature causes the oxygen–hemoglobin bond to become stronger.

An enzyme in red blood cells called **carbonic anhydrase** causes 60% of the carbon dioxide produced by cell metabolism to rapidly combine with water and create carbonic acid. The carbonic acid, in turn, rapidly ionizes in the red blood cells to form bicarbonate and hydrogen ions. Hemoglobin acts as a buffer by combining with the hydrogen ions while the bicarbonate diffuses into the plasma. Some carbon dioxide (30%) also forms a weak bond with hemoglobin (carbaminohemoglobin), which transports it to the alveoli. The remaining 10% of carbon dioxide produced is carried dissolved in the plasma.

Table 48-2 presents laboratory tests to assess various lung functions and their rationales for use.

Table 48-2 Laboratory Tests

Test	Rationale
Arterial blood gases	Evaluates acid-base balance
	Respiratory acidosis: Caused by respiratory depression or pulmonary disease—retention of carbon dioxide decreases pH below 7.35
	Kidneys compensate by increasing the production and retention of bicarbonate

Table 48-2 Laboratory Tests (continued)

Test	Rationale
Arterial blood gases	Respiratory alkalosis: Caused by hyperventilation—carbon dioxide rapidly exhaled, leading to a pH increase above 7.45
	Kidneys compensate by excreting bicarbonate
	Metabolic acidosis: Caused by increased production or retention of hydrogen ions as in shock, ketoacidosis, renal failure—pH decreases, bicarbonate decreases
	Lungs compensate by increasing ventilation rate
	Metabolic alkalosis: Caused by loss of hydrogen ions or ingestion of bicarbonate as in prolonged vomiting or bicarbonate overdose—pH increases, bicarbonate increases
	Lungs compensate by slow ventilation to retain carbon dioxide
Bronchoscopy	Allows for visualization of the larynx, trachea, and bronchi
	Local or general anesthesia or conscious sedation may be used
	Biopsies are collected to test for infection, cancer
	Aspirated foreign objects, such as peanuts, are removed
	Requires NPO status until gag reflex returns
Pulmonary function tests	Measures the amount of air inspired and expired during a normal breath (tidal volume) and after maximum inspiration and/or expiration
	Abnormal readings signal pulmonary disease
	Effectiveness of bronchodilators is evaluated by comparing results before and after their use
Ventilation/perfusion	Perfusion of the pulmonary vessels is determined by scan (V/Q scan) injecting radio-tagged albumin intravenously
	Pulmonary blood flow distributes the albumin
	Ventilation scan detects areas of poor ventilation

Test	Rationale
Ventilation/perfusion	Radio-tagged gas is inhaled and lungs are scanned for gas distribution
	If all lung areas are ventilated and perfused equally, a pulmonary emboli is ruled out
	If the lungs are equally ventilated but not perfused, a pulmonary emboli is suspected

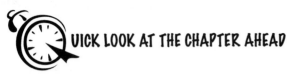

This chapter discusses common causes of airway obstruction, including croup syndromes, bronchitis, bronchiolitis, and pertussis.

49

Respiratory Disorders of the Intrathoracic and Conducting Airways

TERMS
- ☐ Bacterial tracheitis
- ☐ Bronchitis
- ☐ Bronchiolitis
- ☐ Croup syndromes
- ☐ Epiglottitis
- ☐ Pertussis
- ☐ Stridor
- ☐ Syncytia

CROUP SYNDROMES

Croup syndrome is the term used to describe an acute inflammation of the larynx, trachea, and major bronchi. It includes viral croup, epiglottitis, and bacterial tracheitis characterized by inspiratory stridor, cough, hoarseness, and respiratory distress. The signs and symptoms are caused by an edematous airway, mucous production, and loss of ciliary function. Edema leads to stridor as inspired air attempts to pass through the edematous airway.

Viral Croup

A parainfluenza virus is a cause of viral croup, which commonly affects young children 6 months to 3 years of age mainly in the fall and winter months. More boys develop croup than do girls. Other viruses that may cause viral croup include respiratory syncytial virus (RSV), rubeola virus, adenovirus, and other influenza viruses.

The upper airway signs of croup are caused by edema of the subglottic space. Before the barking cough and **stridor** (high-pitched harsh noise) characteristic of croup, the child may have signs of an upper respiratory tract infection. Stridor increases when the child is agitated and crying. As the edema increases, stridor may occur when the child is quiet and resting. The parent/caregiver will also notice retractions, air hunger, and cyanosis. This child needs emergent care. A way to distinguish viral croup from epiglottitis is to assess for a cough and drooling. With croup the child will have a cough but no drooling. Usually, with epiglottitis the child will not cough but will drool.

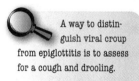

A way to distinguish viral croup from epiglottitis is to assess for a cough and drooling.

The treatment for viral croup is determined by the presenting symptoms. Keeping the child quiet and encouraging fluid intake may be all that is required for a child with mild croup (barking cough but no stridor at rest). Whether or not to use mist therapy is controversial due to the lack of research demonstrating its effectiveness. Children who have stridor at rest require oxygen therapy, glucocorticoids, hospitalization, and possible intubation or tracheostomy.

Epiglottitis

Epiglottitis is most commonly caused by *Haemophilus influenzae* type B and most often affects children aged 2 to 5 years. Other viruses that may cause epiglottitis include *Streptococcus pneumoniae, Streptococcus pyogenes* groups A and C, and *Neisseria meningitides.* Regardless of the causative virus, epiglottitis develops rapidly and can be life threatening because of the resulting upper airway obstruction. The *H. influenzae* type B conjugate vaccine given to infants at 2, 4, and 6 months of age with a booster at 12 to 15 months of age has helped to markedly decrease the incidence of epiglottitis.

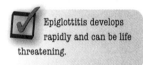 Epiglottitis develops rapidly and can be life threatening.

The child with epiglottitis develops a sudden high fever, difficulty swallowing, drooling, a soft voice quality, inspiratory retractions, cyanosis, agitation, restlessness, and soft stridor. Assessment often finds the child in the "tripod position," sitting upright and leaning forward with the chin thrust out, mouth open, and tongue protruding. If not treated immediately respiratory arrest may result. The nurse *should not attempt to visualize* the mouth and throat because total airway closure may result. If the epiglottis requires visualization, it is usually performed in the operating room by a physician.

 The nurse *should not attempt to visualize* the mouth and throat if epiglottitis is suspected because total airway closure may result.

Epiglottitis requires intubation to maintain the airway. After the intubation, cultures are obtained from the epiglottis and blood and intravenous antibiotics are started. Antibiotics usually produce rapid results, with swelling decreasing within 24 hours and return to a normal epiglottis within 72 hours.

Bacterial Tracheitis

Bacterial tracheitis (pseudomembranous croup) is a severe form of laryngotracheobronchitis. *Staphylococcus aureus, H. influenza* (A), *Streptococcus pyogenes,* and *Neisseria* are usually the causative pathogens. It is thought that bacteria invade the mucosa of children with viral croup and thus cause edema, purulent drainage, and pseudomembranes.

The child with bacterial tracheitis has signs and symptoms similar to the child with viral croup, but instead of getting better the child with bacterial tracheitis will develop a high fever, toxicity, and progressive upper airway obstruction that do not respond to the usual treatments for viral croup. It is not uncommon for a child with bacterial tracheitis to develop sudden respiratory failure/arrest, toxic shock, and acute respiratory distress syndrome. Because of the danger of respiratory arrest coupled with thick purulent secretions, the child with bacterial tracheitis usually requires intubation. Although this is a serious illness, children usually survive.

DISORDERS OF THE INTRATHORACIC AIRWAYS

Bronchitis

Bronchitis may develop as a result of exposure to tobacco smoke, a lower respiratory infection, or because of underlying diseases such as cystic fibrosis. A child with acute bronchitis presents with a cough that started

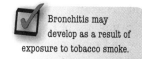

Bronchitis may develop as a result of exposure to tobacco smoke.

out as nonproductive and then became productive, diffuse rhonchi, and a normal white blood cell count. Treatment includes avoiding exposure to irritating agents and symptomatic treatment of viral or bacterial respiratory infections.

Bronchiolitis

Infants and children younger than 1 year of age frequently develop **bronchiolitis**, a common, serious, acute respiratory illness occurring mainly during the winter months. Approximately 125,000, or 33%, of infants and children who develop bronchiolitis each year require hospitalization, and 500 die from the illness.

The most common cause of bronchiolitis is RSV (respiratory syncytial virus), although parainfluenza, influenza viruses, and adenoviruses are also potential causes. Some infants and children develop asthma as a sequela to bronchiolitis. Premature infants, infants under 6 months of age, and those infants and children with underlying chronic diseases such as cystic fibrosis or congenital heart disease are in the most danger for respiratory collapse from bronchiolitis.

Exposure to respiratory secretions through close contact with infected persons or contact with contaminated surfaces or objects spreads RSV. This virus can live on objects such as gloves, countertops, and paper tissues for 6 hours and on skin for 30 minutes. Touching the mucous membranes of the eyes, mouth, or nose after touching a contaminated object or inhalation of respiratory droplets generated by a sneeze or cough can spread RSV.

 RSV can live on objects such as gloves, countertops, and paper tissues for 6 hours and on skin for 30 minutes.

Once the RSV has invaded the epithelial cells of the respiratory tract, swelling occurs and cilia are destroyed. The infected cells fuse with adjacent cells, producing a giant cell with multiple nuclei. This multinucleated mass of protoplasm is termed "**syncytia**." Exudate and mucus fill the bronchioles, causing an obstruction and, in some cases, hyperinflation and atelectasis.

Symptoms of RSV include fever, runny nose, cough, wheezing, shallow and rapid respiratory rate, and respiratory distress. Nasal flaring, cyanosis, retractions, and rales may also be present. Some infants have periods of apnea. Preventative treatment, especially for premature infants and those with underlying chronic illness such as bronchopulmonary dysplasia, consists of monthly intramuscular vaccination with palivizumab. Synagis (palivizumab, an RSV-specific antibody that helps fight RSV infection) is given once a month during the RSV season, generally November to April.

Other preventative measures to prevent the spread of RSV include good and frequent hand washing before touching the infant or child; avoidance of sharing cups, pacifiers, feeding spoons, and so forth; avoidance of crowds and daycare settings if possible; avoidance of contact with other people who have symptoms of a upper respiratory tract infection; avoidance of sharing toys; washing toys with soap and water as often as feasible; and avoidance of tobacco smoke.

Pertussis

Pertussis, a highly contagious bacterial respiratory illness resulting in severe bronchitis caused by *Bordetella pertussis*, is also called whooping cough. The infection is most dangerous for infants before the age of 6 months. Adults may have a mild case of pertussis and infect infants and children with whom they have close contact, such as daycare workers infecting children in their care. In 1976, 1,000 cases of pertussis were reported, contrasting with over 25,000 cases reported in 2004. Approximately 30% of the cases reported in 2003 occurred in older children and adolescents. One reason for the rise in cases is that the original vaccination loses its effectiveness over a 5- to 10-year period, so adolescents vaccinated as young children are now susceptible to the disease.

Pathology

The incubation period for pertussis is usually 7 to 10 days between acquiring the infection and the onset of symptoms, but it can be as long as 21 days. The organism attaches itself to the ciliated epithelial cells of the respiratory tract where it multiplies. Toxins are then produced, resulting in lymphocytosis and other symptoms that follow a predictable course. One to 2 weeks after becoming infected the infant shows signs of a upper respiratory tract infection, namely a runny nose, sneezing, mild, dry, irritating cough, and low-grade fever. Within 2–4 weeks the severe coughing spells begin. The coughing spells, which can last for more than a minute, are paroxysmal in nature, causing 10 to 30 coughs in a row and ending with a loud inspiration, producing the characteristic whooping sound. Vomiting, cyanosis, sweating, and exhaustion follow the spells. The coughing spells may last for months, although they lessen in severity. Complications from pertussis include bronchopneumonia pneumonia from a superinfection, which one in five children under the age of 12 months develop; atelectasis; ear infections; seizures; dehydration; apnea; hypoxia; sudden death during a coughing spell; and frequently fatal encephalopathy.

Diagnosis is made by considering the child's history and physical assessment. A culture of the nose and throat along with blood cultures and a chest x-ray also confirm the disease. Infected people are most contagious during the earliest stages of the illness up to about 2 weeks after the cough begins. Antibiotics shorten the period of *contagiousness* to 5 days from the start of antibiotic treatment but do not affect the course of the disease.

Prevention

To prevent pertussis the child should receive five doses of the DTaP (diphtheria, tetanus, acellular pertussis) vaccine before their 6th birthday. Two new pertussis preventative vaccines were recently made available for older children and adults. Adolescents ages 10 to 18 may receive a booster Tdap vaccine called Boostrix, which contains tetanus, diphtheria, and acellular pertussis. Another option for adolescents and adults ages 11 to 64 is the Adacel booster vaccination, which also contains tetanus, diphtheria, and acellular pertussis. Either vaccine is given as a single-dose vaccination, and both were approved for use in 2005. Active immunity occurs after an infection with pertussis. If people who had pertussis as a child are later reinfected, the illness is usually milder than the original infection.

Exposed family members, children under the age of 2, and health care workers are generally started on a prophylaxis course of erythromycin after contact with an infected infant or child. Erythromycin successfully eradicates *Bordetella pertussis* in the respiratory tract.

Treatment

The treatment for pertussis is a 2-week course of antibiotics, including macrolides, erythromycin, azithromycin and clarithromycin, or ampicillin. These antibiotics stop the transmission of the disease but do not modify the course of the disease unless given before coughing begins. Seventy-five percent of infected infants under age 6 months require hospitalization and supportive respiratory care. Infants or children who are hospitalized are placed in isolation. Corticosteroids are not generally used because they mask the signs of a bacterial superinfection. Likewise, Albuterol is generally avoided because it may cause a bronchospasm and tachycardia. Cough suppressants do not stop the coughing spells.

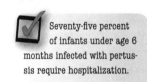 Seventy-five percent of infants under age 6 months infected with pertussis require hospitalization.

Childhood mortality from pneumonia has declined dramatically. **Pneumonia**, which is more common before age 5 than in later childhood, is an inflammatory process that may be caused by numerous infectious agents such as bacteria, viruses, fungi, yeast, or protozoa (Figure 50-1). *Streptococcus pneumoniae* is responsible for up to 75% of all cases of pneumonia. In contrast to bacterial pneumonia, viral pneumonia is usually mild and heals without intervention; however, it can lead to a more virulent bacterial pneumonia.

50

Pneumonia: Acquired Disorders Involving Alveoli

TERMS
- ☐ Atypical pneumonia
- ☐ Bronchopneumonia
- ☐ Lobar pneumonia
- ☐ Nosocomial pneumonia
- ☐ Pneumonia

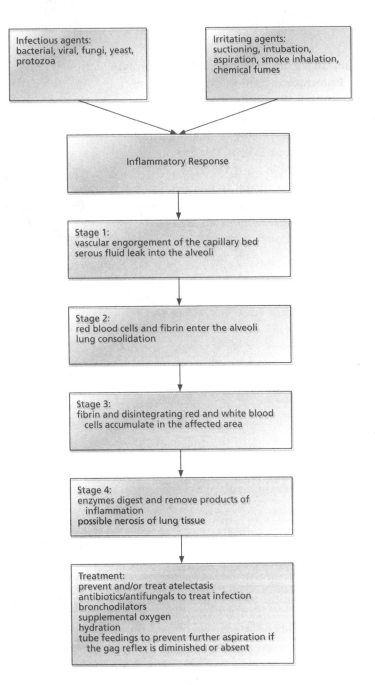

Figure 50-1. Pneumonia.

Irritating agents or events such as suctioning, intubation, aspirated gastric juice, inhalation of smoke, or chemical fumes can also lead to pneumonia. Aspiration pneumonia may occur because the gag reflex is impaired, as in children with seizures or with anatomic abnormalities such as cleft palate, or because a nasogastric tube prevents the lower esophageal sphincter from closing, allowing gastric juice or tube feeding to enter the lungs. Gastric secretions and tube-feeding formulas are irritating to lung tissue and set up an inflammatory response when aspirated.

Other common causes of pneumonia are stasis of respiratory secretions and thickened secretions. Stasis of secretions in a child with cystic fibrosis can lead to pneumonia because bacteria can grow in the static secretions. When respiratory secretions become thick ciliary action cannot remove the bacteria-laden mucus, and pneumonia may result.

Pneumonia may be classified by the agent that causes it or by its location in the lung. **Lobar pneumonia** is confined to a single lobe of the lung, whereas **bronchopneumonia**, the most common type, is described as patchy pneumonia in several lobes. **Atypical pneumonia**, usually caused by viruses (type A/B influenza) or some bacteria (*Legionella*), is also patchy but does not involve the alveoli. Pneumonia may also be classified according to where it was acquired. **Nosocomial pneumonia** is pneumonia acquired while the child was hospitalized, and community-acquired pneumonia is pneumonia acquired outside of a hospital/health care setting.

 ## STAGES OF PNEUMONIA

The inflammatory process is responsible for the four stages of pneumonia. The first stage is the 24-hour congestion stage during which there is vascular engorgement of the capillary bed and serous fluid leak into the alveoli. During this time the child may complain of

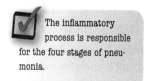
The inflammatory process is responsible for the four stages of pneumonia.

fever, chills, aching chest, malaise, dyspnea (a subjective symptom), and watery phlegm and the white blood cell count begins to rise. Auscultation reveals fine crackles over the affected area.

The second stage is called the red hepatization stage because red blood cells and fibrin enter the alveoli, creating a red firm lung appearance. Lung sounds in the consolidated area are absent. The child may complain of dyspnea and tachypnea.

The third stage is called the gray hepatization stage because fibrin and disintegrating red and white blood cells accumulate in the affected area. The cough may become blood tinged or purulent. The last stage is the resolution stage or "clean-up" stage during which enzymes digest and remove the products of inflammation. The exudate is either coughed up or removed by white blood cells. Necrosis of lung tissue may occur.

Diagnostic tests for pneumonia include a chest x-ray, which shows areas of consolidation, culture, and sensitivity of collected sputum; white blood cell counts and complete blood count; arterial blood gases (determine oxygenation needs, including intubation and ventilation support); and possibly a bronchoscopy to collect samples and/or remove secretions.

BACTERIAL PNEUMONIA

When the cough/gag reflex, mucociliary system, or immune system is compromised, bacteria and other pneumonia-causing agents enter the normally sterile lung fields. Bacteria can enter the lungs by inhalation or via the bloodstream and most commonly presents as unilateral lobar pneumonia. Children with congenital abnormalities such as cleft palate or disorders such as cystic fibrosis or congestive heart failure are prone to develop bacterial pneumonia.

Infants may exhibit few symptoms of bacterial pneumonia, as may older children and those who are immunocompromised. Some children complain of abdominal pain and chest pain, and some have a concurrent 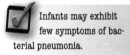 infection caused by the same organism in other areas such as the middle ear or sinuses. An elevated white blood cell count with a high neutrophil count signals bacterial pneumonia.

Infants may exhibit few symptoms of bacterial pneumonia.

Empyema may develop if the causative pathogen was staphylococcal, pneumococcal, or group A β-hemolytic. Sepsis is also a possible complication, especially in children who are immunocompromised.

VIRAL PNEUMONIA

Over 75% of viral pneumonia cases in children are caused by respiratory syncytial virus, parainfluenza, and influenza viruses. The signs and symptoms of viral pneumonia are similar to those found with bacterial pneumonia, although some symptoms such as wheezing, stridor, and low-grade fever are more common with viral pneumonia. Pleural effusion, fever, and lobar consolidation are more common with bacterial pneumonia. Children with viral pneumonia have usually had an upper respiratory tract infection with rhinitis and a cough before the development of the pneumonia.

Complications of viral pneumonia include bronchiolitis obliterans (a plug of granulation tissue found within the terminal and respiratory bronchioles), severe respiratory failure, and persistent reactive airway disease.

 ## CHLAMYDIAL PNEUMONIA

Newborns may develop chlamydial pneumonia during the vaginal birth process if the mother has a chlamydial infection. This type of infant pneumonia has reached epidemic proportions in urban areas of the country and worldwide. Although some infected infants may not appear to be ill, others present with a cough similar to whooping cough, rapid respiratory rate, grunting, nasal flaring, irritability, and an elevated serum IgM. The antibiotic of choice is erythromycin. It may take 7 to 8 years before pulmonary function tests return to normal in an infant who has had this type of pneumonia.

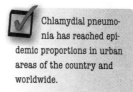

Chlamydial pneumonia has reached epidemic proportions in urban areas of the country and worldwide.

 ## MYCOPLASMA PNEUMONIA

College-aged young adults and children living in group housing such as dormitories commonly develop pneumonia caused by the *Mycoplasma pneumoniae*, a type of community-acquired pneumonia. This type of pneumonia has a long incubation period of up to 3 weeks, with a slow onset of symptoms. Signs and symptoms include fever, headache, cough, and general malaise. Other symptoms include a sore throat and middle ear infection. The white blood cell count is usually within the normal range; however, a chest x-ray is likely to show bronchopneumonic infiltrates. Antibiotic therapy with Cipro or a macrolide is the treatment of choice.

GENERAL MANAGEMENT

Careful and consistent hand washing help to prevent nosocomial infections. Children who are in a high-risk group for community-acquired pneumonia benefit from influenza and pneumococcus vaccines. Once pneumonia develops treatment focuses on eradicating the infection and/or correcting the underlying cause of the inflammation. Bacterial and fungal infectious agents are treated with antibiotic therapy. Few antiviral agents are available at this time. Bronchodilators may be prescribed to reduce or prevent bronchospasm.

Supportive measures include careful monitoring of respiratory and oxygenation status, hydration to thin secretions so they can be expectorated, supplemental oxygen, rest to promote healing, and, in some cases, chest physiotherapy. If aspiration pneumonia occurs, treatment is aimed at eliminating the cause of the aspiration.

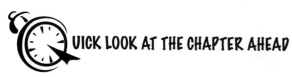
This chapter discusses the etiology and treatment for asthma. **Asthma** is the most common chronic disease of childhood, affecting over 5 million children in the United States and accounting for school absenteeism and restricted activity.

51

Asthma

TERMS
☐ Asthma

INTRODUCTION

Over 80% of children with asthma exhibit signs and symptoms of the disease before age 5. Forty percent of infants and young children who wheeze in response to a viral respiratory infection continue to have asthma symptoms throughout childhood. Since the 1970s morbidity and mortality rates have increased. For children between the ages of 0 and 4 years there has been 160% increase in asthma incidence from 1980 to 1994. Black Americans are hospitalized and die from asthma each year at a higher rate than other ethnic groups. More children aged 11 to 17 are hospitalized each year for asthma than other age groups. Possible explanations for the high rate of childhood asthma and asthma deaths include failure to diagnosis or adequately treat the disease, lack of recognition of severe signs and symptoms resulting in delayed treatment, an increase in air pollution, and failure to follow prescribed treatment plans.

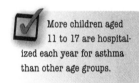
More children aged 11 to 17 are hospitalized each year for asthma than other age groups.

Asthma is characterized by acute airway inflammation, bronchoconstriction, bronchospasm, edema of the bronchioles, and increased production of mucus. Characteristic signs and symptoms of asthma are chest tightness, cough, tachypnea, wheezing, anxiety, and dyspnea caused by airway narrowing. Unless treated promptly, asthma can lead to ineffective gas exchange and death. Status asthmaticus is a severe prolonged asthma attack that does not respond to usual treatment and is life threatening. Signs of severe bronchoconstriction in children include flaring of the nostrils, intercostals and suprasternal retractions, use of accessory muscles, agitation, and lethargy.

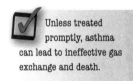
Unless treated promptly, asthma can lead to ineffective gas exchange and death.

Wearing a face mask that warms the air and retains airway humidity is helpful in preventing exercise-induced asthma. Asthma caused by allergens such as dust mites, animal dander, cockroaches, and mold can be managed by removing as much of the offending allergen as possible from the child's environment. Air filters, absence of tobacco smoke, hardwood floors rather than carpeting, and dusting daily are some of the measures used to control dust mites and other allergens. Desensitization treatments are also useful in controlling extrinsic asthma.

PATHOPHYSIOLOGY

Asthma may be classified according to cause, such as extrinsic (allergic), intrinsic (idiopathic), nocturnal, exercise induced, occupational, and drug induced, or more precisely by severity, such as mild intermittent, mild persistent, moderate persistent, and severe persistent (Figure 51-1). Extrinsic asthma is a result of increased IgE synthesis and hypersensitivity of the airways, resulting in mast cell destruction and release of inflammatory mediators. When stimulated by allergens such as house mites, food additives, pollen, animal dander, drugs such as aspirin, or mold spores, mast cells in the bronchial tissue release leukotrienes, which cause bronchoconstriction; histamine, which causes increased vascular permeability; and prostaglandins, which cause increase mucous production. The onset of extrinsic asthma generally occurs before ages 4 or 5 and is more common in boys than in girls until adolescence, when girls have a higher incidence of asthma than boys.

In contrast to extrinsic asthma, intrinsic asthma is triggered by factors other than allergens. Triggers for intrinsic asthma are an upper respiratory infection, air pollution, tobacco smoke, emotional stress, exercise, and exposure to cold air. Exercise-induced asthma is fairly common, affecting approximately 70% of the people who have asthma. In this type of asthma the attack usually begins 5 to 10 minutes after the activity begins. Hypotheses related to exercise-induced asthma focus on increased airway cooling and drying of the mucosa. Children should be encouraged to participate in physical activity that does not trigger an asthma attack. Short-acting β agonists taken before activity are useful in increasing exercise tolerance.

> Short-acting β agonists taken before activity are useful in increasing exercise tolerance.

Teens may develop occupational asthma, which is caused by a reaction to substances such as fumes from plastic, formaldehyde, or cedar dust. Each exposure to the offending substance produces increasingly severe asthma attacks. Time away from work, such as during the weekend, results in clearing of symptoms.

A common cause of drug-induced asthma is acetylsalicylic acid (ASA) and may be fatal. ASA intolerance usually develops in children who have nasal polyps, sinusitis, and asthma. Delayed reactions may occur 12 hours after

> ASA intolerance usually develops in children who have nasal polyps, sinusitis, and asthma.

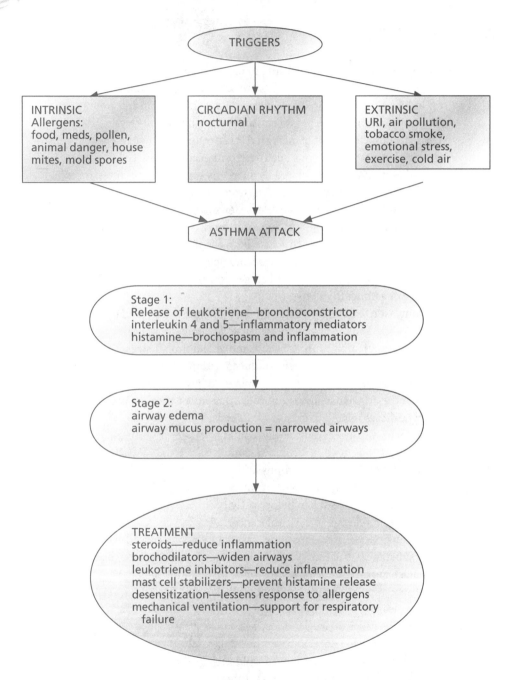

Figure 51-1 Asthma.

the ingestion of ASA or may occur shortly after taking the drug. There appears to be a cross-sensitivity to nonsteroidal anti-inflammatory drugs (NSAID—nonsteroidal drugs) in the person with ASA-induced asthma. Both ASA and nonsteroidal anti-inflammatory drugs prevent the conversion of arachidonic acid to prostaglandins, thereby stimulating leukotriene release, which is a powerful bronchoconstrictor. Food additives, such as yellow dye no. 5 used in pharmaceutical, hair, and food products, and monosodium glutamate, or MSG, have also been indicated in asthma attacks.

Nocturnal asthma, generally occurring between 3 AM and 7 AM, is thought to be related to circadian rhythms. At night, natural cortisol and epinephrine levels decrease and plasma histamine levels increase. Epinephrine is a naturally occurring bronchodilator; thus a decrease in epinephrine release produces bronchoconstriction. Nocturnal airway diameter in asthmatics can decrease by as much as 50%. This narrowing, coupled with airway cooling and drying, impaired mucociliary clearance, increased vagal tone,

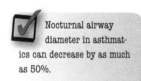

Nocturnal airway diameter in asthmatics can decrease by as much as 50%.

and gastroesophageal reflex disease (GERD) causing microaspiration, are thought to be contributing factors for nocturnal asthma. Also under investigation is the role of late-phase response to allergens that may occur 6 to 12 hours after exposure.

Regardless of classification, asthma attacks are the body's response to bronchial inflammation. Stage one of an acute asthma attack, generally signaled by coughing, is primarily bronchospastic in nature and reaches a peak within 15 to 30 minutes of the beginning of the attack. Chemical inflammatory mediators responsible for stage one include leukotrienes, interleukin-4 and -5, and histamine.

Stage two of an asthma attack peaks within 2–6 hours of onset and is a result of airway edema and mucous production. The mucus produced during stage two is generally thick and contains bronchial casts. Air trapping during expiration with resulting alveolar hyperinflation is common. Bronchospasm, smooth muscle contraction, inflammation, and increased mucous production combine to produce a narrowed airway.

Pulmonary function tests, arterial blood gas analysis, complete blood count, challenge testing, and allergy testing are mainstays of asthma diagnosis. Pulmonary function testing in children with asthma reveals a decreased peak expiratory flow rate indicating trapped air. Arterial blood gas analysis reveals a decreased carbon dioxide level and respiratory alkalosis related to tachypnea. As respiratory exhaustion takes place there is an increase in the arterial carbon dioxide level and a decrease in the oxygen level. Eosinophilia, as reflected in a complete blood count, indicates the body's response to an allergen. Allergy testing is used to pinpoint the offending allergen(s).

 ## MANAGEMENT

Inhaled steroids, nebulizer treatments, inhaled bronchodilators, and leukotriene modifiers are some of the pharmaceutical agents used to control and/or prevent asthma attacks. β Agonists are useful in preventing exercise-induced asthma, as is cromolyn sodium, which is a mast cell stabilizer. Ipratropium bromide, an inhaled anticholinergic, is used to relax bronchial smooth muscle. During status asthmaticus intravenous steroids, intravenous bronchodilators, and mechanical ventilation may be necessary.

Prevention of nocturnal asthma is vital because the majority of asthma-related fatalities occur during the early morning hours. The treatment for nocturnal asthma includes longer acting β agonists and histamine blockers to control gastroesophageal reflex disease. Left untreated, long-term asthma may result in bronchial tissue damage and scarring, which in turn leads to increased hyperreactivity of the airways.

This chapter covers the pathophysiology and treatment of two common pediatric respiratory system health deviations: bronchopulmonary dysplasia and cyctic fibrosis.

52

Bronchopulmonary Dysplasia and Cystic Fibrosis

TERMS
☐ Bronchopulmonary
  dysplasia (BPD)
☐ Cor pulmonale
☐ Cystic fibrosis (CF)

BRONCHOPULMONARY DYSPLASIA

Low-birth-weight infants (less than 1,000 g) who experience acute respiratory distress and require prolonged mechanical ventilation have a 30% chance of developing **bronchopulmonary dysplasia (BPD)**. The National Institutes of Health defines BPD using the following criteria: (1) oxygen therapy longer than 28 days, (2) history of positive pressure ventilation or continuous positive airway pressure, and (3) gestational age.

Although BPD is a common sequelae of hyaline membrane disease, full-term newborns with meconium aspiration or persistent pulmonary hypertension can also develop the disorder. The number of days oxygen therapy is needed plays a role in BPD development. Infants who do not require prolonged mechanical ventilation but do require prolonged oxygen therapy are at risk for BPD. During the first week of life some infants display markers associated with BPD, namely increased airway resistance, altered protease and antiprotease ratios, and increased numbers of inflammatory cells and mediators.

Pathophysiology

The exact cause of BPD is not known. What is known is that a premature infant's lungs do not make enough surfactant, resulting in atelectasis. The immature lung is unable to protect itself from the effects of supplemental oxygen. Increased amounts of oxygen cause toxic metabolites to develop, injuring lung tissue. As a response to prolonged oxygen therapy, an inflammatory response is initiated. The damaged lung tissue becomes fibrosed. More

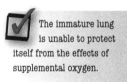

The immature lung is unable to protect itself from the effects of supplemental oxygen.

oxygen therapy is then needed because of a decreased ventilation capacity, leading to a cycle of further toxicity, injury, inflammation, and fibrosis. Other events that compound the need for oxygen therapy include cardiac defects such as patent ductus arteriosus, infection, pulmonary edema, and pulmonary hypertension. Intubated infants are also at risk of developing structural defects such as a high-arched palate and subglottic narrowing. These defects may result in sleep apnea.

Pulmonary edema may develop in response to left-sided congestive heart failure, salt and water retention related to chronic hypoxia and hypercapnia, or because of increased pulmonary vessel permeability related to oxygen toxicity. Diuretic therapy used to treat pulmonary edema carries its own risks as infants may develop fluid volume deficit and electrolyte imbalance.

Pulmonary hypertension may develop as a result of hypoxemia, which causes an increase in pulmonary artery pressure. Low serum oxygen levels cause the pulmonary arteries to constrict. Prolonged pulmonary hypertension, in turn, causes the right ventricle to enlarge (**cor pulmonale**) to have enough force to move blood through the constricted pulmonary arteries. To prevent pulmonary hypertension the Sao_2 should be maintained above 93%.

 To prevent pulmonary hypertension the Sao_2 should be maintained above 93%.

Clinical Course and Treatment

Some infants with BPD require minimal oxygen therapy for a few months, whereas others develop severe BPD and require a tracheostomy and mechanical ventilation for several years and are hospitalized frequently because of lingering respiratory difficulties. Oxygen therapy increases caloric and nutritional needs; therefore careful monitoring of nutritional status is essential for these infants. Additionally, the infant may be nutritionally compromised because of feeding difficulties and gastric reflux. Hypercaloric formulas and a gastric feeding tube may be required.

Although a short course of systemic postnatal glucocorticoids may help in weaning the infant from mechanical ventilation, this drug has been linked to a decrease in alveolar development in animal studies and is therefore a controversial therapy. Cerebral palsy has been linked to longer courses of postnatal glucocorticoids. Inhaled glucocorticoids, rather than systemic steroids, have not been shown to decrease the incidence of BPD. Surfactant therapy given immediately after birth has, however, been shown to decrease the chance of requiring mechanical ventilation and BPD development.

Infants with BPD have increased airway resistance and bronchial hyperreactivity. Inhaled steroids and β-adrenergic agonists are used to decrease the inflammatory response and increase the action of the β-adrenergic agonists. Some infants also require chest percussion to loosen thick secretions that may lead to atelectasis.

CYSTIC FIBROSIS

Pathophysiology

Cystic fibrosis (CF), the most common genetic disease in the United States, is the leading cause of death in early adulthood. Chromosome 7 contains the gene responsible for the production of the cystic fibrosis transmembrane conductance regulator protein (CFTR). This protein is an ion channel that allows salt and water into and out of epithelial cells. Without this protein chloride ions build up in the epithelial cells of the lungs and other organs, drawing water into the cells to dilute the chloride. The normal flow of water and chloride into and out of cells is disrupted and leads to thick and sticky mucous production that blocks the ducts. Another result of CF is excessive salt secretion by the sweat glands.

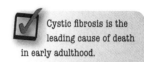
Cystic fibrosis is the leading cause of death in early adulthood.

The infant with CF may have multiple organ involvement including the liver, gastrointestinal system (Table 52-1), male reproductive system (Table 52-2), and lungs. Involvement of the lungs occurs in almost all

Table 52-1 Gastrointestinal and Nutritional Implications in CF

Signs and Symptoms	Pathology	Treatment
Abdominal distention Bulky greasy stools Increased flatulence	Exocrine pancreatic insufficiency and malabsorption	Pancreatic enzyme replacement with each meal and snack
Hypoalbuminemia Anemia Edema	Protein loss in stool Portal hypertension Low serum osmotic pressure secondary to low serum protein levels	Unrestricted diet
Hepatomegaly cirrhosis	Bile duct blockage	
Intestinal blockage	Thick stools	Cathartics and enemas
Fat-soluble vitamin deficiency	Fat loss in stools	Pancreatic enzyme supplements

Signs and Symptoms	Pathology	Treatment
Poor growth	Protein calorie malnutrition	Unrestricted diet
Decreased body fat		High calorie supplements Nighttime nasogastric feedings

Table 52-2 Reproductive Implications in CF

Signs and Symptoms	Pathology	Treatment
Male infertility	Vas deferens are absent or undeveloped	No medical treatment at present

cases of CF and results in chronic infections and loss of pulmonary function (Table 52-3). Most infants with CF live into young adulthood, with a median survival of 33 years.

Diagnosis

At birth approximately 15% of newborns with CF have a meconium ileus. In some infants the ileus is reversed with an enema administered under radiologic observation, whereas other infants require a bowel resection. Almost half of all infants with CF have failure to thrive and respiratory difficulty. Diagnosis of CF is based on presenting symptoms such as meconium ileus, failure to thrive, frequent respiratory infections, and elevated immunoreactive trypsinogen-pancreatic enzyme precursor and is confirmed by a sweat chloride test above 60 mEq/L or genetic testing.

Table 52-3 Pulmonary Implications in CF

Signs and Symptoms	Pathology	Treatment
Cough Tachypnea Rales Wheezing Decreased pulmonary function	Diminished air flow Diminished vital capacity Airway reactivity	Intravenous antibiotics, bronchodilators Aggressive airway clearance therapy
Respiratory syncytial virus (RSV)	Exposure to virus	Vaccination with palivizumab (Synagis), an RSV-specific antibody
Respiratory infection	Stasis of secretions	Antibiotic therapy—inhaled tobramycin
Hemoptysis	Bronchiectasis	
Increased thick secretions	Hyperplasia of mucous glands of the bronchial epithelium	Inhaled DNase (Pulmozyme)

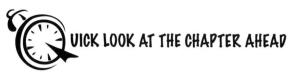

This chapter discusses common causes of apnea in the pediatric population.

53

Disorders of the Control of Breathing

TERMS

- ☐ Apnea of infancy
- ☐ Apparent life-threatening events (ALTEs)
- ☐ Central apnea
- ☐ Obstructive sleep apnea
- ☐ Sudden infant death syndrome (SIDS)

477

PEDIATRIC SLEEP APNEA

Obstructive sleep apnea, defined as the attempt to breathe through an obstructed airway, most commonly occurs in children with craniofacial abnormalities (Crouzon's syndrome, etc.), in those with neuropathies, and in those medicated with hypnotics, sedatives, and anticonvulsants. **Central apnea**, defined as the lack of effort to breathe, occurs mainly in premature infants. Sleep apnea can be life threatening in infants. In toddlers it may present as failure to thrive, hyperactivity, and behavior problems. Mood changes and lethargy may be the presenting symptoms in teenagers.

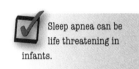
Sleep apnea can be life threatening in infants.

Pediatric sleep disorder clinics are able to provide testing and treatment. Adenotonsillectomy relieves obstructive sleep apnea in many children. Other treatment choices include the use of a Bi-Pap (bilevel positive airway pressure) apparatus during sleep.

APPARENT LIFE-THREATENING EVENTS IN INFANCY

Infants who have **apparent life-threatening events (ALTEs)** commonly do so because of a combination of obstructive and central apnea. During the episode they stop breathing, become cyanotic or very pale, become limp, and may choke or gag. If no apparent reason for the event is discovered the infant is diagnosed as having **apnea of infancy**. This condition is most common in infants 2 to 4 months of age. The risk for sudden infant death syndrome rises if the child has apnea of infancy. The exact cause of ALTEs is unknown. Because these events do not occur past infancy, immaturity of the nervous system, reflexes, and responses to apnea during sleep may be causes (Table 53-1).

Once the cause of ALTEs is identified, therapy is individualized (Table 53-2). Antibiotics are administered for bacterial respiratory infections. Anticonvulsant medications are given to help control a seizure disorder. Structural abnormalities are corrected with surgery. Home monitoring is used to detect bradycardia and apnea when no specific cause for the episodes is found. Parents and caregivers should be taught infant cardiopulmonary resuscitation techniques. If the alarm is not triggered for several months, monitoring is usually discontinued. Other treatments

Table 53-1 Causes of ALTEs

Category	Examples of Specific Causes
Infections	Viral: respiratory syncytial virus and other viruses Bacterial: sepsis, pertussis, *Chlamydia*
Gastrointestinal	Gastroesophageal reflux Discoordinated swallowing Chronic aspiration
Respiratory	Abnormal airway structure Pneumonia
Neurological	Seizures Meningitis, encephalitis Brain tumor Vasovagal response
Cardiovascular	Cardiomyopathy Dysrhythmias
Nonaccidental trauma	Battering—shaken baby syndrome Drug overdose Munchausen-by-proxy syndrome (assess for pinch marks on the nares)
Other	Apnea of infancy Breath-holding while crying

include oxygen therapy to increase serum oxygen saturation and respiratory stimulants such as caffeine and aminophylline to counteract central sleep apnea.

 # SUDDEN INFANT DEATH SYNDROME

Sudden infant death syndrome (SIDS) occurs when an infant less than 12 months of age dies suddenly from an unexplained cause. Most SIDS cases occur between ages 2 and 4 months and between midnight and 8 AM when both the infant and caregivers are sleeping. Infants up to 6 months of age are at greater risk of SIDS than infants 6–12 months of age. All SIDS cases are investigated in-depth by performing a complete

Table 53-2 Diagnostic Tools for ALTEs

Findings	Implications
Elevated white blood cell count	Infection
High serum bicarbonate	Chronic hypoventilation
Decreased serum bicarbonate	Acute acidosis related to hypoxia during the episode
Chronic acidosis	Metabolic disorder
Chest x-ray showing infiltrates	Acute infection or chronic aspiration
Arterial blood gases: low PaO_2 or high $Pa\,CO_2$	Cardiorespiratory disorder
Barium swallow—abnormal	Anatomical abnormalities, i.e., tracheoesophageal fistula Reflux Aspiration

autopsy, examining the death scene, and reviewing the infant's clinical history. Eighty percent of SIDS cases cannot be explained by autopsy results.

Factors associated with SIDS include exposure to maternal smoking, male gender, African-American or Native American ethnic and/or racial group, having a low socioeconomic status, low birth weight, born to a teenage or to a drug-addicted mother, and a family history of SIDS. Recent immunization has not been shown to be a risk factor.

Since 1994 the "Back-to-Sleep" campaign has focused on educating caregivers about SIDS risk factors. Those risk factors that can be modified include infant sleeping positions, mattress firmness, bottle-feeding, prenatal maternal smoking, exposure to smoke after birth, and infant overheating. The recommended sleep position is supine on a firm mattress in a crib that does not contain soft bedding. Both side-lying and prone positions may increase the risk of SIDS because they contribute to decreased arousal during hypoxia and/or sleep, rebreathing of carbon dioxide, or effects on the autonomic nervous system, which in infants is immature.

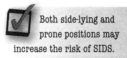 Both side-lying and prone positions may increase the risk of SIDS.

Infants born to mothers who smoked during pregnancy have an increased risk of SIDS due to the effects smoking has on the developing autonomic nervous system and on pulmonary growth. Exposure to smoke after birth has also been shown to increase the risk of SIDS. Studies concerning the risk reduction effects of breast-feeding versus bottle-feeding are inconclusive. Data point to other factors associated with breast-feeding that may reduce the risk of SIDS rather than a component of breast milk that is protective. Overheating infants by tightly swaddling them is also discouraged.

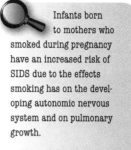

Infants born to mothers who smoked during pregnancy have an increased risk of SIDS due to the effects smoking has on the developing autonomic nervous system and on pulmonary growth.

SECTION XXII • REVIEW QUESTIONS

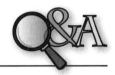

1.   The functions of the respiratory system include (select all that apply):
   a.   Removing carbonic acid from the bloodstream
   b.   Providing oxygen to cells
   c.   Regulating serum pH
   d.   Producing ATP (adenosine triphosphate)

2.   Which of the following statements correctly explains the functional anatomy of the respiratory system?
   a.   Turbinates provide moisture to inspired air.
   b.   Approximately 200 cc of fluid is lost each day in expired air.
   c.   The sinuses are air-filled spaces.
   d.   The epiglottis open during swallowing.

3.   Surfactant is produced by:
   a.   Alveolar type II cells
   b.   Pulmonary capillaries
   c.   The basement membrane
   d.   Pulmonary epithelium

4.   Johnny, a 2½-year-old, has frequent temper tantrums during which time he holds his breath. His father asks the nurse if Johnny can have permanent damage from one of these episodes. The nurse correctly replies that:
   a.   If Johnny holds his breath to the point of unconsciousness, he may develop brain damage.
   b.   At his age Johnny cannot hold his breath long enough to become unconscious and harm himself.
   c.   General cell damage may occur because of lack of oxygen.
   d.   Johnny will lose consciousness if he holds his breath long enough but at that time ventilation will automatically start.

5.   Ventilation occurs because of a:
   a.   Rise in serum pH
   b.   Buildup of serum carbon dioxide
   c.   Elevation of serum oxygen
   d.   Reduction in carbonic acid production

6. In contrast to an adult airway, the airway of an infant or child has a (select all that apply):
   a. Larynx that is more posterior
   b. Floppy epiglottis
   c. Longer trachea
   d. Larger tongue

7. Conditions that cause oxygen to be released easily from hemoglobin include:
   a. Acidosis
   b. Below sea-level altitude
   c. Alkalosis
   d. Subnormal body temperature

8. The enzyme carbonic anhydrase:
   a. Is found in alveoli
   b. Buffers hydrogen ions
   c. Facilitates carbonic acid production
   d. Ionizes red blood cells

9. When explaining croup to Tanisha, whose 8-month-old was diagnosed with viral croup, the nurse correctly states that croup is an acute inflammation of the (select all that apply):
   a. Larynx
   b. Trachea
   c. Major bronchi
   d. Esophagus

10. During the admission process the nurse asks Louisa questions concerning her child, Luis, who was admitted to the hospital with possible viral croup. Which of the following statements by Louisa help confirm the diagnosis of viral croup? (Select all that apply.)
    a. "Luis had a high fever at home."
    b. "Luis has an upper respiratory infection."
    c. "I noticed Luis drooling today."
    d. "Luis has a cough."

11. Which actions should *not* be performed by the nurse caring for Rosita, a 3-year-old who is in the emergency department because of possible epiglottis?
    a. Blood pressure check

b.   Visualization of the mouth and throat

c.   Asking her mother to leave the room during the examination

d.   Placing her in a supine position to listen to her lung sounds

12.   Which description of stridor is *correct*?

a.   Stridor sounds low pitched.

b.   Stridor sounds soft.

c.   Stridor sounds harsh.

d.   Stridor sounds bark-like.

13.   The community health nurse is discussing epiglottitis with a group of parents. One of the parents asks if epiglottitis can be prevented. The nurse correctly replies that the risk of epiglottitis can be reduced if their child:

a.   Received the Hib vaccine

b.   Has a tonsillectomy

c.   Is not exposed to other children who have a cold

d.   Was full-term at birth

14.   A new RN asks her preceptor how she will know if a child recovering from viral croup is developing bacterial tracheitis. The preceptor correctly responds that the child:

a.   With viral croup is highly unlikely to develop a bacterial infection

b.   Will develop sudden respiratory distress

c.   Will have a low-grade fever for 3–5 days

d.   Will drool

15.   The parents of Oliver, a 2-month-old, ask the nurse during a well baby visit how they can reduce the risk of bronchitis. The nurse correctly replies that _____ reduces the risk that Oliver will develop bronchitis.

a.   Supplemental vitamins

b.   Keeping Oliver indoors

c.   Not smoking

d.   Feeding Oliver on a "demand" schedule

16.   Children at risk for respiratory collapse from bronchiolitis include those who (select all that apply):

a.   Are premature

b.   Are over 6 months of age

c.   Attend daycare

d.   Have congenital heart disease

17. The community health nurse visiting a daycare center correctly tells the center's owner that RSV can (select all that apply):
   a. Live on toys for up to 6 hours
   b. Live on skin for up to 30 minutes
   c. Be spread by exposure to respiratory droplets from an infected person
   d. Cause serious illness in infants

18. RSV causes which of the following events?
   a. Multiplication of cilia
   b. Production of a multiple nucleated giant cell
   c. Collapse of the bronchioles
   d. Dehydration of bronchial epithelium

19. The parents of Catherine, a premature infant, ask the nurse if there is anything they can do to prevent Catherine from acquiring RSV. The nurse correctly tells them that to lower Catherine's risk of getting the RSV infection they should (select all that apply):
   a. Have Catherine vaccinated monthly with palivizumab
   b. Follow frequent hand-washing practices
   c. Add multivitamins to her formula
   d. Make sure her Hib vaccination is current

20. The school nurse is presenting a program about pertussis to the PTA. Which of the following facts should the nurse include in the presentation?
   a. Pertussis is a disease of childhood, not adulthood.
   b. Pertussis is most dangerous in children aged 1–3.
   c. The number of cases of pertussis has declined over the past 15 years.
   d. The pertussis vaccine loses its effectiveness after approximately 5–10 years.

21. During a well baby visit the parents of 5-month-old Victoria, who attends daycare, ask the nurse how they can recognizes signs and symptoms of pertussis. The nurse tells them that initial signs and symptoms of pertussis include (select all that apply):
   a. A runny nose
   b. A high fever
   c. Mild cough
   d. Difficulty breathing

22. Parents of 7-year-old Matthew, who has whooping cough, ask the nurse about the disease. The nurse correctly tells them that:
   a.   Antibiotics greatly shorten the course of the disease.
   b.   Matthew will be contagious for 5 days after the antibiotic treatment begins.
   c.   Whooping cough can be confirmed by a sputum culture.
   d.   Matthew is no longer contagious because the coughing has begun.

23. When giving a report to the oncoming nurse about Marisa, a 4-month-old with pertussis, the reporting nurse describes Marisa's coughing spell as:
   a.   Sudden and violent
   b.   Infrequent
   c.   Beginning with a loud inspiration
   d.   Dry and lasting 10 seconds

24. Which of the following statements concerning pertussis is *true*?
   a.   Children should receive three DTaT vaccinations before their 6th birthday.
   b.   Booster vaccines were approved in 2005 for children aged 10–13.
   c.   The Adacel booster vaccine has been approved for adults 18–64.
   d.   Pertussis confers passive immunity.

25. Which of the following statements concerning pneumonia is *correct*?
   a.   Twenty-five percent of pneumonia cases are caused by *Streptococcus pneumoniae.*
   b.   Viral pneumonia is more serious than bacterial pneumonia.
   c.   Tube feeding a premature infant lowers the risk of pneumonia, compared with premature infants who are bottle-fed.
   d.   Pneumonia is an inflammatory process.

26. During the gray hepatization stage of pneumonia:
   a.   The child may cough up blood-tinged mucus.
   b.   Necrosis of lung tissue may occur.
   c.   The affected area will begin to consolidate.
   d.   Red blood cells begin to enter the alveoli.

27. Adina, a 4-year-old, was admitted to the hospital because she has bacterial pneumonia. The nurse caring for Adina can expect to assess:

    a.   High basophil count

    b.   Abdominal pain

    c.   Low neutrophil count

    d.   Low-grade fever

28. Compared with a child with bacterial pneumonia, the child with viral pneumonia is more likely to have:

    a.   Pleural effusion

    b.   Fever

    c.   Lobar consolidation

    d.   Wheezing

29. Infant Danielle was diagnosed with chlamydial pneumonia. The nurse should explain to Danielle's parents that:

    a.   This type of pneumonia is rare.

    b.   Danielle will have a cough that sounds like whooping cough.

    c.   Danielle may have abnormal pulmonary function tests for years.

    d.   This type of pneumonia is most frequently caused by exposure to ill children at daycare.

30. Tori, a college freshman, has developed mycoplasma pneumonia. The infirmary nurse explains to Tori that this type of pneumonia:

    a.   Has a short incubation period

    b.   Causes an elevated white blood cell count

    c.   Is usually treated with intravenous antibiotics for 4 weeks

    d.   Causes symptoms such as sore throat and headache

31. When discussing asthma with teachers the nurse should stress that:

    a.   Asthma generally develops between ages 5 and 11.

    b.   African-American children are more likely to be hospitalized because of asthma than children in other ethnic groups.

    c.   Mortality rates from asthma have declined.

    d.   Asthma is the third most common chronic disease of childhood.

32. The community health nurse discussing asthma at a town meeting stresses that pediatric deaths from asthma are thought to be attributed to the (select all that apply):
    a. Failure to diagnose asthma
    b. Failure to treat asthma
    c. Lack of recognition of the signs and symptoms requiring immediate intervention
    d. Environmental increase in pollution

33. The teacher asks the school nurse how to recognize when Clarise, a girl in her first grade class, is beginning to have an asthma attack. The nurse tells her that _____ is the first sign of an asthma attack.
    a. Coughing
    b. Slowed deep respirations
    c. Lethargy
    d. Air hunger

34. Extrinsic asthma may be caused by (select all that apply):
    a. Aspirin
    b. Food additives
    c. Inspired cold air
    d. Upper respiratory infection

35. Nocturnal asthma is thought to be due to (select all that apply):
    a. Increase of epinephrine levels
    b. Microaspiration related to GERD
    c. Increased cortisol levels
    d. Late-phase response to allergens

36. The parents of John, a 6-year-old recently diagnosed with asthma, ask the nurse to explain what happens in an asthma attack. The nurse tells them that during an asthma attack the (select all that apply):
    a. Large airways become hyperinflated
    b. Airway becomes dry
    c. Airway becomes inflamed
    d. Bronchioles become edematous

37. Which of the following statements concerning bronchopulmonary dysplasia is correct?
    a. BPD most commonly affects infants who weigh less than 1,350 grams.
    b. BPD affects virtually all infants who require mechanical ventilation.
    c. BPD is associated with the number of days an infant needs oxygen therapy.
    d. BPD affects only premature infants.

38. When explaining BPD to a new RN orienting to the unit, the preceptor should state that supplemental oxygen may cause (select all that apply):
    a. Pulmonary hypertension
    b. Sleep apnea
    c. Increased pulmonary vessel permeability
    d. Toxic metabolites

39. To prevent Tara, a premature infant requiring supplemental oxygen therapy, from developing pulmonary hypertension the nurse should keep the Sao_2 above:
    a. 80%
    b. 93%
    c. 78%
    d. 85%

40. The nurse caring for Simon, an infant with BPD, should question which of the following orders?
    a. Hypercaloric formula
    b. Glucocorticoids
    c. Chest percussion
    d. β-Adrenergic agonist

41. Which of the following statements about cystic fibrosis is *correct*? Cystic fibrosis is the:
    a. leading cause of death in early adulthood in the United States.
    b. second most common genetic disorder in the United States.
    c. result of a defective gene on chromosome 6.
    d. result of excessive cystic fibrosis transmembrane conductance regulator protein production.

42. The parents of Shanese, an infant thought to have cystic fibrosis, ask how the disease is suspected or confirmed. The nurse correctly tells them that the diagnosis is based on the following items (select all that apply):

    a.   Sweat chloride test results above 48 mEq/l

    b.   Meconium ileus at birth

    c.   Respiratory difficulty

    d.   Decreased immunoreactive trypsinogen-pancreatic enzyme precursor

43. The parents of Michael, an infant with CF, ask the nurse what they can expect when they bring Michael home. The nurse tells them that Michael:

    a.   Will have thin bowel movements

    b.   May have a vitamin D deficiency

    c.   Should meet growth and development milestones on time

    d.   May have frequent respiratory infections

44. The nurse practitioner tells Mary's parents that she suspects the toddler has central apnea. Signs and symptoms of central apnea include (select all that apply):

    a.   Failure to thrive

    b.   Lethargy

    c.   Behavior problems

    d.   Craniofacial abnormalities

45. Sara, a 2-month-old infant, has been diagnosed with idiopathic apnea of infancy. Which of the following statements about this condition is *correct*?

    a.   Idiopathic apnea of infancy will likely persist until Sara is an adolescent.

    b.   Idiopathic apnea of infancy requires home monitoring.

    c.   Idiopathic apnea of infancy requires that apnea monitoring equipment be used until Sara is of school age.

    d.   Idiopathic apnea of infancy has been linked to aminophylline therapy.

46. The nurse presenting a community health education program about sudden infant death syndrome (SIDS) should make which of the following statements?

a. "SIDS is most common in infants between 12 and 18 months of age."

b. "Approximately 60% of SIDS deaths can be explained following autopsy."

c. "Male babies born to teenaged mothers or to mothers who smoke have an increased risk of SIDS."

d. "Most cases of SIDS follow a recent immunization."

47. During a prenatal class a mother-to-be asks if she can do anything to lower her baby's risk of SIDS. The nurse tells the group that _____has been shown to lower SIDS risk.

a. Putting the baby in a side-lying position for sleep

b. Not smoking during pregnancy

c. Tight swaddling to keep the baby warm

d. Bottle feeding

ANSWERS AND RATIONALES

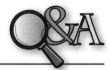

1. **The answers are b and c.** Rationale: Carbon dioxide is removed from the bloodstream, and mitochondria produce ATP by oxidative phosphorylation.

2. **The answer is c.** Rationale: Turbinates provide air turbulence, approximately 1 pint (2 cups or 480 ml) of fluid is lost via ventilation each day, and the epiglottis closes over the trachea during swallowing.

3. **The answer is a.**

4. **The answer is d.** Rationale: If a child holds his or her breath long enough, he or she will become unconscious at which time breathing will automatically resume; cell damage will not occur.

5. **The answer is b.** Rationale: Ventilation is stimulated by a rise in serum carbon dioxide, decrease in serum pH, a drop in arterial oxygen, or a drop in cerebrospinal fluid pH.

6. **The answers are b and d.** Rationale: In contrast to the airway of an adult, the infant or child has a long floppy epiglottis, larger tongue, shorter trachea and neck, and a larynx that is more anterior.

7. **The answer is a.** Rationale: Acidosis, high altitude, heart failure, anemia, and hypercapnia all cause hemoglobin desaturation easily.

8. **The answer is c.** Rationale: Carbonic anhydrase causes 60% of the carbon dioxide produced by cells to combine with water to form carbonic acid.

9. **The answers are a, b, and c.**

10. **The answers are b and d.** Rationale: A high fever and drooling are signs of epiglottitis, not viral croup.

11. **The answers are b, c, and d.** Rationale: Crying (initiated by separating Rosita from her mother), visualization of the mouth and throat, and placing her supine may cause total closure of the airway.

12. The answer is c.

13. The answer is a.

14. **The answer is b.** Rationale: A bacterial infection can develop when a child also has a viral infection because of a weakened immune system; bacterial tracheitis develops suddenly; and the child will have a high fever, toxicity, and respiratory distress.

15. **The answer is c.** Rationale: Exposure to tobacco smoke, lower respiratory infection, and chronic illness increase the likelihood that a child will develop bronchitis.

16. **The answers are a and d.** Rationale: Infants under 6 months of age and those who are premature and/or who have chronic diseases or congenital heart disease are at greatest risk for developing respiratory collapse from bronchiolitis.

17. **The answers are a, b, c, and d.**

18. **The answer is b.** Rationale: RSV causes respiratory tract edema, cilia death, and syncytia (cells fuse together to form a large cell with many nuclei).

19. **The answers are a and b.**

20. **The answer is d.** Rationale: People of all ages can acquire pertussis, although it is most dangerous in children under the age of 6 months; the number of cases has been rising in recent years because the pertussis vaccine loses effectiveness after 5–10 years.

21. **The answers are a and c.** Rationale: Initially, pertussis causes upper respiratory tract infection–like symptoms (runny nose, sneezing, mild, dry cough, and low-grade fever); after 2–4 weeks the characteristic coughing spells begin.

22. **The answer is b.** Rationale: Antibiotics shorten the period during which someone is contagious but do not alter the course of the disease; people are contagious from the onset of symptoms until about 2 weeks after the cough begins.

23. **The answer is a.** Rationale: Whooping cough spells are sudden and violent, lasting more than a minute and having 10–30 coughs in a row ending in a loud inspiration.

24. **The answer is c.** Rationale: Children should receive five doses of the DTaP vaccine before their 6th birthday, Boostrix booster vaccine is for adolescents ages 10–18, and pertussis confers active immunity.

25. **The answer is d.** Rationale: 75% of pneumonia cases are caused by *Streptococcus pneumoniae*, bacterial pneumonia is more serious than viral pneumonia, and tube feeding raises the risk of aspiration pneumonia.

26. **The answer is a.** Rationale: During the red hepatization stage the affected area is consolidated and red blood cells and fibrin enter the alveoli; tissue necrosis may occur during the resolution stage.

27. **The answer is b.** Rationale: Abdominal and chest pain, elevated white blood cell count, high neutrophil count, and fever are signs of bacterial pneumonia.

28. **The answer is d.** Rationale: Pleural effusion, fever, and lobar consolidation are more common with bacterial pneumonia; however, wheezing and stridor are more common with viral pneumonia.

29. **The answer is c.** Rationale: Chlamydial pneumonia is passed to the infant during a vaginal birth if the mother has the infection, some infants are asymptomatic, and this type of pneumonia has reached epidemic proportions in some areas of the country and world.

30. **The answer is d.** Rationale: Mycoplasma pneumonia has a long incubation period, does not usually elevate the white blood cell count, is treated with an oral antibiotic, and causes symptoms such as fever, headache, sore throat, middle ear infection, cough, and malaise.

31. **The answer is b.** Rationale: Children between 0 and 5 years of age are more likely to develop asthma than other age groups, the mortality rate has increased, and asthma is the most common chronic disease of childhood.

32. **The answers are a, b, c, and d.**

33. **The answer is a.** Rationale: Coughing is an early sign of an asthma attack.

34. **The answers are a and b.** Rationale: Extrinsic (allergic) asthma is caused by allergens such as medication, animals, and pollen, whereas intrinsic asthma (idiopathic) is triggered by factors other than allergens, such as exercise, upper respiratory tract infection, and exposure to tobacco smoke.

35. **The answers are b and d.** Rationale: Cortisol and epinephrine levels decrease during the night and histamine levels increase.

36. **The answers are c and d.** Rationale: During an asthma attack mucous production and bronchoconstriction occur.

37. **The answer is c.** Rationale: Infants weighing less than 1,000 grams who require oxygen therapy longer than 28 days are at risk to develop BPD; full-term infants who have aspirated meconium or who have persistent pulmonary hypertension are also at risk for developing BPD.

38. **The answers are c and d.** Rationale: Sleep apnea may result from structural defects caused by intubation; hypoxia may cause pulmonary hypertension because during hypoxia the pulmonary arteries constrict.

39. **The answer is b.**

40. **The answer is b.** Rationale: The use of postnatal glucocorticoids for BPD is questioned because of its link to cerebral palsy.

41. **The answer is a.** Rationale: Cystic fibrosis is the most common genetic disease in the United States; a defect in the gene on chromosome 7, which regulates the production of cystic fibrosis transmembrane conductance regulator protein, causes the disease.

42. **The answers are b and c.** Rationale: Meconium ileus, failure to thrive, frequent respiratory infections, and elevated immunoreactive trypsinogen-pancreatic enzyme precursor are indications of CF, and a sweat chloride test above 60 mEq/l confirms the diagnosis.

43. **The answer is d.** Rationale: Infants and children with CF may have bulky greasy stools, poor growth, fat-soluble vitamin deficiency, and frequent respiratory infections.

44. **The answers are a and c.** Rationale: Toddlers with central apnea may exhibit failure to thrive, hyperactivity, and behavior problems; teenagers may exhibit mood changes and lethargy; and craniofacial abnormalities cause obstructive sleep apnea.

45. **The answer is b.** Rationale: Idiopathic apnea of infancy is most common in infants 2–4 months of age and usually resolves once the infant matures; aminophylline is a respiratory stimulant and is a treatment for this type of apnea.

46. **The answer is c.** Rationale: Immunization has not been shown to be a risk factor for SIDS, most cases occur between 2 and 4 months of age, and 80% cannot be explained by autopsy results.

47. **The answer is b.** Rationale: Maternal smoking during pregnancy, placing the infant in a prone or a side-lying position for sleep, and bottle-feeding are modifiable risk factors for SIDS.

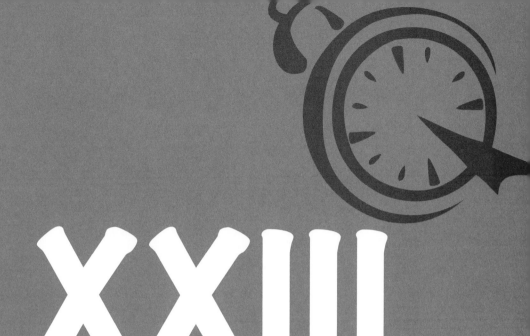

XXIII

Rheumatic Disease

- Early recognition and diagnosis of Lyme disease can prevent long-term complications.

- Approximately 30% of children with juvenile rheumatoid arthritis will have progressive arthritis into adulthood.

- There are three phases to Kawasaki disease, which can last 6–8 weeks after onset of symptoms.

54

Rheumatic Diseases

TERMS
- ☐ Juvenile rheumatoid arthritis (JRA)
  Kawasaki disease
- ☐ Lyme disease

499

JUVENILE RHEUMATOID ARTHRITIS

Juvenile rheumatoid arthritis (JRA) is a chronic disease that affects 60,000 to 200,000 children in the United States. In 1997 the International League of Association for Rheumatology suggested renaming juvenile rheumatoid arthritis as juvenile idiopathic arthritis to encompass criteria for all classifications, but for this chapter we use JRA.

Chronic arthritis in children is thought to have both an environmental and a genetic component. Factors such as familial, seasonal, and ethnic differences account for some of the environmental factors. Certain human leukocyte antigen alleles are associated with disease occurrence from a genetic perspective. Although JRA is rarely life threatening, long-term outcomes for children are hard to predict.

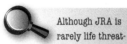

Although JRA is rarely life threatening, long-term outcomes for children are hard to predict.

Pathophysiology

Current literature suggests that T cells are activated and cause development of antigen–antibody complexes that release cytokines into specific organs such as joints and skin. JRA is characterized by inflammation of the synovium with joint effusion and eventual destruction of the articular cartilage lasting 6 weeks or longer. Classification depends on the number of joints involved and other coexisting symptoms. Joint swelling, stiffness, and restriction of motion usually are present. The three types of JRA are systemic, pauciarticular, and polyarticular (Table 54-1).

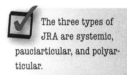

The three types of JRA are systemic, pauciarticular, and polyarticular.

Treatment

There is no cure for JRA. However, in 85% of the cases disease activity diminishes with age and ceases by puberty. Problems later in life are usually associated with residual joint damage. Treatment for JRA consists of controlling the pain, preserving joint range of motion, minimizing the effects of inflammation, and promoting optimal growth and development. Several medications are used to treat JRA:

- Nonsteroidal anti-inflammatory drugs
- Slower acting antirheumatic drugs
- Corticosteroids
- Etanercept or Remicade (a new biological agent)
- Cytotoxic agents

Other treatment modalities are as follows:

- Physical therapy
- Splints
- Moist heat
- Swimming

Table 54-1 Characteristics of Juvenile Rheumatoid Arthritis Related to Type of Onset

	Systemic (Variable Joint Involvement)	**Pauciarticular (Types I and II) (< 4 Joints)**	**Polyarticular (> 5 Joints)**
Percent	30%	45%	25%
Incidence Age, Sex	1–3 8–10 1.5:1 (f:m)	Type I: < 10 Almost all female Type II: > 10 1:9 (f:m)	> 10 Mostly female
Laboratory findings	Anemia, elevated ESR, ANA rarely (+), leukocytosis, RF negative	Elevated ESR, ANA positive Type I: HLA-DRW5 positive Type II: HLA-B27 positive	Elevated ESR Type I: RF positive Type II: RF negative
Prognosis	Mortality 1–2% Joint destruction in 40%	Continuous disease Eventual remission 60% Type I: functional blindness Type II: ankylosing spondylitis	Longer duration, more crippling Type I: high incidence of disabling arthritis Type II: less crippling

ANA, antinuclear antibodies; ESR, erythrocyte sedimentation rate; RF, rheumatoid factor.

KAWASAKI DISEASE

Kawasaki disease, also referred to as mucocutaneous lymph node syndrome, is an acute febrile disease of young children. It is the most common cause of acquired heart disease in young children. Kawasaki disease is seen more often in boys than in girls, and 80% of the cases occur in children younger than 5 years of age. Peak incidences occur in the winter and spring.

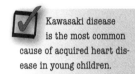
Kawasaki disease is the most common cause of acquired heart disease in young children.

Pathophysiology

Kawasaki disease is thought to affect young children by triggering the immune response in a susceptible child, causing multisystem vasculitis. There are three phases of the illness. During the acute phase there is acute onset of fever and progressive inflammation of the small vessels. Other symptoms that begin to appear are conjunctival inflammation, the characteristic "strawberry tongue," a rash, cervical lymphadenopathy, and edematous hands and feet. The vasculitis progresses to the medium-sized muscular arteries and finally to the coronary arteries.

The subacute phase begins with resolution of the fever and lasts until all clinical symptoms resolve (day 10 to day 40). It is during this period that coronary artery aneurysm can occur.

The convalescent stage begins when all symptoms have resolved, yet laboratory values may still be altered. This phase is complete by about 6–8 weeks after onset when all laboratory values have returned to normal.

Treatment

Diagnosis is confirmed by the existence of several clinical symptoms. These include a fever that lasts for more than 5 days and at least four of the five other characteristics: changes in extremities, cervical lymphadenopathy, bilateral conjunctival inflammation, polymorphous rash, and changes in oral mucous membranes.

Along with the above symptoms, several laboratory tests may assist in making a definitive diagnosis: anemia, an elevated erythrocyte sedimentation rate, and transient elevated liver enzymes. Often, a baseline echocardiogram may be done to monitor for cardiac involvement.

Treatment consists of high-dose intravenous immune globulin along with salicylate therapy. This therapy is aimed at decreasing the incidence of coronary artery dilation and aneurysm formation and is most effective if given within the first 10 days of illness. Children who have suffered from Kawasaki disease may be at a higher risk for developing coronary artery disease as adults.

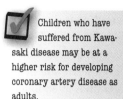 Children who have suffered from Kawasaki disease may be at a higher risk for developing coronary artery disease as adults.

LYME DISEASE

Lyme disease was first identified in 1975 in a town in southeastern Connecticut after which it is named. It is the most common tick-borne disorder in the United States. It is caused by the spirochete, *Borrelia burgdorferi*, that enters the bloodstream through the salvia and feces of ticks. Because the ticks are so small their bite is often unrecognized, and treatment may be delayed.

Pathophysiology

There are three stages to Lyme disease. The first or acute stage is characterized by the "bull's eye rash," which is erythema chronicum migrans. The rash has a clear center at the bite site surrounded by a red ring. It may appear from 1 to 28 days after the bite. The rash may be warm to touch, pruritic, and have a burning sensation. This may be accompanied by other flu-like symptoms such as malaise, fever, headache, and chills.

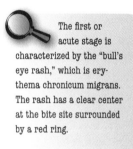 The first or acute stage is characterized by the "bull's eye rash," which is erythema chronicum migrans. The rash has a clear center at the bite site surrounded by a red ring.

If untreated or undetected, the second stage that occurs 2 to 3 months later consists of arthritis, neurological manifestations, and cardiac disease. Headache is the most common symptom early on, followed later by cranial nerve palsies, meningoencephalitis, and peripheral radiculoneuritis. During stage three musculoskeletal pains, chronic arthritis, and late neurological problems such as deafness and chronic encephalopathy may occur. Diagnosis is made by clinical manifestations and history.

Treatment

Prevention is the best treatment. When outdoors in wooded or in tick-infested areas,
use repellants containing DEET, wear long-
sleeved shirts and pants, and check skin and
extremities as soon as possible after returning inside.

Treatment for diagnosed Lyme disease
consists of oral doxycycline or amoxicillin
for 14–21 days. If undetected and additional
symptoms appear, such as neurological, car-
diac, or arthritic symptoms, intravenous or intramuscular injections of
ceftriaxone or penicillin G may be administered.

Prevention is the
best treatment.
When outdoors in wooded or
in tick-infested areas, use
repellants containing DEET,
wear long-sleeved shirts and
pants, and check skin and
extremities as soon as possible after returning inside.

SECTION XXIII · REVIEW QUESTIONS

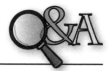

1. A child presents in the pediatric clinic where it is determined that he has Lyme disease in stage II. You would expect to see?
   a. Bull's eye rash
   b. Fever
   c. Neurological changes
   d. Lethargy

2. What classification of drugs is commonly used to treat JRA?
   a. Steroids
   b. Nonsteroidal anti-inflammatory drugs
   c. Antibiotics
   d. Hormones

3. Children who are treated for Kawasaki's disease may be seen by what type of specialist?
   a. Gastroenterologist
   b. Urologist
   c. Cardiologist
   d. Hematologist

4. Sam, a 10-year-old, is being treated for Lyme disease. When he asks his nurse what causes Lyme disease, she correctly answers:
   a. Mosquitos
   b. Deer
   c. Parasites
   d. Spirochete

5. When caring for a child who has been admitted for Kawasaki's disease, you would expect which of the following?
   a. Decreased urine output and diuretics
   b. Joint swelling and anti-inflammatories
   c. Aspirin treatment
   d. Steroid treatment

6. Diagnostic criteria for JRA includes:
   a. Butterfly rash on the face
   b. Inflammation of the joints lasting longer than 6 weeks
   c. Inability to get out of bed in the morning
   d. Chronic headaches lasting longer than 1 month

7. Dad is concerned about getting John ready for school in the morning because of his JRA. You suggest that he:
   a. Ask the principal if he can bring John in later
   b. Do everything for him so John can get ready faster and catch the bus
   c. Stay home and not go to school until he feels better
   d. Start with a warm bath and gentle range-of-motion exercises

ANSWERS AND RATIONALES

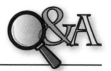

1. **The answer is c.** Rationale: If left untreated, Lyme disease progresses to stage II where neurological symptoms present.

2. **The answer is b.** Rationale: The most successful pharmacological intervention to date is nonsteroidal anti-inflammatory drugs, along with other supportive interventions.

3. **The answer is c.** Rationale: Kawasaki's disease primarily affects the cardiac system and might be overseen by a cardiologist.

4. **The answer is d.** Rationale: Lyme disease is caused by a spirochete that enters the bloodstream through the salvia and feces of ticks.

5. **The answer is c.** Rationale: The use of high-dose aspirin and intravenous immunoglobulin during the acute phase has greatly reduced the complications of Kawasaki's disease.

6. **The answer is b.** Rationale: Inflammation of the joints lasting longer than 6 weeks is one of the diagnostic criteria for JRA.

7. **The answer is d.** Rationale: Children with JRA should be encouraged to maintain independence and participation in activities. Moist heat has been shown to be beneficial to relieving pain and stiffness.

References

REFERENCES

Section I

Ladewig, P. W., London, M. L., & Davidson, M. R. (2006). *Contemporary maternal-newborn nursing care* (6th ed.). Upper Saddle River, NJ: Pearson Prentice Hall.

Littleton, L. Y., & Engelbretson, J. C. (2005). *Maternity nursing care* (1st ed.). Clifton Park, NJ: Pearson Prentice Hall.

Lowdermilk, D. L., & Perry, S. E. (2004). *Maternity and women's health care* (8th ed.). St. Louis: Mosby.

McKinney, E. S., James, S. R., Murray, S. S., & Ashwill, J. W. (2005). *Maternal-child nursing* (2nd ed.). St. Louis: Elsevier Saunders.

O'Toole, M. T. (2003). *Miller-Keane encyclopedia and dictionary of medicine, nursing, and allied health* (7th ed.). Philadelphia: Saunders.

Pillitteri, A. (2007). *Maternal and child health nursing care of the child-bearing and childrearing family* (5th ed.). Philadelphia: Lippincott Williams & Wilkins.

Reeder, S. J., Martin, L. L., & Koniak-Griffin, D. (1997). *Maternity nursing family, newborn and women's health care* (18th ed.). Philadelphia: Lippincott Williams & Wilkins.

Ricci, S. S. (2007). *Essentials of maternity, newborn, and women's health nursing* (1st ed.). Philadelphia: Lippincott Williams & Wilkins.

Section II

ACOG Practice Bulletin. (2005). *Intrauterine devices.* No. 59, January 2005.

Dominguez, L., Moore, A., & Wysocki, S. (2005). The extended-cycle oral contraceptive: Six seasons and counting. *The American Journal for Nurse Practitioners, 9*(3), 55–64.

Freeman, S. (2003). The contraceptive vaginal ring: A novel option in contraception. *The American Journal for Nurse Practitioners, 7*(6), 31–38.

Freeman, S. (2004). Lower-dose hormone therapy for postmenopausal women. *The American Journal for Nurse Practitioners, 8*(3), 9–21.

Hatcher, R., Trussell, J., Stewart, F., Nelson, A., Cates, W. L., Guest, F., & Kowal, D. (2004). *Contraceptive technology* (18th ed.). New York: Ardent Media.

Minkin, M., & Wright, C. (2005). *A woman's guide to sexual health.* New Haven, CT: Yale University Press.

Murphy, P. (2005). Recent innovations in vaginal barrier contraception. *Women's Health Care: A Practical Journal for Nurse Practitioners, 4*(5), 21–30.

Schreiber, C., & Creinin, M. (2005). The health benefits of hormonal contraceptives. *The Female Patient,* April Supplement, 19–34.

Stein Pollack, J., & Moriarty Daley, A. (2003). Improve adolescents' access to emergency contraception. *The Nurse Practitioner, 28*(8), 11–23.

Youngkin, E., & Davis, M. (2004). *Women's health: a primary care clinical guide* (3rd ed.). New Jersey: Pearson Prentice Hall.

Section III

Ladewig, P. W., London, M. L., & Davidson, M. R. (2006*). Contemporary maternal-newborn nursing care* (6th ed.). Upper Saddle River, NJ: Pearson Prentice Hall.

Littleton, L. Y., & Engelbretson, J. C. (2005). *Maternity nursing care* (1st ed.). Clifton Park, NJ: Pearson Prentice Hall.

Lowdermilk, D. L., & Perry, S. E. (2004). *Maternity and women's health care* (8th ed.). St. Louis: Mosby.

McKinney, E. S., James, S. R., Murray, S. S., & Ashwill, J. W. (2005). *Maternal-child nursing* (2nd ed.). St. Louis: Elsevier Saunders.

O'Toole, M. T. (2003). *Miller-Keane encyclopedia and dictionary of medicine, nursing, and allied health* (7th ed.). Philadelphia: Saunders.

Pillitteri, A. (2007). *Maternal and child health nursing care of the childbearing and childrearing family* (5th ed.). Philadelphia: Lippincott Williams & Wilkins.

Reeder, S. J., Martin, L. L., & Koniak-Griffin, D. (1997). *Maternity nursing family, newborn and women's health care* (18th ed.). Philadelphia: Lippincott Williams & Wilkins.

Ricci, S. S. (2007). *Essentials of maternity, newborn, and women's health nursing* (1st ed.). Philadelphia: Lippincott Williams & Wilkins.

Section IV

Ladewig, P. W., London, M. L., & Davidson, M. R. (2006*). Contemporary maternal-newborn nursing care* (6th ed.). Upper Saddle River, NJ: Pearson Prentice Hall.

Littleton, L. Y., & Engelbretson, J. C. (2005). *Maternity nursing care* (1st ed.). Clifton Park, NJ: Pearson Prentice Hall.

Lowdermilk, D. L., & Perry, S. E. (2004). *Maternity and women's health care* (8th ed.). St. Louis: Mosby.

McKinney, E. S., James, S. R., Murray, S. S., & Ashwill, J. W. (2005). *Maternal-child nursing* (2nd ed.). St. Louis: Elsevier Saunders.

O'Toole, M. T. (2003). *Miller-Keane encyclopedia and dictionary of medicine, nursing, and allied health* (7th ed.). Philadelphia: Saunders.

Pillitteri, A. (2007). *Maternal and child health nursing care of the child-bearing and childrearing family* (5th ed.). Philadelphia: Lippincott Williams & Wilkins.

Reeder, S. J., Martin, L. L., & Koniak-Griffin, D. (1997). *Maternity nursing family, newborn and women's health care* (18th ed.). Philadelphia: Lippincott Williams & Wilkins.

Ricci, S. S. (2007). *Essentials of maternity, newborn, and women's health nursing* (1st ed.). Philadelphia: Lippincott Williams & Wilkins.

Section V

Freeman, S. (2002). Polycystic ovary syndrome: Diagnosis and management. *Women's Health Care: A Practical Journal for Nurse Practitioners, 1*(4), 15–20.

Hill, K. (2003). Update: The pathogenesis and treatment of PCOS. *The Nurse Practitioner, 28*(7), 8–23.

Lowdermilk, D., & Perry, S. (2004). *Maternity and women's health care* (8th ed.). St. Louis: Mosby.

Women's health: A guide to health promotion and disorder management (2005). Philadelphia: Lippincott Williams & Wilkins.

Youngkin, E., & Davis, M. (2004). *Women's health: A primary care clinical guide* (3rd ed.). New Jersey: Pearson Prentice Hall.

Section VI

Crowther, C. A., Hiller, J. E., Moss, J. R., McPhee, A. J., Jeffries, W. S., & Robinson, J. S. (2005). Effect of treatment of gestational diabetes mellitus on pregnancy outcomes. *New England Journal of Medicine, 352,* 2477–2486.

Hatcher, R., Trussell, J., Stewart, F., Nelson, A., Cates, W. I., Guest, F., & Kowal, D. (2004). *Contraceptive technology* (18th ed.). New York: Ardent Media.

Kahn, R. (1993). *Medical management of pregnancy complicated by diabetes.* Alexandria, VA: The American Diabetes Association.

Littleton, L., & Engebretson, J. (2005). *Maternity nursing care.* Canada: Thomson Delmar Learning.

Lowdermilk, D., & Perry, S. (2004). *Maternity and women's health care* (8th ed.). St. Louis: Mosby.

Mulcahy, K., & Lumbar, T. (2004). *The diabetes ready reference for health professionals* (2nd ed.). Alexandria, VA: The American Diabetes Association.

Padden, M. (1999). HELLP syndrome: Recognition and perinatal management. *American Family Physician, 60*(3), 829–836, 839.

Reece, E., Coustan D., & Gabbe, S. (2004). *Diabetes in women* (3rd ed.). Philadelphia: Lippincott Williams & Wilkins.

Schuiling, K., & Likis, F. (2006). *Women's gynecological health.* Sudbury, MA: Jones and Bartlett.

Women's health: A guide to health promotion and disorder management (2005). Philadelphia: Lippincott, Williams and Wilkins.

Youngkin, E. Q., & Szmania Davis, M. (2004). *Women's health: A primary care clinical guide* (3rd ed.). Upper Saddle River, NJ: Pearson Education, Inc.

Section VII

Freeman, S., Moore, A., & Wysocki, S. (2004). Menopause hormone therapy: Where do we go from here? A focus on the estrogen component. *Women's Health Care: A Practical Journal for Nurse Practitioners, 3*(4), 8–17.

Minkin, M., & Wright, C. (2005). *A woman's guide to menopause and perimenopause.* New Haven, CT: Yale University Press.

Woodward, J. (2005). Hormone therapy in menopause: A review of evidenced-based guidelines. *Clinician Reviews, 15*(4), 45–51.

Wysocki, S., & Alexander, I. (2005). Bioidentical hormones for menopause hormone therapy: An overview. *Women's Health Care: A Practical Journal for Nurse Practitioners, 4*(2), 9–17.

Section VIII

Centers for Disease Control and Prevention: http://www.cdc.gov/std

Davidson, M. (2004). Sexually transmitted infections: Screening and counseling. *Clinician Reviews, 14*(6), 55–61.

Mark, H., Hanahan, A., & Stender, S. (2003). Herpes simplex virus type 2: An update. *The Nurse Practitioner, 28*(11), 34–41.

Morrow, R. (2003). Diagnosis: Infections and the nature of the disease. *The Female Patient*, Supplement, April 2003, 3–7

Sandhaus, S. (2001). Genital herpes in pregnant and nonpregnant women. *The Nurse Practitioner*, *26*(4), 15–27.

Section IX

Allen, P., & Vessey, J. (2004). *Primary care of the child with a chronic condition* (4th ed.). St. Louis: Mosby.

Ball, J. W., & Bindler, R. (2006). *Child health nursing: Partnering with children and families*. Upper Saddle River, NJ: Pearson Prentice Hall.

Fochtman, D., & Foley, G. (1982). *Nursing care of the child with cancer*. Boston: Little, Brown and Company.

Hockenberry, M., Wilson, D., Winkelstein, M., & Kline, N. (2003). *Nursing care of infants and children* (7th ed.). St. Louis: Mosby.

McCance, K., & Huether, S. (2006). *Pathophysiology: The biologic basis for disease in adults and children*. St. Louis: Elsevier.

Porth, C. M. (2005). *Pathophysiology: Concepts of altered health states* (7th ed.). Philadelphia: Lippincott Williams & Wilkins.

Potts, N., & Mandleco, B. (2007). *Pediatric nursing: Caring for children and their families* (2nd ed.). Albany, NY: Thomson Delmar Learning.

Section X

Ball, J. W., & Bindler, R. C. (2006). *Child health nursing: Partnering with children and families*. Upper Saddle River, NJ: Pearson Prentice Hall.

Bullock, B. A., & Henze, R. L. (2000). *Focus on pathophysiology*. Philadelphia: Lippincott Williams & Wilkins.

Hay, W. W., Levin, M. J., Sondheimer, J. M., & Deterding, R. R. (2005). *Current pediatric diagnosis and treatment* (17th ed.). New York: McGraw-Hill.

Hockenberry, M. J. (2003). *Wong's nursing care of infants and children* (7th ed.). St. Louis: Mosby.

Huether, S. E., & McCance, K. L. (2004). *Understanding pathophysiology* (3rd ed.). St. Louis: Mosby.

McKinney, E. S., James, S. R., Murray, S. S., & Ashwill, J. W. (2005). *Maternal-child Nursing* (2nd.ed.). St. Louis: Elsevier Saunders.

McPhee, S. J., Lingappa, V. R., Ganong, W. F., & Langee, J. D. (2000). *Pathophysiology of disease* (3rd ed.). New York: McGraw-Hill.

Porth, C. M. (2005). *Pathophysiology-concepts of altered health states* (7th ed.). Philadelphia: Lippincott Williams & Wilkins.

Thomas, D. O., & Bernardo, L. M. (2003). *Core curriculum for pediatric emergency nursing.* Sudbury, MA: Jones and Bartlett.

White, L. (2005). *Foundations of maternal & pediatric nursing* (2nd ed.). Albany, NY: Thomson Delmar Learning.

Section XI

Ball, J. W., & Bindler, R. C. (2006). *Child health nursing: Partnering with children and families.* Upper Saddle River, NJ: Pearson Prentice Hall.

Bullock, B. A., & Henze, R. L. (2000). *Focus on pathophysiology.* Philadelphia: Lippincott Williams & Wilkins.

Hay, W. W., Levin, M. J., Sondheimer, J. M., & Deterding, R. R. (2005). *Current pediatric diagnosis and treatment* (17th ed.). New York: McGraw-Hill.

Hockenberry, M. J. (2003). *Wong's nursing care of infants and children* (7th ed.). St. Louis: Mosby.

Huether, S. E., & McCance, K. L. (2004). *Understanding pathophysiology* (3rd ed.). St. Louis: Mosby.

McKinney, E. S., James, S. R., Murray, S. S., & Ashwill, J. W. (2005). *Maternal-child Nursing* (2nd ed.). St. Louis: Elsevier Saunders.

McPhee, S. J., Lingappa, V. R., Ganong, W. F., & Langee, J. D. (2000). *Pathophysiology of disease* (3rd ed.). New York: McGraw-Hill.

Porth, C. M. (2005). *Pathophysiology-concepts of altered health states* (7th ed.). Philadelphia: Lippincott Williams & Wilkins.

Thomas, D. O., & Bernardo, L. M. (2003). *Core curriculum for pediatric emergency nursing.* Sudbury, MA: Jones and Bartlett.

White, L. (2005). *Foundations of maternal & pediatric nursing* (2nd ed.). Albany, NY: Thomson Delmar Learning.

Section XII

Ball, J. W., & Bindler, R. C. (2006). *Child health nursing: Partnering with children and families.* Upper Saddle River, NJ: Pearson Prentice Hall.

Bullock, B. A., & Henze, R. L. (2000). *Focus on pathophysiology.* Philadelphia: Lippincott Williams & Wilkins.

Hay, W. W., Levin, M. J., Sondheimer, J. M., & Deterding, R. R. (2005). *Current pediatric diagnosis and treatment* (17th ed.). New York: McGraw-Hill.

Hockenberry, M. J. (2003). *Wong's nursing care of infants and children* (7th ed.). St. Louis: Mosby.

Huether, S. E., & McCance, K. L. (2004). *Understanding pathophysiology* (3rd ed.). St. Louis: Mosby.

McKinney, E. S., James, S. R., Murray, S. S., & Ashwill, J. W. (2005). *Maternal-child Nursing* (2nd ed.). St. Louis: Elsevier Saunders.

McPhee, S. J., Lingappa, V. R., Ganong, W. F., & Langee, J. D. (2000). *Pathophysiology of disease* (3rd ed.). New York: McGraw-Hill.

Porth, C. M. (2005). *Pathophysiology-concepts of altered health states* (7th ed.). Philadelphia: Lippincott Williams & Wilkins.

Thomas, D. O., & Bernardo, L. M. (2003). *Core curriculum for pediatric emergency nursing.* Sudbury, MA: Jones and Bartlett.

White, L. (2005). *Foundations of maternal & pediatric nursing* (2nd ed.). Albany, NY: Thomson Delmar Learning.

Section XIII

Allen, P., & Vessey, J. (2004). *Primary care of the child with a chronic condition* (4th ed.). St. Louis: Mosby.

Ball, J. W., & Bindler, R. (2006). *Child health nursing: Partnering with children and families.* Upper Saddle River, NJ: Pearson Prentice Hall.

Hockenberry, M., Wilson, D., Winkelstein, M., & Kline, N. (2003). *Nursing care of infants and children* (7th ed.). St. Louis: Mosby.

McCance, K., & Huether, S. (2006). *Pathophysiology: The biologic basis for disease in adults and children.* St. Louis: Elsevier.

Porth, C. M. (2005). *Pathophysiology: Concepts of altered health states* (7th ed.). Philadelphia: Lippincott Williams & Wilkins.

Potts, N., & Mandleco, B. (2007). *Pediatric nursing: Caring for children and their families* (2nd ed.). Albany, NY: Thomson Delmar Learning.

Section XIV

Ball, J. W., & Bindler, R. (2006). *Child health nursing: Partnering with children and families.* Upper Saddle River, NJ: Pearson Prentice Hall.

Hay, W. W. Jr., Levin, M. J., Sondheimer, J. M., & Deterding, R. R. (2005). *Current pediatric diagnosis & treatment* (7th ed.). New York: Lange Medical Books/McGraw-Hill.

Hockenberry, M., Wilson, D., Winkelstein, M., & Kline, N. (2003). *Nursing care of infants and children* (7th ed.). St. Louis: Mosby.

Jackson Allen, P., & Vessey, J. A. (2000). *Primary care of the child with a chronic condition* (4th ed.). St. Louis: Mosby.

McCance, K., & Huether, S. (2006). *Pathophysiology: The biologic basis for disease in adults and children.* St. Louis: Elsevier.

Porth, C. M. (2005). *Pathophysiology: Concepts of altered health states* (7th ed.). Philadelphia: Lippincott Williams & Wilkins.

Potts, N., & Mandleco, B. (2007). *Pediatric nursing: Caring for children and their families* (2nd ed.). Albany, NY: Thomson Delmar Learning.

Sickle Cell Advisory Committee of the Genetic Network of New York, Puerto Rico and the Virgin Islands. (2002). *Guidelines for the treatment of people with sickle cell disease.* Project MCJ-361004 MCHB, HRSA, DHHS. New York: Author.

Wong, D. L. Hockenbury, M. J., Wilson, D., Perry S. E., & Lowdermilk, D. L. (2006). *Maternal child nursing care* (3rd ed.). St. Louis: Mosby Elsevier.

Section XV

Ball, J. W., & Bindler, R. C. (2006). *Child health nursing: Partnering with children and families.* Upper Saddle River, NJ: Pearson Prentice Hall.

Bullock, B. A., & Henze, R. L. (2000). *Focus on pathophysiology.* Philadelphia: Lippincott Williams & Wilkins.

Hay, W. W., Levin, M. J., Sondheimer, J. M., & Deterding, R. R. (2005). *Current pediatric diagnosis and treatment* (17th ed.). New York: McGraw-Hill.

Hockenberry, M. J. (2003). *Wong's nursing care of infants and children* (7th ed.). St. Louis: Mosby.

Huether, S. E., & McCance, K. L. (2004). *Understanding pathophysiology* (3rd ed.). St. Louis: Mosby.

McKinney, E. S., James, S. R., Murray, S. S., & Ashwill, J. W. (2005). *Maternal-child nursing* (2nd ed.). St. Louis: Elsevier Saunders.

McPhee, S. J., Lingappa, V. R., Ganong, W. F., & Langee, J. D. (2000). *Pathophysiology of disease* (3rd ed.). New York: McGraw-Hill.

Porth, C. M. (2005). *Pathophysiology-concepts of altered health states* (7th ed.). Philadelphia: Lippincott Williams & Wilkins.

Thomas, D. O., & Bernardo, L. M. (2003). *Core curriculum for pediatric emergency nursing.* Sudbury, MA: Jones and Bartlett.

White, L. (2005). *Foundations of maternal & pediatric nursing* (2nd ed.). Albany, NY: Thomson Delmar Learning.

Section XVI

Ball, J. W., & Bindler, R. C. (2006). *Child health nursing: Partnering with children and families.* Upper Saddle River, NJ: Pearson Prentice Hall.

Bullock, B. A., & Henze, R. L. (2000). *Focus on pathophysiology.* Philadelphia: Lippincott Williams & Wilkins.

Hay, W. W., Levin, M. J., Sondheimer, J. M., & Deterding, R. R. (2005). *Current pediatric diagnosis and treatment* (17th ed.). New York: McGraw-Hill.

Huether, S. E., & McCance, K. L. (2004). *Understanding pathophysiology* (3rd ed.). St. Louis: Mosby.

McKinney, E. S., James, S. R., Murray, S. S., & Ashwill, J. W. (2005). *Maternal-child nursing* (2nd ed.). St. Louis: Elsevier Saunders.

Porth, C. M. (2005). *Pathophysiology-concepts of altered health states* (7th ed.). Philadelphia: Lippincott Williams & Wilkins.

Section XVII

Ball, J. W., & Bindler, R. C. (2006). *Child health nursing: Partnering with children and families.* Upper Saddle River, NJ: Pearson Prentice Hall.

Bullock, B. A., & Henze, R. L. (2000). *Focus on pathophysiology.* Philadelphia: Lippincott Williams & Wilkins.

Hay, W. W., Levin, M. J., Sondheimer, J. M., & Deterding, R. R. (2005). *Current pediatric diagnosis and treatment* (17th ed.). New York: McGraw-Hill.

Hockenberry, M. J. (2003). *Wong's nursing care of infants and children* (7th ed.). St. Louis: Mosby.

Huether, S. E., & McCance, K. L. (2004). *Understanding pathophysiology* (3rd ed.). St. Louis: Mosby.

McKinney, E. S., James, S. R., Murray, S. S., & Ashwill, J. W. (2005). *Maternal-child nursing* (2nd ed.). St. Louis: Elsevier Saunders.

McPhee, S. J., Lingappa, V. R., Ganong, W. F., & Langee, J. D. (2000). *Pathophysiology of disease* (3rd ed.). New York: McGraw-Hill.

Porth, C. M. (2005). *Pathophysiology-concepts of altered health states* (7th ed.). Philadelphia: Lippincott Williams & Wilkins.

Rothenberg, M. A. (2001). *Pathophysiology—A plain English approach.* Eau Claire, WI: Pesi Healthcare.

Thomas, D. O., & Bernardo, L. M. (2003). *Core curriculum for pediatric emergency nursing.* Sudbury, MA: Jones and Bartlett.

White, L. (2005). *Foundations of maternal & pediatric nursing* (2nd ed.). Albany, NY: Thomson Delmar Learning.

Section XVIII

Ball, J. W., & Bindler, R. C. (2006). *Child health nursing: Partnering with children and families.* Upper Saddle River, NJ: Pearson Prentice Hall.

Hay, W. W., Levin, M. J., Sondheimer, J. M., & Deterding, R. R. (2005). *Current pediatric diagnosis and treatment* (17th ed.). New York: McGraw-Hill.

Hockenberry, M. J. (2003). *Wong's nursing care of infants and children* (7th ed.). St. Louis: Mosby.

McKinney, E. S., James, S. R., Murray, S. S., & Ashwill, J. W. (2005). *Maternal-child nursing* (2nd ed.). St. Louis: Elsevier Saunders.

Porth, C. M. (2005). *Pathophysiology-concepts of altered health states* (7th ed.). Philadelphia: Lippincott Williams & Wilkins.

White, L. (2005). *Foundations of maternal & pediatric nursing* (2nd ed.). Albany, NY: Thomson Delmar Learning.

Section XIX

Ball, J., & Bindler, R. (2006). *Child health nursing: Partnering with children and families.* Upper Saddle River, NJ: Prentice Hall.

Broughton, N. S., & Menelaus, M. B. (1998). *Menenalus' orthopaedic management of spina bifida cystica* (3rd ed.). London: W. B. Saunders.

Capute, A. J., & Accardo, P. J. (1996). *Developmental disabilities in infancy and childhood* (2nd ed., Volumes I & II). Baltimore: Paul H. Brookes.

Edwards, P. A., Hertzberg, D. L., Hays, S. R., & Youngblood, N. M. (1999). *Pediatric rehabilitation nursing.* Philadelphia: W. B. Saunders.

Hay, W. W. Jr., Levin, M. J., Sondheimer, J. M., & Deterding, R. R. (2005). *Current pediatric diagnosis & treatment* (7th ed.). New York: Lange Medical Books/McGraw-Hill.

Jackson Allen, P., & Vessey, J. A. (2000). *Primary care of the child with a chronic condition* (4th ed.). St. Louis: Mosby.

Potts, N., & Mandleco, B. (2007). *Pediatric nursing: Caring for children and their families.* Clifton Park, NY: Thomson Delmar Learning.

Wong, D. L. Hockenberry, M. J., Wilson, D., Perry, S. E., & Lowdermilk, D. L. (2006). *Maternal child nursing care* (3rd ed.). St. Louis: Mosby Elsevier.

Section XX

Ball, J., & Bindler, R. (2006). *Child health nursing: Partnering with children and families.* Upper Saddle River, NJ: Pearson Prentice Hall.

DiFazio, R., & Atkinson, C. (2005). Extremity fractures in children: When is it an emergency? *Journal of Pediatric Nursing, 20*(4), 298–304.

Hay, W., Levin, M., Sondheimer, J., & Deterding, R. (2005). *Current pediatric diagnosis and treatment* (17th ed.). New York: McGraw-Hill.

Hockenberry, M., Wilson, D., Winkelstein, M., & Kline, N. (2003). *Wong's nursing care of infants and children* (7th ed.). St. Louis: Mosby.

McCance, K., & Huether, S. (2006). *Pathophysiology: The biologic basis for disease in adults and children.* St. Louis: Mosby.

Porth, C. (2005). *Pathophysiology: Concepts of altered health states* (7th ed.). Philadelphia: Lippincott Williams & Wilkins.

Potts, N., & Mandleco, B. (2007). *Pediatric nursing: Caring for children and their families* (2nd ed.). Clifton Parks, NY: Thomson/ Delmar Learning.

Section XXI

Ball, J. W., & Bindler, R. C. (2006). *Child health nursing: Partnering with children and families.* Upper Saddle River, NJ: Pearson Prentice Hall.

Bullock, B. A., & Henze, R. L. (2000). *Focus on pathophysiology.* Philadelphia: Lippincott Williams & Wilkins.

Hay, W. W., Levin, M. J., Sondheimer, J. M., & Deterding, R. R. (2005). *Current pediatric diagnosis and treatment* (17th ed.). New York: McGraw-Hill.

Hockenberry, M. J. (2003). *Wong's nursing care of infants and children* (7th ed.). St. Louis: Mosby.

Huether, S. E., & McCance, K. L. (2004). *Understanding pathophysiology* (3rd ed.). St. Louis: Mosby.

McKinney, E. S., James, S. R., Murray, S. S., & Ashwill, J. W. (2005). *Maternal-child nursing* (2nd ed.). St. Louis: Elsevier Saunders.

McPhee, S. J., Lingappa, V. R., Ganong, W. F., & Langee, J. D. (2000). *Pathophysiology of disease* (3rd ed.). New York: McGraw-Hill.

Porth, C. M. (2005). *Pathophysiology-concepts of altered health states* (7th ed.). Philadelphia: Lippincott Williams & Wilkins.

Thomas, D. O., & Bernardo, L. M. (2003). *Core curriculum for pediatric emergency nursing.* Sudbury, MA: Jones and Bartlett.

White, L. (2005). *Foundations of maternal & pediatric nursing* (2nd ed.). Albany, NY: Thomson Delmar Learning.

Section XXII

Ball, J. W., & Bindler, R. C. (2006). *Child health nursing: Partnering with children and families.* Upper Saddle River, NJ: Pearson Prentice Hall.

Bullock, B. A., & Henze, R. L. (2000). *Focus on pathophysiology.* Philadelphia: Lippincott Williams & Wilkins.

Hay, W. W., Levin, M. J., Sondheimer, J. M., & Deterding, R. R. (2005). *Current pediatric diagnosis and treatment* (17th ed.). New York: McGraw-Hill.

Hockenberry, M. J. (2003). *Wong's nursing care of infants and children* (7th ed.). St. Louis: Mosby.

Huether, S. E., & McCance, K. L. (2004). *Understanding pathophysiology* (3rd ed.). St. Louis: Mosby.

McKinney, E. S., James, S. R., Murray, S. S., & Ashwill, J. W. (2005). *Maternal-child nursing* (2nd ed.). St. Louis: Elsevier Saunders.

McPhee, S. J., Lingappa, V. R., Ganong, W. F., & Langee, J. D. (2000). *Pathophysiology of disease* (3rd ed.). New York: McGraw-Hill.

Porth, C. M. (2005). *Pathophysiology-concepts of altered health states* (7th ed.). Philadelphia: Lippincott Williams & Wilkins.

Thomas, D. O., & Bernardo, L. M. (2003). *Core curriculum for pediatric emergency nursing.* Sudbury, MA: Jones and Bartlett.

White, L. (2005). *Foundations of maternal & pediatric nursing* (2nd ed.). Albany, NY: Thomson Delmar Learning.

Section XXIII

Allen, P., & Vessey, J. (2004) *Primary care of the child with a chronic condition* (4th ed.). St. Louis: Mosby.

Ball, J., & Bindler, R. (2006). *Child health nursing: Partnering with children and families.* Upper Saddle River, NJ: Pearson Prentice Hall.

Hay, W., Levin, M., Sondheimer, J., & Deterding, R. (2005). *Current pediatric diagnosis & treatment* (17th ed.). New York: McGraw-Hill.

Hockenberry, M., Wilson, D., Winkelstein, M., & Kline, N. (2003). *Wong's nursing care of infants and children* (7th ed.). St. Louis: Mosby.

McCance, K., & Huether, S. (2006). *Pathophysiology: The biologic basis for disease in adults and children.* St. Louis: Mosby.

Porth, C. (2005). *Pathophysiology: Concepts of altered health states* (7th ed.). Philadelphia: Lippincott Williams & Wilkins.

Potts, N., & Mandleco, B. (2007). *Pediatric nursing: Caring for children and their families* (2nd ed.). Clifton Parks, NY: Thomson Delmar Learning.

Glossary

GLOSSARY

ABO incompatibility: Occurs when a mother is blood type O and her infant is either blood type A, B, or AB.

Abruptio placentae: The premature separation of a normally implanted placenta.

Acanthosis nigricans: When skin over the posterior neck, armpits, and elbows is thick and dark.

Accessory muscles: Muscles used during dyspnea to assist in ventilation and include the sternocleidomastoid and scalenus muscles in the neck and possibly facial muscles.

Acne neonatorum: Acne in infants; may occur when the infant is 4 to 6 weeks old and may persist for 6 months to a year until spontaneous resolution occurs.

Acquired glaucoma: Another type of secondary glaucoma that may be caused by trauma, infection, or cataract removal.

Acquired immunodeficiency syndrome (AIDS): A chronic progressive disease affecting multiple organs. AIDS is caused by a viral infection with the human immunodeficiency virus (HIV) that affects the helper T lymphocytes, monocytes, and macrophages.

Acute renal failure (ARF): Renal failure which begins abruptly and is generally reversible.

Afterload: The vascular resistance to receiving the blood pumped by the left ventricle.

Amniocentesis: A test used to evaluate the condition of the fetus.

Amnion: Innermost of the two fetal membranes and containing the amniotic fluid.

Amniotic cavity: A fluid-filled sac inside the amnion that contains the developing embryo.

Anemia: A reduction in the total number of erythrocytes in the circulating blood or a reduction in the quality or quantity of hemoglobin. The most common blood disorder in children.

Angle-closure glaucoma (also acute, closed angle, or narrow angle): The anterior chamber is narrowed or closed, preventing the outflow of aqueous humor.

Apgar score: Evaluation of a newborn's physical status by assigning numerical values to five criteria: heart rate, respiratory effort, muscle tone, reflex irritability, and skin color.

Apnea of infancy: A respiratory condition most common in infants 2 to 4 months of age. The risk for sudden infant death syndrome rises if the child has apnea of infancy.

Apocrine glands: Located in the groin area and axilla. As the fluid secreted by apocrine glands breaks down, body odor results. These glands become functional at puberty.

Apparent life-threatening events (ALTEs): A respiratory disorder in which the exact cause is unknown. Because these events do not occur past infancy, immaturity of the nervous system, reflexes, and responses to apnea during sleep may be causes.

Aqueous humor: A thin watery fluid continually produced by the ciliary body that fills the space between the cornea and the iris (anterior chamber). Its functions include feeding the cornea and lens and giving the front of the eye shape.

Arial-septal defect (ASD): A defect located near the foramen ovale that results in blood flowing between the right and left atria, causing an enlarged right atrium and ventricle and an increased blood flow to the pulmonary artery.

Artificial insemination: Sperm is artificially inserted into the female reproductive tract to aid conception. With intracervical insemination, sperm are inserted into the cervix, and with intrauterine insemination sperm are inserted into the uterus. A husband's sperm or a donor's sperm can be used.

Asthma: Characterized by acute airway inflammation, bronchoconstriction, bronchospasm, edema of the bronchioles, and increased production of mucus. Asthma is characterized as exercise induced, occupational, drug induced or more precisely by severity: mild intermittent, mild persistent, moderate persistent, and severe persistent.

Astigmatism: An irregularly shaped cornea or lens.

Atrial natriuretic peptide: A hormone discovered in 1981 that causes the vasodilation of afferent arterioles, which lead into the glomerulus, and efferent arterioles, which lead out of the glomerulus, resulting in an increased glomerular filtration rate. Atrial natriuretic peptide also inhibits aldosterone secretion and sodium reabsorption from the collecting tubules. This hormone is released from muscle cells in the atria when the atrial walls are stretched.

Atypical pneumonia: A type of patchy pneumonia, usually caused by viruses (type A/B influenza) or some bacteria (*Legionella*), that does not involve the alveoli.

Autonomic Nervous System (ANS): Regulates activity of the visceral organs of the body to maintain a steady state. These organs and activities include the actions of the smooth muscles of the heart, gastrointestinal system, genitourinary system, blood vessels, bronchi, and actions of the secretory glands. There are components of the ANS in both the central and peripheral nervous systems that provide complementary, opposing, or synergistic actions to keep the body regulated.

Azotemia: Buildup of nitrogenous waste products in the blood.

Bacterial tracheitis: Also know as pseudomembranous croup, this is a severe form of laryngotracheobronchitis.

Barkan membrane: A membrane covering the trabecular channels.

Barrier contraception: A nonhormonal coitus-dependent form of birth control that provides a barrier between the penis and the vagina and cervix.

Bicuspid valve or mitral valve: The left atrioventricular valve has two cusps or leaflets and is called this because when it is closed it resembles a bishop's hat (miter).

Blastocyst: The phase where large cells collect at the periphery of the ball with a fluid space surrounding an inner cell mass.

Blepharitis: Inflammation of the lid margin that may be caused by bacterial infections (commonly *Staphylococcus*), louse infestation (*Phthirus pubis*), and localized infections of the sebaceous glands of the eyelid (hordeolum) and/or of the oil-secreting glands of the eyelid (chalazion).

Bloody show: Discharge of the mucous plug that fills the cervical canal during pregnancy. The exposed cervical capillaries release a small amount of blood that mixes with the mucus, resulting in red-tinged secretions.

Bronchiolitis: Inflammation of the bronchioles.

Bronchitis: Inflammation of the major conducting airways within the lung—trachea and bronchi.

Bronchopneumonia: The most common type of pneumonia, characterized by patchy pneumonia in several lobes.

Bronchopulmonary dysplasia (BPD): premature infant's lungs do not make enough surfactant resulting in atelectasis. The National Institutes of Health defines BPD using the following criteria: (1) oxygen therapy longer than 28 days, (2) history of positive pressure ventilation or continuous positive airway pressure, and (3) gestational age.

Bullous impetigo (impetigo neonatorum): A superficial skin infection of neonates that usually affects the buttocks, perineum, trunk, face, and extremities.

Buphthalmos: Enlargement of the globe of the eye.

C-peptide: Amino acid molecule which indicates the amount of insulin produced daily by the beta cells.

Capacitation: A prerequisite for a sperm to fertilize an ovum.

Capillary malformations: Flat vascular birthmarks that appear either light red–orange or dark red–bluish red.

Carbonic anhydrase: An enzyme in red blood cells that causes 60% of the carbon dioxide produced by cell metabolism to rapidly combine with water and create carbonic acid.

Cardiac output: The amount of blood pumped to the general circulation from the left ventricle each minute.

Cardiomyopathy: A condition in which the heart muscle stretches and becomes weak, resulting in congestive heart failure.

Carnitine: Acts as a transport for long-chain fatty acids so they can enter the mitochondria of muscle and heart cells, resulting in energy production.

Cataracts: Cloudiness of the eye lens.

Cell differentiation: The process in which dividing cells become more specialized, acquiring the structure and function of the cells they replace.

Central apnea: Lack of effort to breathe, occurring mainly in premature infants.

Central nervous system (CNS): The CNS comprises the brain and spinal cord and the soft (dura mater, arachnoid membrane, and pia mater) and bony (skull and vertebral spine) tissue protection. The brain includes the cerebral cortex, cerebellum, and glandular system (thalamus, pituitary, and hypothalamus) and is the nerve center.

Chlamydia: A sexually transmitted bacterial infection, caused by *Chlamydia trachomatis*.

Chordae tendineae: Strong, inelastic, tendon-like cords attached on one end to the ventricular surface of an atrioventricular cusp and on the other end to a small protrusion on the ventricular myocardium (papillary muscle) to hold the closed atrioventricular valves in place.

Chorion: The outermost of the two fetal membranes.

Chorionic villi: These villi develop out of the trophoblast and manifest "finger-like projections" and continue to burrow into the blood-filled spaces of the endometrium. They obtain oxygen and nutrients from the maternal bloodstream and dispose of carbon dioxide and waste products into the maternal blood.

Cleft lip: Described as unilateral or bilateral and incomplete or complete. This classification is dependant on whether or not the cleft extends into the nasal cavity. Cleft lip is usually below the center of one nostril.

Closed/narrow angle: Acute glaucoma.

Closed fracture: A type of bone fracture that has no contact outside the skin surface.

Colostrum: A form of breast milk produced during the first 48–72 hours of breast-feeding. Colostrum is a natural laxative which encourages the passage of meconium which is high in bilirubin.

Congenital glaucoma: An inherited disorder that occurs in 1 in 5,000 to 10,000 births.

Congestive heart failure (CHF): Occurs when the heart fails as a pump and is therefore unable to meet the circulatory and metabolic requirements of the body.

Conjunctiva: A thin transparent mucous membrane that lines the posterior surface of the eyelids and anterior surface of the cornea. When this area becomes inflamed in response to exposure to viruses, bacteria, chemicals, or allergens, it is called conjunctivitis.

Cor pulmonale: Prolonged pulmonary hypertension that causes the right ventricle to enlarge.

Corona radiata: Elongated follicle cells surrounding the zona pellucida of the ovum.

Corpus luteum: After rupture of the Graafian follicle at ovulation, the follicle develops into a yellow structure that secretes progesterone and some estrogen in the second half of the menstrual cycle.

Croup syndromes: A term used to describe an acute inflammation of the larynx, trachea, and major bronchi. It includes viral croup, epiglottis, and bacterial tracheitis characterized by inspiratory stridor, cough, hoarseness, and respiratory distress.

Culdocentesis: A procedure performed to determine intraperitoneal bleeding by insertion of a needle into the cul-de-sac between the rectum and the posterior wall of the uterus.

Cystic fibrosis (CF): The most common genetic disease in the United States and the leading cause of death in early adulthood. Chromosome 7 contains the gene responsible for the production of the cystic fibrosis transmembrane conductance regulator protein (CFTR). This protein is an ion channel that allows salt and water into and out of epithelial cells. Without this protein chloride ions build up in the epithelial cells of the lungs and other organs, drawing water into the cells to dilute the chloride. The normal flow of water and chloride into and out of cells is disrupted and leads to thick and sticky mucous production that blocks the ducts.

Cystitis: A urinary tract infection that indicates inflammation of the bladder.

Cytomegalovirus (CMV): A DNA virus in the herpes family that is transmitted maternally through sexual contact, blood transfusions, or respiratory contact.

Decidua basalis: What the endometrium is called once implantation has taken place (7–8 days).

Depolarization: The process of sodium flowing into the cells and potassium moving out of the cells during the cardiac cycle.

Depot medroxyprogesterone acetate (DMPA): An injectable progesterone birth control method that inhibits ovulation by suppressing follicle-stimulating hormone and luteinizing hormone production.

Deprivation amblyopia: A condition in which a dense cataract or complete ptosis occurs and prevents the retina of the affected eye from receiving an image.

Dermatitis: Presents as an area of edema, redness, oozing, and crusting and possibly lichenification defined as thickened skin with a shiny surface and deep skin markings caused by chronic rubbing and scratching.

Dermatophytes: A type of fungi that causes tinea infections.

Dermis: One of the three major layers of the skin, it is a flexible but strong and tough matrix of loose connective tissue that contains hair follicles, sweat and sebaceous glands, blood vessels, sensory nerves, and lymphatic vessels. Also called the corium.

Diabetic ketoacidosis: Develops when there is a lack of insulin, resulting in the inability to use glucose for energy.

Diastole: Ventricular relaxation. During diastole, blood trickles from the atria to the ventricles through the atrioventricular (AV) valves.

Dilated cardiomyopathy: A condition in which the heart muscle stretches and becomes weak resulting in heart failure.

Direct Coombs test: Determines whether there are maternal antibodies in fetal cord blood.

Dislocatable hip: A hip that can be manually displaced but returns to the acetabulum with release of pressure.

Dislocated hip: Characterized by a complete loss of contact of the femoral head with the acetabulum.

Diurnal enuresis: Daytime wetting. More common in shy children or those with attention deficit hyperactivity disorder and may signal the onset of diabetes mellitus.

Dysarthria: Impaired, stammering, or slurred speech pattern.

Dysphagia: Swallowing difficulty resulting in drooling that may be associated with cerebral palsy.

Eccrine glands: Help regulate body temperature by producing sweat. These glands are found in the highest numbers in the palms, forehead, and soles of the feet and do not mature until ages 2 or 3 years.

Eclampsia: Final phase of untreated pre-eclampsia causing seizures in a pregnant woman who has no other metabolic or physiological reason for seizure activity, such as epilepsy or a brain mass.

Ectoderm: One of three embryonic layers of cells; this upper layer forms the central nervous system, special senses, skin, nails, hair, and glands. See also endoderm and mesoderm.

Ectopic pregnancy: The implantation of a fertilized ovum outside of the endometrial cavity, fallopian tube, ovary, cervix, or abdominal cavity.

Eczema: Acute weeping dermatosis.

ELISA: An enzyme-linked immunosorbent assay used to diagnosis conditions such as HIV infection.

End-diastolic volume: The amount of blood each ventricle contains at the end of its filling period.

Endocardium: The internal lining of the myocardium that is continuous with the endothelium that lines all blood vessels, creating one continuous circuit.

Endoderm: One of three embryonic layers of cells; this lower layer forms the respiratory system, liver, pancreas, and digestive system. See also ectoderm and mesoderm.

Endometriosis: The implantation of uterine endometrium outside the uterus.

Enterocolitis: Inflammation of the small intestine and colon.

Enuresis: A condition during which the child has either voluntary or involuntary wetting either at night or during the day. Bed wetting may last until late childhood.

Enzyme-linked immunosorbent assay (ELISA): A serologic assay used to diagnose human immunodeficiency virus infection by detecting the presence of human immunodeficiency virus antibodies (seroconversion) in blood and blood products.

Enzymes: Specific proteins that increase or decrease the speed of a chemical reaction but do not change themselves.

Epidermis: One of the three major layers of the skin; it is composed of the stratum germinativum, stratum spinosum, stratum granulosum, stratum lucidum (on the palms of the hands and soles of the feet), and stratum corneum.

Epiglottitis: The inflammation and edema of the epiglottis and arytenoids; the small muscles of the larynx.

Epithelization: Also called the reconstruction stage, it is the second stage in wound healing, lasting 4 to 14 days. During this stage epithelial cells grow into the injured area as capillaries establish blood flow and natural enzymes dissolve the clot or scab that has formed over the injury.

Epstein pearls: Milia that occur in the oral cavity. Epstein pearls rupture spontaneously and disappear.

Erythema toxicum: Blotchy red macules, usually found on the chest, back, face, or, less commonly, the extremities, that occur in up to 50% of all full-term infants 24 to 48 hours after birth. Usually the macules begin to fade in one to two days and are gone by one week. Although serum eosinophilia may occur, the macules are not caused by microorganisms.

Erythropoietin: A hormone that stimulates the bone marrow to produce red blood cells in response to hypoxia from conditions such as anemia or from cardiac and/or pulmonary disease.

Estrogenic phase: The ovarian function of the menstrual cycle. The endometrium within the uterus becomes thickened, succulent, and extremely rich in blood supply. Also referred to as the proliferative phase.

Eustachian tube: A narrow tube composed of membrane and cartilage that allows air to enter behind the sealed eardrum from the back of the nose and replace the air that is normally absorbed by the body from the middle ear.

Ewing's sarcoma: A primary bone tumor that arises from immature cells within the bone marrow space, causing bone destruction within.

Exotropia: Outward deviation of the eye.

External method: Noninvasive fetal monitoring using external transducers placed on the maternal abdomen to assess fetal heart rate and uterine activity.

Fertility-awareness methods (FAMs): A nonhormonal form of birth control. Also called natural family planning, this method requires familiarity of bodily changes during the menstrual cycle and periodic abstinence or use of barrier methods during ovulation if pregnancy is not desirable.

Fibrous pericardium: The outer-most layer of the heart wall composed of fibrous connective tissue.

Fistula: A tube-like passage that may develop between the gastrointestinal tract and adjoining areas such as the bladder, vagina, urethra, or other segments of the gastrointestinal tract.

Follicle-stimulating hormone: Hormones released by the anterior pituitary that stimulate the ovaries resulting in production of estrogen and progesterone.

Follicular phase: The ovarian function of the menstrual cycle that extends from the end of menstruation to ovulation.

Foramen ovale: One-way valve that permits shunting of blood from the inferior vena cava through the right atrium to the left atrium.

Gamete intrafallopian transfer (GIFT): A technique that is done with the laparoscope by placing both ova and sperm into the fimbriated end (open end) of the fallopian tube. Fertilization occurs in the fallopian tube.

Gastroenteritis: An inflammation of the mucous membranes of the stomach and intestines caused by infectious agents that comes on quickly, often with few other symptoms.

Gestational diabetes mellitus (GDM): The onset of impaired glucose or carbohydrate metabolism that is diagnosed during pregnancy.

Giant pigmented nervus: A birthmark with an irregular dark brown–black plaque that covers at least 5% of the body. Malignant changes may occur in these lesions.

Glaucoma: A disease of the eye in which there is increasing intraocular pressure, damaging the optic nerve. Generally classified as open angle (also chronic or simple) or angle closure (also acute, closed angle, or narrow angle).

Glomerulus: Plasma-filtering capillary tuft created by the efferent and afferent arterioles that deposits its filtrate into a thin double-walled capsule called Bowman's capsule.

Glucogenesis: The process wherein between meals the liver releases glycogen, which is broken down into glucose.

Gluconeogenesis: The liver manufactures glucose from amino acids, glycerol, and lactic acid.

Glucosuria: A condition in which excess glucose spills into the urine because the kidneys are unable to reabsorb all the glucose when the serum level rises above 180 mg/dl.

Glucuronyl transferase: An enzyme used to conjugate bilirubin.

Glycogen: Glucose from each meal that is stored in the liver.

Gonorrhea: A sexually transmitted infection caused by the bacteria *Neisseria gonorrhoeae,* a gram-negative intracellular diplococcus.

Gravida: Any pregnancy, regardless of duration.

Greenstick fracture: A partial break in the bone with bending on the opposite side.

Group B streptococcus (GBS): A gram-positive bacterium normally found in the vaginas of nonpregnant women and approximately 9–23% of healthy pregnant women. It causes vertical transmission (from mother to infant) during birth and is the leading cause of neonatal infections in the United States.

Guttate: A type of psoriasis that develops 2 to 3 weeks after streptococcal pharyngitis or an upper respiratory tract infection. Latin for "drop-like."

HELLP syndrome: A syndrome of hemolysis (H), elevated liver enzymes (EL), and low platelets (LP) believed to occur when fragmented red blood cells pass through vessels that have endothelial damage and deposits of fibrin. It is a severe variant of preeclampsia.

Hemangioma: A benign tumor of capillary endothelial cells that is red in color and rubbery with a rough surface.

Hemodilution: Increased water load in the bloodstream that dilutes serum sodium levels.

Hemolysis: Destruction of the fetal red blood cells.

Hemophilia: An inherited disorder of blood coagulation characterized by a permanent tendency to hemorrhage due to a defect in the blood-coagulating mechanism. Typical clinical features of hemophilia include bruising and bleeding episodes involving skin, mucosa, muscles, joints, and organs which occur spontaneously or following tissue trauma or injury.

Hepatitis B and C: Considered sexually transmitted infections due to their transmission during intimate sexual activity.

Herpes labialis: A virus caused by the herpes simplex virus type 1. Commonly called "cold sores" or "fever blisters," as type I is most frequently found on the lips or mouth area.

Herpes simplex virus: A virus that causes recurrent, incurable infections, characterized by painful vesicles on skin and mucosal surfaces. There are two types: HSV-1 and HSV-2.

Hirschsprung's disease: A motility disorder that commonly coexists with other congenital anomalies, particularly Down's syndrome. Also called congenital aganglionic megacolon, this disease results from an absence of ganglion cells in one or more segments of the colon.

Hodgkin's disease: One of two types of malignant lymphomas found in young adults.

HSV-1 infections: Herpes simplex virus type 1 infection that generally involves the gingival, lips and/or the periorbital region, or the thumb in children who suck their thumbs.

HSV-2 infections: Herpes simplex virus type 2 infection that is usually found in the genital area; primarily a sexually transmitted infection.

Human chorionic gonadotropin (hCG): A hormone secreted by the chorionic villi of the placenta, found in urine or blood serum of the pregnant woman.

Human immunodeficiency virus (HIV): An infection that can result in acquired immunodeficiency syndrome (AIDS) that is transmitted sexually, through sharing of needles, and through vertical transmission from mother to fetus. HIV replicates by invading T cells and other immune system cells, thus weakening the system.

Human papilloma virus (HPV): Genital or venereal warts. Also referred to as condylomata acuminata and as genital or venereal warts.

Human placental lactogen (HPL): Maternally produced by the placenta to assist with appropriate regulation of glucose. Human placental lactogen decreases the sensitivity of maternal cells to insulin.

Hyaluronidase: An enzyme that helps the sperm penetrate the protective layers around the ovum.

Hydralazine (Apresoline): A Pregnancy Category A vasodilator used to control high blood pressure.

Hydatidiform mole: An overproduction of placental cells that forms a tumor in the uterus and can be mistaken for an early pregnancy.

Hydralazine (Apresoline): A pregnancy Category A vasodilator that is used to control high blood pressure.

Hydrocephalus: Either a congenital anomaly or a traumatic or acquired encephalopathy (inflammation, neoplasm, or bleed) that disrupts the anatomy or physiology of the central nervous system and the balance between the formation and absorption of the cerebrospinal fluid.

Hyperbilirubinemia: Excessive amounts of bilirubin in the blood.

Hyperglycemia: High blood sugar levels that result when glucose is unable to enter the cells, remaining in the bloodstream.

Hyperopia (farsightedness): When distant objects can be seen clearly but closer objects are blurred because light rays focus behind the retina.

Hypertrophic cardiomyopathy: Ventricular hypertrophy and ventricular septum hypertrophy that causes an outflow obstruction.

Hypoglycemia: Insulin reaction.

Hyponatremia: Low serum sodium that occurs because water is pulled into the bloodstream in response to a high glucose load (high serum osmolarity).

Hysterosalpingogram: An x-ray procedure performed to assess for tubal patency and health.

Idiopathic scoliosis: A lateral curvature of the spine that occurs most often in girls and often presents during the preadolescent growth spurt.

Impetigo contagiosa: A common, highly contagious, superficial skin infection caused by staphylococci (*Staphylococcus aureus*) and/or streptococci (*Streptococcus pyogenes*) bacteria.

In vitro fertilization: An assisted reproductive technique whereby mature oocytes (one or more) via laparoscopy are removed from the woman's ovary, fertilized in the laboratory, and then transferred to the woman's uterus. Commonly used with a woman who has blocked fallopian tubes, endometriosis, pelvic adhesions, or if the man has a low sperm count.

Inborn errors of metabolism (IEMs): Disorders caused by single faulty genes resulting in the inability of the normal metabolic pathway to function and correctly synthesize or breakdown proteins, carbohydrates, or fats.

Infantile eczema: The first of three phases of atopic dermatitis, which begins around ages 1–4 months and ends at ages 18–24 months.

Infertility: The inability to conceive a child after 1 year of regular sexual intercourse without using any method of contraception or the inability to carry a pregnancy to term.

Internal method: A spiral electrode is applied to the fetal presenting part to assess the fetal electrocardiogram and an intrauterine pressure catheter is inserted to assess uterine activity and pressure.

Intrarenal ARF: An intrinsic type of acute renal failure that results from injury to the kidney itself.

Intrauterine device (IUD): A "T"-shaped device that is inserted into the uterus by a health care provider during the first 5 days of menses that provides immediate protection against pregnancy.

Intrauterine pressure catheter (IUPC): A device used to measure frequency, duration, and intensity of uterine contractions.

Intussusception: Occurs in the lower gastrointestinal tract as one segment of the bowel telescopes into the lumen of the adjacent section of intestine. The walls of the bowel press against each other, become inflamed and edematous, and may cause bleeding.

Juvenile glaucoma: A type of open-angle glaucoma that develops after age 3 but before age 20.

Juvenile rheumatoid arthritis (JRA): A chronic disease that affects 60,000 to 200,000 children in the United States characterized by inflammation of the synovium with joint effusion and eventual destruction of the articular cartilage lasting 6 weeks or longer.

Kawasaki's disease: An acute febrile disease of young children. It is also referred to as mucocutaneous lymph node syndrome.

Ketonemia: A condition that results when the serum ketone level is above 1.0 mmol/l.

Ketonuria: A condition that results when moderate or significant ketones in the urine are detected.

Kussmaul respirations: Deep, rapid respirations.

Kyphosis: An increased convex curve, normally in the thoracic region, that may be postural, congenital, or secondary to other disorders. Kyphosis may also be associated with chronic diseases such as muscle disease, cerebral palsy, and spinal muscle atrophy.

Labor: A series of processes by which the products of conception are expelled from the mothers' body.

Labyrinthitis: Infection of the inner ear.

Laparoscopy: A procedure using an endoscope to view the peritoneal cavity. It is usually done early in the menstrual cycle. If a woman is infertile, it may reveal endometriosis, fibroids, pelvic adhesions, polycystic ovaries, and tubal occulsion. This method is also used in reproductive technology to retrieve eggs.

Leukemia: The most common malignancy in children under the age of 15. It is a broad classification of malignant neoplasms of cells that arise from the hematopoietic stem cell.

Letting-go phase: After giving birth, in this phase the mother reestablishes relationships with others outside the immediate family circle.

She is comfortable in the motherhood role and with the care and responsibility of her newborn.

LH (luteinizing hormone): Hormones synthesized by the anterior pituitary that stimulate the ovaries to produce estrogen and progesterone.

The L/S ratio (lecithin/sphingomyelin): Determines the maturity of the fetal lungs, especially useful in pre-term labor, as well as other complications.

Lightening: When the fetal presenting part descends into the true pelvis.

Lobar pneumonia: Pneumonia that is confined to a single lobe of the lung.

Lochia alba: A discharge from the vagina after childbirth that follows lochia serosa and continues for approximately 2 to 6 weeks after delivery. It contains leukocytes, mucus, serum, and decidual cells.

Lochia rubra: A discharge from the vagina after childbirth that appears immediately after the delivery of the placenta and is bright red in color and composed of blood, decidual and trophoblastic debris, and bacteria.

Lochia serosa: A discharge from the vagina after childbirth that follows lochia rubra and continues from days 4 to 10 days after delivery. It contains serous fluids, old blood, leukocytes, and tissue debris.

Logan's bow: A small metal strip used after surgery to correct a cleft lip that protects the suture line, along with arm restraints, to prevent the child from touching and pulling at the incision.

Lordosis: A curvature of the spine in which there is an increased concave curve, normally in the lumbar region. With lordosis the muscles of the spine are unable to support themselves in an erect position.

L/S ratio (lecithin/sphingomyelin): A ratio to determine the maturity of the fetal lungs; especially useful in preterm labor, as well as other complications.

Luteinizing hormone (LH): Hormones synthesized by the anterior pituitary that stimulate the ovaries to produce estrogen and progesterone.

Lyme disease: A disease caused by the spirochete, *Borrelia burgdorferi*, which enters the bloodstream through the salvia and feces of ticks.

Lymphoblast: An immature white cell that crowds out normal cells, resulting in pancytopenia and immunosuppression.

Macrosomia: A large for gestational age infant that weighs about 4,000 g and can cause vaginal trauma if not delivered via cesarean birth.

Magnesium sulfate (MgSO$_4$): A Pregnancy Category A anticonvulsant medication used to prevent or control seizures and acts as a smooth muscle relaxant to decrease vasoconstriction.

Malignant brain tumors: The second leading cause of cancer after leukemia. Although no known cause of brain tumors exists, there are suggestions that environmental and hereditary factors may play a role.

Malignant hyperthermia: A complication of anesthesia that occurs in Duchenne's muscular dystophy and other muscular dystrophies.

Mastoiditis: Infection of the mastoid bone.

Maturation stage: A mature scar forms and becomes strong.

Medical/surgical history: Based on any present conditions a pregnant woman may have and their effects on pregnancy.

Melanin: A pigment which is the primary determinant of skin color.

Menarche: The first menstrual period of puberty.

Meningitis: Inflammation of the membranes of the brain or spinal cord at the level of the lining (meninges) caused by an infectious process.

Menopause: The cessation of menses for 12 consecutive months. It is also referred to as the climacteric phase of a woman's life.

Menstrual phase (menses): Periodic vaginal discharge of bloody fluid from the nonpregnant uterus that occurs from the age of puberty to menopause.

Mesoderm: One of three embryonic layers of cells, this middle layer forms the skeletal, urinary, circulatory, spleen, and reproductive organs. See also endoderm and ectoderm.

Middle ear: A pea-sized, sealed, air-filled cavity that gives the paper-thin eardrum the ability to vibrate easily (compliance) and transmit sound waves from the three tiny bones in the middle ear to the inner ear and then to the brain for processing.

Milia: Occurs in 40% of infants as 1-mm-diameter papules scattered over the forehead, nose, and cheeks. They are caused by superficial epidermal cysts.

Miliaria: Eccrine sweat duct obstructions caused by exposure to heat and high humidity that resolve when the infant is moved to a cooler, drier environment.

Mongolian spot: A bluish black macule appearing on the lumbosacral area caused by pigment cells deep in the dermis.

Morula: A cluster of cells that forms as cell division continues after the ovum is fertilized.

Multigravida: A woman who is pregnant with her second child or any subsequent pregnancy.

Multipara: A woman who has had two or more births at more than 20 weeks' gestation.

Myocardial contractility: How forcefully the ventricle contracts.

Myocardium: The muscle that forms the chambers of the heart (atria and ventricles).

Myopia (nearsightedness): When close objects can be seen clearly but more distant objects are blurred because light rays focus in front of the retina.

Natriuretic peptides: Peptide hormones that are antagonists to the renin-aldosterone-angiotensin system and limit aldosterone secretion and promote salt and water loss.

Negatively inotropic: Any factor that weakens the contraction force of the ventricles, such as hypoxia.

Neonatal period: The first 28 days of life.

Nephrons: The functional units of the kidneys; each kidney has approximately 1.2 million nephrons.

Non-Hodgkin's lymphoma (NHL): A malignant tumor that may originate in any lymphatic tissue in the body, has rapid onset, and presents with widespread involvement at the time of diagnosis.

Nosocomial pneumonia: Pneumonia acquired while hospitalized.

Nuchal cord: An umbilical cord which is wrapped around the fetal neck.

Nuchal rigidity: Stiff neck.

Nutritional history: An extremely important assessment because the developing embryo/fetus relies on nutrition for proper growth and development.

Oblique fracture: A fracture that occurs diagonally across the long bone.

Obstetric/gynecological history: Reviews the age of menarche, menstrual history, contraceptive practices, infertility, gynecological problems, sexually transmitted infections, and all pregnancies as well as their outcomes.

Obstructive sleep apnea: The attempt to breathe through an obstructed airway; most commonly occurs in children with craniofacial abnormalities (Crouzon's syndrome, etc.), in those with neuropathies, and in those medicated with hypnotics, sedatives, and anticonvulsants.

Open-angle glaucoma (also chronic or simple): A type of glaucoma in which the anterior chamber angle is open but there is an obstruction in the trabecular mesh leading to the canal of Schlemm.

Open fracture: A fracture that breaks through the skin.

Oral contraceptives: Birth control taken orally containing hormones that inhibit ovulation.

Osteogenic sarcoma: A primary bone tumor that arises from the mesenchymal matrix-forming cells of the bone, causing bone destruction and osteoid tissue formation. Also called osteosarcoma.

Osteomyelitis: An infection in the bone that occurs most often in the lower extremities and may occur after trauma or puncture to an infected area (exogenous), after surgery, or by spread of infection to the bone through the bloodstream from elsewhere in the body (hematogenous).

Otitis externa: Inflammation of the skin lining the ear canal and surrounding soft tissue.

Otitis media: Inflammation of the middle ear.

Overflow incontinence (paradoxic incontinence): involves a deficient detrusor muscle or bladder outlet obstruction. In this type of incontinence the bladder does not empty completely because of detrusor muscle malfunction as occurs with multiple sclerosis or from blockage of the bladder outlet from conditions such as a urethral stricture

Ovulation predictor kit: A urine test used to predict ovulation based on the luteinizing hormone that is measured in the urine.

Ovulatory phase: The ovary function of the menstrual cycle.

Oxyhemoglobin: Oxygen and hemoglobin combined in the lungs.

p24 assay: A test that detects the p24 antigen, an indication of active human immunodeficiency virus replication, within 2 to 6 weeks of human immunodeficiency virus infection.

Para: Birth after 20 weeks' gestation, regardless of whether the infant is alive or dead.

Parietal pericardium: A serous membrane that lines the inner surface of the fibrous pericardium.

Parietal pleura: Part of the double-layered membrane that surrounds the lung that lines the inside of the thoracic cavity.

Patent ductus arteriosus (PDA): During fetal life blood is shunted from the pulmonary artery to the aorta (fetal gas exchange takes place at the placenta, not by breathing).

Percutaneous umbilical blood sampling: A method that directly takes a sample of fetal blood from the umbilical cord to determine whether the fetus is severely compromised.

Pericardial sac: The fibrous pericardium and parietal pericardium surrounding the heart.

Peripheral nervous system (PNS): There are 31 pairs of spinal nerves that extend out from the spinal cord to the organs of the body divided into the autonomic nervous system, that regulates the internal organs, and the somatic nervous system, that regulates motor control.

Peristalsis: Wave-like motion that moves digested food through the intestinal track.

Peritonitis: Inflammation of the peritoneum caused by events such as bowel perforation.

Pertussis: A highly contagious bacterial respiratory illness caused by *Bordetella pertussis* that results in severe bronchitis. Also called whooping cough.

Phototherapy: A therapy that exposes the newborn to high-intensity light (in the blue-light spectrum) and decreases serum bilirubin levels in the skin.

Placenta previa: An abnormally implanted placenta in which the placenta is implanted in the lower uterine segment instead of the upper uterine segment.

Plantar warts: Warts that appear on the bottom (sole) of the foot.

Pleural effusion: Accumulation of excess pleural fluid.

Pneumonia: An inflammatory process that may be caused by numerous infectious agents such as bacteria, viruses, fungi, yeast, or protozoa. Community-acquired pneumonia is pneumonia acquired outside of a hospital/health care setting.

Polydipsia: Excessive thirst.

Polyhydramnios: Occurs when there is more than 200 ml of amniotic fluid.

Polymerase chain reaction (PCR): A nucleic acid amplification procedure that uses an in vitro replication of target nucleic acid sequences, thereby identifying specific human immunodeficiency virus genetic information.

Polyuria: Excessive urination.

Port wine stains: The dark red–bluish red macules of capillary malformations. They may occur anywhere on the body, but the location of the port wine stain may signal certain syndromes.

Positively inotropic: Any factor that strengthens the force of a ventricular contraction such as digoxin, sympathetic nervous stimulation, and epinephrine.

Postcoital test: A test to evaluate the cervical mucus to determine the receptivity of the cervical mucus to sperm and the ability of the sperm to travel within it.

Postpartum period: The period from the birth of the newborn (and placenta) to about 6 weeks after the delivery. Also called the puerperium and the fourth trimester.

Postrenal or obstructive ARF: A type of acute renal failure that results from urinary tract outflow obstruction by renal calculi, tumors, trauma resulting in hematoma, neurogenic bladder, or structural abnormalities, such as ureterovesical junction stricture.

Preload: The amount of blood in the ventricle at the end of diastole.

Prerenal factors: Factors that occur before blood being filtered by the kidneys, and may be caused by anything which promotes renal hypoperfusion. Prerenal factors include shock, congestive heart failure, volume depletion from vomiting/diarrhea, or diabetic acidosis.

Preterm: Labor that occurs after 20 weeks' but before the completion of 37 weeks' gestation.

Primigravida: A woman who is pregnant for the first time.

Probable signs of pregnancy: Because pregnancy tests are only 95% accurate in diagnosing pregnancy, they are considered only probable signs of pregnancy.

Progestational phase: Refers to the ovary. See luteal phase.

Proinsulin: A molecule composed of 81 amino acids from which insulin is derived.

Proliferative phase: The uterine function of the menstrual cycle.

Psoriasis: A type of papulosquamous eruption that presents as red papules covered by thick white scales.

Psychosocial history: A history that includes the spouse/partner, family situation, and any history of domestic violence.

Pulmonary stenosis: The membrane formed when the pulmonic valve leaflets (cusps) are fused together.

Pyloric stenosis: The most common upper gastrointestinal disorder requiring surgery during the neonatal period. An example of an obstructive disorder, it occurs when the muscle at the pylorus narrows and thickens due to an increase in cell size and cell number.

Pyloromyotomy: The surgical treatment for pyloric stenosis in which the muscles are split and separated.

Reflex incontinence: A form of incontinence caused by trauma or damage to the nervous system, as seen in spinal cord injury above S2-4 or diabetes mellitus.

Refractive amblyopia: Decreased vision that may occur in one or both eyes if a refractive error is not corrected.

Remission: A state in which there is no detectable sign of leukemia on physical examination or laboratory results.

Renal failure: The inability to concentrate water, balance electrolytes, and remove waste products; classified as acute or chronic.

Renal insufficiency: Denotes a 20% to 50% reduction in the glomerular filtration rate.

Renal osteodystrophy: Demineralization of bone from three major causes: the inability of the kidneys to activate vitamin D, which results in decreased absorption of calcium from food; decreased excretion of parathyroid hormone, which leads to demineralization of bones and teeth; and retention of phosphate, which leads to increased renal excretion of calcium.

Renin-angiotensin-aldosterone system: A hormone system that helps regulate long-term blood pressure and extracellular volume in the body.

Respiration: The exchange of oxygen and carbon dioxide between cells, alveoli, and environment.

Restless leg syndrome (spontaneous movement of the feet and legs): Altered sensation, weakness and diminished deep tendon reflexes occur because of neurotoxicity caused by uremia.

Restrictive cardiomyopathy: A condition in which the atria enlarge and the ventricles become stiff and rigid.

Rh incompatibility: A sensitization that occurs when an Rh-negative (blood type) mother delivers an Rh-positive (blood type) infant.

Rubella: Also known as German measles, it is caused by the rubella virus.

Scabies: A superficial skin infestation caused by *Sarcoptes scabiei*, a parasitic mite.

Scoliosis: A lateral curvature of the spine where the vertebral curve increases the ribs and the spine rotates toward the convex portion of the curve.

Secondary enuresis: Wetting after the child has had a long period of time during which bladder control was achieved.

Secondary glaucoma: Glaucoma that occurs after 3 years of age.

Secretory phase: The uterine function when the Graafian follicle fills with the corpus luteum.

Seizure disorders: Also called epilepsy, this is a disorder where abnormal electrical discharges from the brain trigger alterations or interruptions in sensory, motor, and/or cognition.

Semen analysis: A primary indicator of male fertility, the semen is analyzed to assess the sperm for volume, motility, number, viscosity, shape, and viability.

Semilunar valves: Valves that prevent the backflow of blood from the aorta and pulmonary artery to the right and left ventricles.

Sexually transmitted infections (STIs): Infections that are transmitted through direct intimate contact with an infected person. Also referred to as sexually transmitted diseases, or STDs.

Sickle cell anemia: A homozygous condition that results from inheriting a sickle cell gene (Hb S) from both parents. It is the most common hemoglobinopathy variant seen worldwide and primarily affects people of African and southwest Asian decent.

Sickle cell disease (SCD): The umbrella term for a number of inherited symptomatic disorders of the oxygen capacity of the red blood cell (erythrocytes) due to the abnormalities in the protein hemoglobin.

Sickle cell trait: The heterozygous carrier state where one receives a normal hemoglobin gene (Hb A) from one parent and an abnormal variant gene from the other parent.

Spiral fracture: A fracture line that circles around the bone; often seen in child abuse.

Spontaneous abortions: The loss or termination of a pregnancy before 20 weeks' gestation.

Sterilization: A surgical, nonhormonal form of birth control performed on both men and women that is considered a permanent means of contraception. It can be performed on both men and women.

Stillbirth: A fetus born dead after 20 weeks' gestation.

Strabismic amblyopia: Decreased vision that occurs when one eye becomes stronger, subduing the image of the weaker eye. Commonly called "lazy eye."

Strabismus: Misalignment of the eyes, classified as esotropia (inward deviation, or "crossed eyes") or exotropia (outward deviation).

Stress incontinence: A form of incontinence that involves a weak urethral sphincter.

Stridor: A high-pitched harsh noise characteristic of croup.

Stroke volume: The amount of blood pumped from the ventricle during one contraction.

Subcutaneous tissues: One of the three major layers of the skin, it is composed of both fat and slender elastic fibers, connects to the muscles, acts as a heat insulator, provides some shock absorption, and stores calories.

Subluxated hip: A hip in which the femoral head remains in the acetabulum but comes partially out of the joint with manipulation.

Substrates: Substances upon which enzymes exert their effects.

Subvalvular aortic stenosis: A condition in which a fibrous ring develops just below the aortic valve.

Sucking blisters: Occur in response to vigorous sucking in the womb. They may occur on the forearms, wrists, thumbs, or upper lip and resolve on their own.

Sudden infant death syndrome (SIDS): Occurs when an infant less than 12 months of age dies suddenly from an unexplained cause. Most SIDS cases occur between ages 2 and 4 months and between midnight and 8 AM when both the infant and caregivers are sleeping.

Supravalvular aortic stenosis: A genetic condition that occurs when the ascending aorta is constricted just above the coronary arteries.

Surfactant: A fluid that coats the inner surface of each alveoli and allows them to remain partially opened during exhalation.

Surrogate embryo transfer: An assisted reproductive technique whereby a donor's ovum is fertilized by the recipient woman's partner's sperm (or donor sperm) and placed in the recipient woman's uterus.

Sweat chloride test: A test used to help disgnose cystic fibrosis.

Syncytia: A multinucleated mass of protoplasm.

Syphilis: One of the oldest known STIs. A chronic and systemic sexually transmitted disease caused by *Treponema pallidum*, a motile spirochete. Characterized by periods of active symptoms and latency. It has four stages: primary, secondary, latent, and tertiary.

Systole: Ventricular contraction.

Taking-hold phase: After giving birth, in this phase the mother becomes preoccupied with the present. This phase starts on the 3rd postpartum day and continues for several weeks.

Taking-in phase: After giving birth, in this phase the mother is more passive and relies on the nurse to help her make decisions. This phase takes place immediately after delivery and lasts about 2 days.

Tetralogy of Fallot (ToF): Comprises four structural abnormalities: a ventricular-septal defect, pulmonary stenosis, an overriding aorta, and right ventricular hypertrophy as a result of the pulmonary stenosis.

Tinea: A fungal infection of the skin, also called ringworm because of the red rings that appear on the affected area.

Tinea capitis: A fungal infection of the skin that affects the scalp, producing bald spots. It is more common in African-American children than in other groups.

Tinea cruris: Commonly referred to as jock itch, this fungal infection of the skin affects the inner thighs, inguinal creases, or perianal area.

Tinea pedis: Commonly referred to as athlete's foot, this fungal infection of the skin affects the webbed areas of the toes and feet.

TORCH: An acronym for a collection of infections that are capable of crossing the placenta and causing adverse effects on the developing fetus. The infections include *T*oxoplasmosis, *O*ther infections, *R*ubella, *C*ytomegalovirus, and *H*erpes simplex virus.

Toxoplasmosis: A disease caused by the protozoan parasite *Toxoplasma gondii* that is associated with eating raw or undercooked meat and with handling infected cat feces and infected mice or farm animals.

Transdermal patch: A hormonal form of birth control that is a beige matrix patch with an adhesive that affixes to the skin.

Transposition of the great arteries (TGA): Occurs three times more often in males than in females and is the second most common cyanotic congenital heart defect in newborns.

Transverse fracture: A fracture that occurs on the shaft of the bone, breaking straight across.

Trichomoniasis: A sexually transmitted infection caused by infection with a species of anaerobic one-celled protozoan with flagellate, *Trichomonas vaginalis.*

Tricuspid valve: The right atrioventricular valve that has three cusps or leaflets.

Trophoblasts: The outer layers of cells surrounding the blastocyst cavity.

Tubal ligation: Female sterilization that involves surgical severance and electrocoagulation or suturing of the fallopian tubes.

Turbinates: Tissue protrusions in each nostril that create air turbulence.

Type 1 diabetes: A chronic disease of altered fuel metabolism, classified as an immune-mediated diabetes (formerly called juvenile diabetes or insulin-dependent diabetes mellitus-IDDM), in which there is a lack of insulin production and ketosis.

Type 2 diabetes: A disease that results in a decreased sensitivity to insulin (formerly called non–insulin-dependent diabetes mellitus (NIDDM)).

Ultrasonography: A non-invasive technique used to evaluate fetal growth.

Uremia (urine in the blood): A symptom complex indicating a toxic condition resulting from azotemia involving multiple organ system dysfunction.

Urethritis: A urinary tract infection that involves inflammation of the urethra.

Urge incontinence: A type of chronic incontinence caused by inappropriate, repetitive, strong contractions of the detrusor muscle that eventually overcome urethral sphincter control. Also called instability incontinence or detrusor hyperreflexia.

Urinary tract infection (UTI): A significant amount of bacteria in the urinary tract; classified as lower or upper tract infections.

Vaginal ring: A hormonal form of birth control that is a flexible ring containing both estrogen and progestin.

Valvular aortic stenosis: A condition that occurs when the aortic valve contains one cusp diaphragm-like structure without defining commissures.

Varicella (chickenpox): A viral infection in the family of all herpesviruses. Once exposed, the virus can remain dormant in the dorsal root of the ganglia for many years before reactivating.

Vasectomy: Male sterilization, an in-office procedure performed by an urologist, is a sterilization procedure in which the vas deferens is severed, preventing sperm from traveling from the testes to the penis. It is not considered successful until 3 ejaculate specimens reveal no sperm. Once successful, its failure rate is less than 1%.

Vasoocclusive crises: Also called "sickling" or "sickle cell crisis," this occurs when the membrane of the red blood cells becomes hard, sticky, and sickle-shaped, causing clumping of the red blood cells in small vessels, blockage and interruption in blood flow, pain episodes, and progressive and irreversible cell and organ damage if not medically managed.

Ventilation: The movement of air denoting inhalation and exhalation.

Ventricular-septal defects (VSD): Small and moderate defects (less than 3–5 mm in diameter) that are asymptomatic.

Viability: The capacity to live outside the uterus; this occurs at about 20 weeks' gestation or when the fetal weight exceeds 500 grams or 1 pound, 1 ounce.

Viral load: The number of viral particles per millimeter of blood; an indicator of clinical progression of human immunodeficiency virus disease.

Viral sexually transmitted infections: Incurable viral infections that can cause recurrent episodes and remain in the patient's body for life. There are no known cures for viral infections.

Visceral pericardium: A serous membrane that covers the heart's surface.

Visceral pleura: Part of the double-layered membrane surrounding the lungs that lines the outside of the lungs.

von Willebrand disease: A disease in which there is both a prolonged bleeding time and low plasma factor VIII levels due to a defect in platelet aggregation.

Warts: An infection with the human papillomavirus that has entered the body through a break in the skin.

Wharton's jelly: Connective tissue wrapped around the umbilical cord that prevents compression of the blood vessels.

Wilms' tumor: An encapsulated tumor of the kidney that is the most common malignant kidney tumor in children. They are rapidly growing large lesions that may reach a considerable size before being diagnosed.

Wood lamp: Ultraviolet light.

Zona pellucida: The thick membranous envelope that encases the ovum during the menstrual cycle when the Graafian follicle ruptures and an ovum is ejected from the ovary into the fallopian tube.

Zygote: The divided fertilized ovum.

Zygote intrafallopian transfer (ZIFT): An assisted reproductive technique in which the oocyte is placed in culture media, inseminated, and then the fertilized eggs are transferred into the fimbriated edges of the fallopian tube. This process is different from GIFT because fertilization takes place outside the body.

INDEX